T0319085

Handbook of Gastrointestinal Motility and Functional Disorders

Handbook of Gastrointestinal Motility and Functional Disorders

Edited by

Satish S. C. Rao, MD, PhD, FRCP
Professor of Medicine
Chief, Gastroenterology/Hepatology
Director, Digestive Health Center
Medical College of Georgia
Georgia Regents University

Henry P. Parkman, MD
Professor of Medicine
Head of GI Motility Laboratory
Gastrointestinal Section
Department of Medicine
Temple University Hospital

Richard W. McCallum, MD, FACP, FRACP (AUST), FACG, AGAF
Professor of Medicine and Founding Chair,
Department of Internal Medicine
Director, Center for Neurogastroenterology and GI Motility
Texas Tech University Health Sciences Center
Paul L. Foster School of Medicine

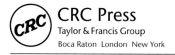

CRC Press
Taylor & Francis Group
Boca Raton London New York

CRC Press is an imprint of the
Taylor & Francis Group, an **informa** business

First published 2015 by SLACK Incorporated

Published 2024 by CRC Press
2385 NW Executive Center Drive, Suite 320, Boca Raton FL 33431

and by CRC Press
4 Park Square, Milton Park, Abingdon, Oxon, OX14 4RN

CRC Press is an imprint of Taylor & Francis Group, LLC

© 2015 Taylor & Francis Group, LLC

Library of Congress Cataloging-in-Publication Data

Handbook of gastrointestinal motility and functional disorders / [edited by] Satish S.C. Rao, Henry P. Parkman, Richard W. McCallum.
  p. ; cm.
Includes bibliographical references.
ISBN 978-1-61711-818-0 (alk. paper)
I. Rao, Satish S. C., editor. II. Parkman, Henry P., editor. III. McCallum, Richard W., editor.
[DNLM: 1. Gastrointestinal Diseases--Handbooks. 2. Gastrointestinal Motility--Handbooks. WI 39]
RC802
616.3'3--dc23
                    2015004809

ISBN: 9781617118180 (pbk)
ISBN: 9781003524519 (ebk)

DOI: 10.1201/9781003524519

DEDICATION

We dedicate this book to our wives Sheila, Martha, and Mary Beth, and our children for generously giving up family time to help us put together this book, as the work involved was often performed outside of the usual business hours, nights, and weekends. We also dedicate this book to our GI motility laboratory personnel — nurses and technicians who skillfully organize and perform our diagnostic studies so efficiently, and provide such a noble service to our patients. We also thank the American Neurogastroenterology and Motility Society for sponsoring the Clinical Training Program that has allowed GI fellows to visit our centers of excellence for GI motility testing in which we have participated. This program has helped each of us grow individually as mentors for the next generation of neurogastroenterologists who are needed by the patients who have the problems we discuss in this handbook. Finally, this book, which covers the many practical aspects of GI motility and functional GI disorders, is dedicated to the pioneers and researchers who have painstakingly developed many technologies, and the nurses and medical assistants who passionately perform these procedures in the GI motility laboratory. Through their hard work and pursuit of excellence, we and others have gained new knowledge of GI motility and functional bowel disorders, and have developed innovative tools that have enabled us to better understand motility disorders and novel treatment approaches. These advances have benefited our patients immensely, who constantly remind us of the unmet needs of the field of neurogastroenterology.

Each of the editors would like to thank their mentors in the field of GI motility. Satish Rao would like to thank Professor Nick Read and Dr. Derek Holdsworth, Sheffield, UK, who have instilled in him the seeds of inquisitiveness and discovery and mentored his research career, as well as Drs. James Christensen, Robert Summers, Konrad Schulze, and Jeffrey Conklin at the University of Iowa, Iowa City for their unwavering support and guidance over the past 20 years.

Henry Parkman would like to thank James C. Reynolds for introducing him to the area of GI motility, Sidney Cohen for his helpful advice in career decisions, Joseph H. Szurszewski for allowing him to work in his laboratory to gain knowledge in the scientific aspects of GI motility, and Robert S. Fisher who "gave" the running of the Temple University GI Motility laboratory to him.

Richard McCallum would like to recognize the late Jon Isenberg, his first Chief of GI at Wadsworth VA Medical Center and UCLA and the late Dick Sturdevant who introduced him to the field of GI Motility; the late Dr. Howard Spiro, his GI Chief at Yale, for his faith in recruiting him and for his wise advice and observations on GI and life in general. He is particularly indebted to the late Edward Hook, his Chair of Medicine at University of Virginia who recruited him as Chief of GI and gave him the tools, the free reins, and the trust to develop a world class Division of Gastroenterology, Hepatology and Nutrition. He also wants to recognize his colleagues in the NIH funded National Gastroparesis Consortium who have helped him grow also in the molecular and translational research aspects of GI motility and neurogastroenterology over the last 8 years. He is very grateful to Dr. Irene Sarosiek, his mentee for the past 20 years and now a co-investigator and faculty colleague, for her loyalty and dedication to their research and patient care.

CONTENTS

ABOUT THE EDITORS

Satish S.C. Rao, MD, PhD, FRCP graduated from Osmania Medical College in Hyderabad, India. Subsequently, he completed his graduate medical education and GI Fellowship and Clinical Research training at several UK hospitals, notably Royal Hallamshire Hospital, Sheffield, and Royal Liverpool Hospitals before becoming a Fellow of the Royal College of Physicians in London. He earned his PhD from the University of Sheffield in the United Kingdom. He joined the faculty at the University of Iowa in 1991 where he participated in many National Institutes of Health (NIH)–funded research projects and cofounded the Pelvic Floor Group. In 2011, Dr. Rao was recruited to the Medical College of Georgia, Georgia Regents University, Augusta, Georgia, to serve as professor of medicine, chief of the Section of Gastroenterology/Hepatology, and the new founding director of the Digestive Health Center and the GI Service Line.

In this role, he is leading an aggressive initiative to expand the university's capabilities in treating digestive disorders that includes a brand-new Digestive Health Center and a state-of-the-art, 5-room neurogastroenterology and motility suite. He plans to work closely with colleagues in surgery, urology, otolaryngology, and neurology to create a model system of interdisciplinary care for GI motility patients.

Dr. Rao is past president of the American Neurogastroenterology and Motility Society. He received the 3 highest honors from the American Gastroenterological Association: the Distinguished Clinician Award, the Masters Award for Outstanding Clinical Research, and the Distinguished Educator Award. He received the Auxiliary Research Award from the American College of Gastroenterology and several international awards for his research and teaching. He serves on the editorial board of several journals, is cochair of AGA Council on Neurogastroentrology and GI Motility, has published over 300 articles, and has edited 5 books on GI motility.

Henry P. Parkman, MD joined the faculty of Temple University School of Medicine in 1990, and has been actively involved in studying GI motility at both the basic science and clinical levels. His clinical focus has been treating patients with GI motility disorders, primarily gastroparesis. Clinically at Temple, Dr. Parkman is in charge of the GI Motility Laboratory that assesses GI motility dysfunction in patients. His clinical laboratory has developed expertise in a comprehensive array of GI motility tests for clinical evaluation of patients, including specialized tests of esophageal and gastric motility. This is a referral center for the evaluation and treatment of GI motility disorders.

Dr. Parkman was funded for 10 years with an NIH K24 Midcareer Investigator Award in Patient-Oriented Research entitled "Novel Evaluation & Treatment of Gastric Dysmotility," which, in addition to funding research in gastric motility, provided time for him to mentor young investigators in clinical research. Through this research, studies were performed on novel ways to assess gastric emptying.

Dr. Parkman is currently a funded member of the NIH Gastroparesis Clinical Research Consortium, now in its second 5-year cycle, established by the NIDDK to enhance the understanding of gastroparesis. This research has better defined the syndromes of diabetic and idiopathic gastroparesis, and the consortium is now conducting clinical trials to help better treat patients with their refractory symptoms of nausea and vomiting. His manuscript on the use of nortriptyline for nausea and abdominal pain in gastroparesis recently appeared in *JAMA*. He is currently studying the neurokinin receptor antagonist aprepitant as a treatment for the nausea and vomiting seen in gastroparesis.

During his presidency of the American Neurogastroenterological and Motility Society, Dr. Parkman helped standardize the radionuclide gastric emptying study and make it a more standardized test that can be done at different institutions in a uniform fashion. He remains active with an initiative to develop a patient-reported outcome (PRO) for gastroparesis that meets the approval of the Food and Drug Administration (FDA). This would help ease the study of treatments for gastroparesis, which are greatly needed.

Richard W. McCallum, MD, FACP, FRACP (AUST), FACG, AGAF is professor and founding chairman of the Department of Internal Medicine, Texas Tech University Health Sciences Center at El Paso. Dr. McCallum also serves as director of the Center for Neurogastroenterology and GI Motility and Functional Bowel Disorders, a referral and research center for patients locally, regionally, and nationally.

After completing his undergraduate studies at the University of Queensland, he earned his medical degree at the Queensland Medical School in Brisbane, Australia. Dr. McCallum completed gastroenterology fellowship training at the University of California in Los Angeles and Wadsworth VA Medical Center. He joined the faculty of Yale University School of Medicine in 1996. Dr. McCallum was professor of medicine chief and program director of the Division of Gastroenterology, Hepatology, and Nutrition at the University of Virginia School of Medicine, Charlottesville, Virginia, from 1985 to 1996, where he was awarded the Paul Janssen Endowed Chair and Professorship. From 1996 to 2004, Dr. McCallum was chief and program director, Division of Gastroenterology and Hepatology, University of Kansas Medical Center, Kansas City, and then became director of the Center for GI Nerve and Muscle Function and chief of Division of GI Motility, University of Kansas School of Medicine from 2004 to 2009 before being recruited as the founding chair of the new Paul L. Foster School of Medicine in El Paso in 2009.

Among his professional honors and memberships are Fellow of the American College of Physicians, Fellow of the Royal Australiasian College of Physicians, Fellow of the American College of Gastroenterology, Fellow of the American Gastroenterology Association, member of the American Society for Clinical Investigation, President and Founders Medal Recipient of the Southern Society for Clinical Investigation, Moreton Award for Original Research in Medicine, and the CURE Award for Diabetes Research, and the Chancellor's Distinguished Research Award at Texas Tech University. He is currently President of the International Gastrointestinal Electrophysiology Society.

Dr. McCallum's area of clinical interest and research is the field of GI motility, neurogastroenterology, and functional bowel disorders. He has been focused on advancing knowledge related to pathophysiology, diagnostic approaches, pharmacology, and device technology. He is a pioneer in the area of gut electrophysiology and developed the concept of electrical "pacing" of the stomach to treat gastroparesis and nausea and vomiting, particularly related to diabetes mellitus. Recently, he has contributed to major advances in understanding and management of cyclic vomiting syndrome in adults, "dumping syndrome," and rumination syndrome and has potentially revolutionized the field of gastroparesis and functional dyspepsia by developing and reporting a new technique to nonsurgically obtain gastric smooth muscle tissue by endoscopic ultrasound biopsy.

Dr. McCallum's research has been funded by the American Diabetes Association VA Medical Centers and NIH. Currently, he is funded by the NIH Gastroparesis Clinical Research Consortium. Established by NIDDK and initiated in 2008, it has been renewed for a further 5 years. The program has developed the world's largest database of gastroparesis patients and conducts cutting-edge basic translational and therapeutic research. Dr. McCallum was recently awarded funding from the International Foundation for Functional Gastrointestinal Diseases (IFFDG) to study a new therapy, transcutaneous electrical stimulation, in patients with nausea, vomiting, and idiopathic gastroparesis. He has published over 400 articles in peer-reviewed scientific journals, more than 100 chapters in textbooks, edited 15 textbooks, and has 3 active patents on GI therapies.

ACKNOWLEDGMENTS

We thank Carrie Kotlar of SLACK Incorporated, whose infectious zeal and enthusiasm and tremendous support throughout the production of this book was the single most important reason this beautiful volume is in your hands. Carrie was instrumental in persuading us to follow up on our well-received book *Gastrointestinal Motility Testing: Laboratory and Office Handbook*, a comprehensive and practical handbook for performing and properly interpreting gastrointestinal motility tests, and to embark on this new journey and fill the knowledge gap by writing this volume using a new format.

We also thank each chapter author for his or her superb contribution to this volume.

CONTRIBUTING AUTHORS

Abimbola O. Aderinto-Adike, MD (Chapter 16)
Division of Gastroenterology and Hepatology
Department of Medicine
Weill Cornell Medical College and Houston Methodist Hospital
Houston, Texas

Patrick Berg, BS (Chapter 10)
Fourth-year medical student at Texas Tech University Health Sciences Center
Paul L. Foster School of Medicine
El Paso, Texas

Deborah M. Bethards, MD (Chapter 24)
Hershey Medical Center
Hershey, Pennsylvania

Wojciech Blonski, MD, PhD (Chapter 2)
Division of Digestive Diseases
University of South Florida College of Medicine
Tampa, Florida

Lin Chang, MD (Chapter 18)
Oppenheimer Family Medical Center for Neurobiology of Stress
David Geffen School of Medicine at University of California - Los Angeles (UCLA)
Los Angeles, California

Giuseppe Chiarioni, MD (Chapter 21)
Gastrointestinal Rehabilitation Division
Valeggio sul Mincio Hospital
Azienda Ospedaliera
University of Verona
Valeggio sul Mincio, Italy

Jeffrey L. Conklin, MD (Chapter 5)
Division of Digestive Diseases
David Geffen School of Medicine at UCLA
Los Angeles, California

Chad J. Cooper, MD (Chapter 12)
Senior Internal Medicine Resident
Texas Tech University Health Sciences Center
Paul L. Foster School of Medicine
El Paso, Texas

Sameer Dhalla, MD, MHS (Chapter 8)
The Johns Hopkins School of Medicine
Division of Gastroenterology and Hepatology
Baltimore, Maryland

Douglas A. Drossman, MD (Chapter 25)
Center for Education and Practice of Biopsychosocial Care
Center for Functional GI and Motility Disorders at the University of North Carolina Drossman
    Gastroenterology, PLLC

Ronnie Fass, MD (Chapter 6)
Director, Division of Gastroenterology and Hepatology
MetroHealth Medical Center
Head, Esophageal and Swallowing Center
Professor of Medicine
Case Western Reserve University
Cleveland, Ohio

Mark R. Fox, MD, MA, FRCP (Chapter 4)
Division of Gastroenterology and Hepatology
University Hospital Zurich
Zurich, Switzerland

Andrew J. Gawron, MD, PhD, MS (Chapter 3)
Assistant Professor
Division of Gastroenterology, Hepatology, and Nutrition
University of Utah
Salt Lake City, Utah

Kevin A. Ghassemi, MD (Chapter 5)
Division of Digestive Diseases
David Geffen School of Medicine at UCLA
Los Angeles, California

C. Prakash Gyawali, MD, MRCP (Chapter 1)
Division of Gastroenterology
Washington University School of Medicine
St. Louis, Missouri

William L. Hasler, MD (Chapter 7)
Professor, Division of Gastroenterology
University of Michigan Health System
Ann Arbor, Michigan

Steve Heymen, PhD (Chapter 21)
UNC Center for Functional Gastrointestinal and Motility Disorders
University of North Carolina at Chapel Hill
Chapel Hill, North Carolina

Michael Horowitz, MBBS, PhD, FRACP (Chapter 23)
Discipline of Medicine
University of Adelaide, Australia
Centre of Research Excellence in Translating Nutritional Science to Good Health University of Adelaide, Australia
Endocrine and Metabolic Unit
Royal Adelaide Hospital, Australia

Karen L. Jones, Dip App Sci (Nuc Med), PhD (Chapter 23)
Discipline of Medicine
University of Adelaide, Australia
Centre of Research Excellence in Translating Nutritional Science to Good Health University of Adelaide, Australia

Carolina Malagelada, PhD, MD (Chapter 13)
Department of Gastroenterology and Digestive System Research Unit
Hospital Universitari Vall d'Hebron
Autonomous University of Barcelona
Barcelona, Spain

Juan R. Malagelada, MD (Chapter 13)
Department of Gastroenterology and Digestive System Research Unit
Hospital Universitari Vall d'Hebron
Autonomous University of Barcelona
Barcelona, Spain

Baha Moshiree, MD (Chapter 15)
Division of Gastroenterology
University of Miami School of Medicine
Miami, Florida

Ann Ouyang, MD (Chapter 24)
Hershey Medical Center
Hershey, Pennsylvania

John E. Pandolfino, MD, MSCI (Chapter 3)
Hans Popper Professor of Medicine
Division Chief, Gastroenterology and Hepatology
Department of Medicine
Feinberg School of Medicine, Northwestern University
Northwestern Memorial Hospital

Pankaj Jay Pasricha, MD (Chapter 8)
The Johns Hopkins School of Medicine
Division of Gastroenterology and Hepatology
Baltimore, Maryland

Eamonn M.M. Quigley, MD, FRCP, FACP, FACG, FRCPI (Chapter 16)
Division of Gastroenterology and Hepatology
Department of Medicine
Weill Cornell Medical College and Houston Methodist Hospital
Houston, Texas

Kulthep Rattanakovit, MD (Chapter 22)
Section of Gastroenterology and Hepatology
Georgia Regents University
Augusta, Georgia

Christopher K. Rayner, MBBS, PhD, FRACP (Chapter 23)
Discipline of Medicine
University of Adelaide, Australia
Centre of Research Excellence in Translating Nutritional Science to Good Health University of
    Adelaide, Australia
Department of Gastroenterology and Hepatology
Royal Adelaide Hospital, Australia

Jose M. Remes-Troche, MD (Chapter 6)
Digestive Physiology and Gastrointestinal Motility Laboratory
Medical-Biological Research Institute (IIMB)
Universidad Veracruzana, Veracruz
Veracruz, Mexico
College of Medicine Miguel Aleman Valdes, Veracruz
Veracruz, Mexico

Joel E. Richter, MD, PhD, MACG (Chapter 2)
Division of Digestive Diseases and Nutrition
The Joy McCann Culverhouse Center for Swallowing Disorders
University of South Florida Morsani College of Medicine
Tampa, Florida

Yehuda Ringel, MD, AGAF, FACG (Chapter 15)
Professor of Medicine
Chief, Division of Gastroenterology
Rabin Medical Center, Beilinson Hospital
Israel

Richard J. Saad, MD, MS (Chapter 19)
Assistant Professor
Division of Gastroenterology
University of Michigan Hospital and Health Systems

Gina Sam, MD, MPH (Chapter 20)
Division of Gastroenterology
Icahn School of Medicine at Mount Sinai
New York, New York

Erica A. Samuel, MD (Chapter 11)
Division of Gastroenterology and Hepatology
Medical College of Wisconsin
Milwaukee, Wisconsin

Maria Samuel, MD (Chapter 1)
Division of Gastroenterology
Washington University School of Medicine
St. Louis, Missouri

Lawrence R. Schiller, MD (Chapter 17)
Professor of Internal Medicine
Texas A&M University College of Medicine, Dallas Campus
Program Director
Gastroenterology Fellowship, Baylor University Medical Center, Dallas
Digestive Health Associates of Texas

Marc Schwartz, MD (Chapter 25)
Department of Medicine
Section of Gastroenterology, Hepatology, and Nutrition
University of Pittsburgh
Pittsburgh, Pennsylvania

Robert M. Siwiec, MD (Chapter 14)
Assistant Professor of Medicine
Division of Gastroenterology & Hepatology
Indiana University School of Medicine
Indianapolis, Indiana

Joseph K. Sunny, Jr., MD (Chapter 12)
Senior Gastroenterology Fellow
Texas Tech University Health Sciences Center
Paul L. Foster School of Medicine
El Paso, Texas

Rami Sweis, MD, PhD, MRCP (Chapter 4)
Department of Gastroenterology
University College Hospital
London, United Kingdom

Eva Szigethy, MD, PhD (Chapter 25)
Departments of Psychiatry, Medicine, and Pediatrics
University of Pittsburgh
Pittsburgh, Pennsylvania

Jan Tack, MD, PhD (Chapter 9)
Translational Research Center for Gastrointestinal Disorders (TARGID)
University of Leuven
Leuven, Belgium

Thangam Venkatesan, MD (Chapter 11)
Division of Gastroenterology and Hepatology
Medical College of Wisconsin
Milwaukee, Wisconsin

Elizabeth J. Videlock, MD (Chapter 18)
Oppenheimer Family Medical Center for Neurobiology of Stress
David Geffen School of Medicine at University of California - Los Angeles (UCLA)
Los Angeles, California

William E. Whitehead, PhD (Chapter 21)
UNC Center for Functional Gastrointestinal and Motility Disorders
University of North Carolina at Chapel Hill
Chapel Hill, North Carolina

John M. Wo, MD (Chapter 14)
Professor of Medicine
Division of Gastroenterology & Hepatology
Indiana University School of Medicine
Indianapolis, Indiana

PREFACE

Handbook of Gastrointestinal Motility and Functional Disorders fills the void in the GI literature for a short and concise go-to book for GI motility and functional GI disorders. The authors have been instrumental in teaching the concepts of GI motility disorders through their involvement in setting up the biennial ANMS GI Motility courses for the practitioners. This was followed with the creation of the ANMS Clinical Training Program where outside fellows visit one of the 10 centers of excellence to learn about GI motility testing. Each of these endeavors has allowed more individuals to learn the concepts about GI motility and/or functional GI disorders. Many of the chapter authors of this book are mentors in the American Neurogastroenterology and Motility Society, and others are internationally renowned investigators and educators in the field of gastrointestinal motility.

FOREWORD

Gastrointestinal motility refers to the motor activity in the gastrointestinal tract that moves the luminal contents in an aboral direction. This motor activity is controlled by events in the enteric nervous system mediated by a balance between neuroendocrine effects with some input from the central nervous system. When the system is functioning normally, solid foods and liquid traverse the entire 30 feet of the gastrointestinal tract effortlessly and without generating symptoms. However, disorders of gastrointestinal motility are common especially if we include functional gastrointestinal disorders such as functional dyspepsia, irritable bowel syndrome, and small intestinal dysmotility that may contribute to symptoms produced by bacteria within the colon or displaced into the small intestine (SIBO).

There have been many advances in our ability to investigate gastrointestinal motility and dysmotility. Luminal pressure measurement has advanced from non-perfused catheters to perfused catheters to catheters that employ solid state transducers to systems that combine solid state pressure and impedance transducers and can produce high resolution, 3-dimensional depiction of gastrointestinal motor activity. Quantitation of gastrointestinal transit has evolved from standard barium x-ray techniques, to physiologic scintigraphic methods to breath testing that can be performed in the doctor's office or at the bedside.

Over the years, we have come to appreciate that gut motility is influenced by diet, visceral sensitivity, central nervous system neuroendocrine activity, gut permeability, the gut microbiota, bowel infection, and psychological factors. This textbook edited by Satish Rao, MD, PhD, FRCP; Henry Parkman, MD; and Richard W. McCallum, MD, FACP, FRACP(AUST), FACG, AGAF integrates all of this material into 25 easy-to-read chapters. Rao, Parkman, and McCallum are experts in gastrointestinal motility and its disorders. Henry Parkman has focused mostly on the upper gastrointestinal tract, Satish Rao on the colon and intestinal gas, and Richard McCallum on the entire gastrointestinal tract. As editors, they have been able to recruit world expert clinicians/investigators as authors. Chapters are divided into symptom-based, disorder-based, and/or organ-based to enhance the utility of the chapters to the reader. Symptoms as well as epidemiology, pathophysiology, diagnosis, and treatment of gastrointestinal motor disorders are included.

This textbook provides an up-to-date comprehensive review of gastrointestinal motility and its disorders; it will be useful to clinicians, gastroenterologists, and investigators as well as to medical students and trainees. Many useful algorithms are included.

Robert S. Fisher, MD
Professor of Medicine
Temple University School of Medicine
Philadelphia, Pennsylvania

INTRODUCTION

Handbook of Gastrointestinal Motility and Functional Disorders is a user-friendly handbook that reviews the latest and most up-to-date information on the evaluation of symptoms and the usefulness of diagnostic tests of GI motility and functional GI disorders. It also provides a practical approach on how to treat these disorders. Each chapter is written by an international expert in the field who was carefully chosen for their renowned scientific and clinical expertise. The book brings together the essence of science and art in the practice of neurogastroenterology and GI motility.

The chapters are short in text, but enriched with algorithms, tables, and figures to enhance learning and readability. Each chapter follows a specific outline; chapters on symptoms follow the format of definition, pathophysiology, and evaluation of the symptoms, whereas the chapters on specific disorders follow the format of definition, diagnosis, and treatment. This allows for quick reading of the various chapters and helps readers gain up-to-date knowledge of the respective topic. The book will be useful for practicing physicians, junior academicians, GI fellows, young faculty, motility laboratory personnel, surgeons, internists, physician assistants, family practitioners, and nurse practitioners who all encounter the common problems of dysphagia, heartburn, nausea, vomiting, gastroparesis, abdominal pain, irritable bowel syndrome, constipation, and fecal incontinence in their daily practice.

This publication addresses a void in the GI literature and serves as a useful reference manual. The book also details the armamentarium of tests that are commonly performed in a modern GI motility and neurogastroenterology laboratory and elaborates on the specific entities that can be identified and treated. The update on management and therapy completes this text and explains how to integrate this diagnostic information into decision making and how to translate this to day-to-day patient care.

Satish S.C. Rao, MD, PhD, FRCP
Henry P. Parkman, MD
Richard W. McCallum, MD, FACP, FRACP (AUST), FACG, AGAF

Section I

Esophageal Disorders

1

Esophageal Symptoms
Dysphagia, Heartburn, and Esophageal Chest Pain

Maria Samuel, MD and C. Prakash Gyawali, MD, MRCP

KEY POINTS

- Dysphagia, chest pain, and heartburn are commonly encountered esophageal symptoms in medical practice.

- The most common causes of these esophageal symptoms may include neuromuscular, structural, and neoplastic disorders, in addition to gastroesophageal reflux, infectious esophagitis, and motility disorders.

- Commonly used diagnostic modalities for the evaluation of esophageal symptoms include barium swallow, upper endoscopy, and esophageal manometry. The initial diagnostic approach is dependent on a detailed clinical history, physical examination, and the presence or absence of alarm symptoms.

- An understanding of the pathophysiologic processes and causes involved in symptom generation in coordination with a systematic diagnostic evaluation, directs management of these common symptoms.

Dysphagia, heartburn, and chest pain are the most common esophageal symptoms encountered in medical practice. An understanding of their pathophysiologic basis and etiology guides both the evaluation and management of these symptoms. Commonly utilized investigative measures, such as upper endoscopy, barium swallow, and high-resolution esophageal manometry, facilitates an accurate diagnosis of the various conditions associated with these symptoms.

Rao SSC, Parkman HP, McCallum RW, eds.
Handbook of Gastrointestinal Motility and Functional Disorders (pp 3-17).

DYSPHAGIA

Definition

Dysphagia is derived from the Greek *dys* meaning "difficulty or disordered," and *phagia*, meaning "to eat." Dysphagia refers to difficulty in the transfer of food from the mouth to the stomach. This can result from dysfunction in bolus transfer from the mouth into the proximal esophagus (oropharyngeal dysphagia) or from the abnormal bolus transit in the tubular esophagus (esophageal dysphagia).[1,2] Dysphagia has a prevalence of 5% to 8% in individuals over 50 years, and 16% in the elderly, with the highest prevalence in nursing home residents.[3]

Pathophysiology

Swallowing involves three distinct processes: 1) the oral preparatory phase, lasting a few seconds when the food bolus is chewed to an appropriate consistency and size; 2) the pharyngeal phase, wherein pharyngeal peristalsis pushes the bolus from the pharynx into the esophagus over <1 second; and 3) the esophageal phase, when the bolus is propelled through the tubular esophagus through a relaxed lower esophageal sphincter (LES). Defects in neurological control mechanisms (central or peripheral), strength and coordination of oropharyngeal and esophageal musculature, and luminal obstructive processes can all result in dysphagia.[1,2]

Dysphagia can be characterized as oropharyngeal or esophageal in origin, depending on the location and mechanism of the defect.[1]

Oropharyngeal Dysphagia

Oropharyngeal dysphagia is defined as an inability to propel a food bolus from the oral cavity through the upper esophageal sphincter (UES) into the esophagus.[1] The musculature of the oropharynx is composed of striated muscle that is controlled by the cerebral cortex and medulla. The oropharyngeal stage begins with contractions of the tongue and the striated muscles of mastication, under control of the motor nuclei of cranial nerves V, VII, and XII.[4] Coordination of the pharyngeal swallow involves multiple processes, including 1) elevation of the soft palate for nasopharyngeal closure, 2) UES opening, 3) laryngeal closure, 4) tongue loading, 5) tongue pulsion, and 6) pharyngeal clearance. Sensory afferent fibers, which travel centrally via the internal branch of the superior laryngeal nerve and the glossopharyngeal nerve, recognize the food bolus and initiate the processes of oropharyngeal swallowing described earlier.[1]

Patients with oropharyngeal dysphagia often describe a sensation of choking or coughing on attempted swallowing, resulting in drooling or nasal regurgitation.[2] These symptoms occur within 1 second of initiating a swallow.[2,5] Symptoms are localized to the back of the throat or the high neck. Patients may also report finding pills or solid boluses retained in the oropharynx after attempted swallowing. Table 1-1 lists disorders that may be associated with oropharyngeal dysphagia. Neuromuscular causes are most frequent; hence, investigation serves to evaluate and exclude these disorders first.

Esophageal Dysphagia

Patients with esophageal dysphagia localize their symptoms to the base of the neck, retrosternal area, or epigastric region. In 30% of cases, the perceived localization is above the suprasternal notch when the actual location of hold-up is within the distal esophageal body.[2,5] Esophageal structural disorders, whether intrinsic, intramural, or extrinsic, are the most common causes of esophageal dysphagia; neuromuscular disorders, including disorders of motor function, are less common.[1] Table 1-1 summarizes etiologies of esophageal dysphagia.

TABLE 1-1
CAUSES OF DYSPHAGIA

OROPHARYNGEAL DYSPHAGIA	ESOPHAGEAL DYSPHAGIA
Neuromuscular Causes	*Structural Causes*
Cerebrovascular accident	Benign stricture
Parkinson's disease	Gastroesophageal reflux disease
Amyotrophic lateral sclerosis	Eosinophilic esophagitis
Brain tumors	Infectious esophagitis
Poliomyelitis	Foreign bodies
Myasthenia gravis	Extrinsic compression
Muscular dystrophies	Esophageal cancer
Polymyositis and dermatomyositis	
Upper esophageal sphincter dysfunction	*Neuromuscular Causes*
	Achalasia spectrum disorders
Structural Causes	Scleroderma esophagus
Pharyngitis	Esophageal spastic disorders
Radiation injury	Chagas disease
Cervical hyperostosis	Nonrelaxing lower esophageal sphincter
Head and neck cancer	
Thyromegaly	

Evaluation and Diagnostic Testing

Clinical History and Physical Examination

The first step is to distinguish between oropharyngeal and esophageal dysphagia, as investigative tests are different for the two types of dysphagia (Figure 1-1).[2] Dysphagia occurring within 1 second of attempting a swallow, aspiration, or nasal regurgitation during attempted swallowing, as well as coexisting neurologic symptoms pertaining to cortical or brainstem dysfunction, suggest oropharyngeal dysphagia.[2,6] With esophageal dysphagia, patients typically report food sticking retrosternally; regurgitation and chest pain may be associated symptoms.

A thorough clinical history is essential in determining the etiology of dysphagia.[1,2] Symptom onset, duration, and progression provide diagnostic information. For instance, a gradual onset of dysphagia to solids associated with heartburn may indicate a peptic process, including peptic stricture. Association with weight loss is concerning for an evolving obstructive process, such as achalasia spectrum disorders or neoplasia. Intermittent, nonprogressive dysphagia to solids only may suggest an esophageal web or ring, the most recognizable of which is the Schatzki ring at the esophagogastric junction (EGJ). Dysphagia of rapid, abrupt onset in association with neurologic deficits is indicative of oropharyngeal dysphagia, perhaps due to a stroke or other central process. Concurrent symptoms of bulbar or brainstem dysfunction, including vertigo and diplopia, also suggest oropharyngeal dysphagia.[2,6]

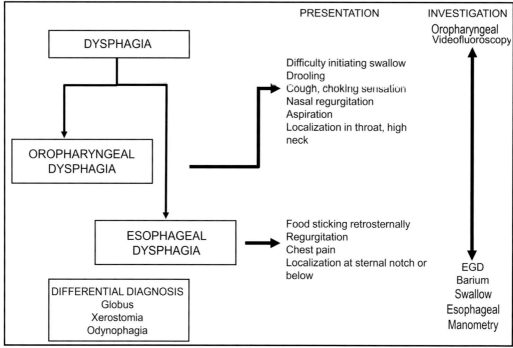

Figure 1-1. Algorithm for the evaluation of dysphagia. The first step is to decide whether the patient has oropharyngeal dysphagia or esophageal dysphagia based on careful history and physical examination. Globus, xerostomia, and odynophagia need to be considered, because these can mimic dysphagia symptoms. Evaluation of oropharyngeal dysphagia starts with videofluoroscopy to ascertain characteristics of oropharyngeal neuromuscular dysfunction and to assess the risk of aspiration with foods of varying consistency. Esophageal dysphagia is first assessed with endoscopy and biopsy, because the most frequent causes relate to mucosal abnormalities. Barium studies may provide complementary information in select situations. If a structural etiology is not identified, esophageal manometry is indicated to exclude a motor abnormality.

Other important historical factors include history of atopic disorders and asthma, raising suspicion for eosinophilic esophagitis; history of collagen vascular disease or scleroderma, suggesting esophageal hypomotility and reflux disease; and certain medications (eg, tetracyclines, doxycycline, bisphosphonates, quinine) that have been implicated in pill esophagitis. Localization of dysphagia; prior history of radiation; and symptoms of coughing, choking, heartburn, chest pain, or regurgitation are also helpful in further assessing dysphagia.[2]

The physical examination should include a full neurological evaluation, as well as a skin exam to assess for features of connective tissue diseases such as scleroderma and CREST syndrome (calcinosis, Raynaud phenomenon, esophageal dysmotility, sclerodactyly, and telangiectasia). Features of malnutrition, weight loss, muscle weakness and atrophy, and pulmonary aspiration should also be considered.

Diagnostic Testing

If oropharyngeal dysphagia is suspected:

- Videofluoroscopy or modified barium swallow provides lateral and anteroposterior views of the oral and pharyngeal phases of swallowing (Table 1-2). Not only is this helpful in identifying the location and severity of pharyngeal neuromuscular dysfunction, but this also defines the influence of bolus consistency (ie, thin liquids, thick liquids, barium cookies, or a cracker) and posture on bolus flow and clearance.[1,6] Identification of these mechanisms is particularly helpful in deciding specific swallow therapies and potential need for enteral feeding. Barium

TABLE 1-2 EVALUATION OF DYSPHAGIA	
OROPHARYNGEAL DYSPHAGIA	**ESOPHAGEAL DYSPHAGIA**
Oropharyngeal videofluoroscopy	Upper endoscopy
Fiberoptic endoscopy with sensory testing	Barium swallow
Cross-sectional imaging	Esophageal manometry (with or without stationary impedance)
Esophageal manometry (preferably high-resolution manometry)	Radionuclide transit studies
Serologic tests for polymyositis, dermatomyositis	Endoscopic functional luminal imaging probe
Serologic tests for myasthenia gravis	
Thyroid function testing	

studies are also utilized in the diagnosis of Zenker diverticulum, which is typically associated with UES dysfunction.

- Transnasal fiberoptic endoscopy, also referred to as fiberoptic endoscopic examination of swallowing (FEES), is useful in identifying mucosal abnormalities and neoplasia in the oropharynx and larynx. This provides indirect information on the pharyngeal swallow response and likelihood of pulmonary aspiration. If structural lesions are suspected, laryngoscopy may also be useful in this setting.[1,2,6]

- High-resolution esophageal manometry, especially when combined with stationary impedance, may be useful in evaluating and assessing UES relaxation and coordination of pharyngeal contraction with UES relaxation.[8] Detection of failed UES relaxation or elevated pharyngeal intrabolus pressures may help guide management, especially the need for cricopharyngeal dilation or myotomy.

If esophageal dysphagia is suspected:

- Whenever possible, upper endoscopy should be the initial test for the evaluation of esophageal dysphagia (Table 1-2). It allows for the evaluation of structural lesions, visual inspection of the mucosa, biopsies for diagnosis of eosinophilic esophagitis, and therapeutic dilation of structural lesions when indicated (Figure 1-2).[7]

- Esophagram (barium swallow) is also utilized in identifying structural abnormalities such as webs, diverticula, strictures, and tumors.[4-7] This is most useful where subtle strictures or narrowings are suspected, in which instance a solid bolus barium swallow can be performed. Esophagograms provide a roadmap for the therapeutic endoscopist when tight and long strictures are suspected. Timed upright barium swallow, which involves administration of 200 mL of barium standing the patient upright; and obtaining films at 1, 2, and 5 minutes, is useful in the assessment of esophageal emptying after therapeutic intervention for achalasia.

- Esophageal manometry involves recording the esophageal lumen pressures, which are surrogate markers for esophageal peristalsis and sphincter function, using mostly solid-state sensors on an esophageal catheter. Esophageal manometry is indicated in esophageal dysphagia with no structural lesions on upper endoscopy and/or barium swallow. In the past decade, high-resolution manometry (HRM) has revolutionized the diagnosis of esophageal outflow

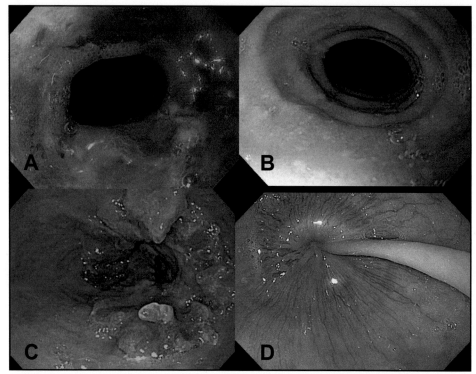

Figure 1-2. Examples of endoscopic findings in patients with esophageal dysphagia. (A) Peptic stricture associated with gastroesophageal reflux disease. (B) Concentric rings in a patient with eosinophilic esophagitis. (C) Circumferential exophytic esophageal cancer with elevated and rolled-out margins. (D) Puckered and tight lower esophageal sphincter that does not open on air insufflation in achalasia.

obstruction and achalasia spectrum disorders in particular, with higher sensitivity and specificity compared to previously utilized conventional manometry.[8,9]

Management

Oropharyngeal Dysphagia

Identifying the risk of pulmonary aspiration is paramount in managing oropharyngeal dysphagia. In addition, a careful assessment of nutritional status, weight, and caloric intake is undertaken. The combination of speech pathologists, diet changes, incorporation of softer foods, and postural measures is helpful in managing oropharyngeal dysphagia. If there is a high risk for aspiration or if oral intake does not provide adequate caloric intake, enteral feeding using percutaneous gastrostomy or jejunostomy tubes is considered.[2,4,6] Management is directed toward treatable underlying causes whenever possible, for example, disorders such as Parkinson's disease, thyrotoxicosis, and myasthenia gravis.[4] Surgical treatments aimed at relieving spastic causes of dysphagia, such as cricopharyngeal myotomy, are most often utilized in the presence of a Zenker diverticulum.

Esophageal Dysphagia

Because esophageal strictures or rings, usually related to reflux disease, constitute the most frequent etiologies for esophageal dysphagia (see Figure 1-2), endoscopy with bougie or balloon dilation and acid suppression with proton pump inhibitors (PPIs) constitute the most common measures for the management of esophageal dysphagia. The recognition of eosinophilic

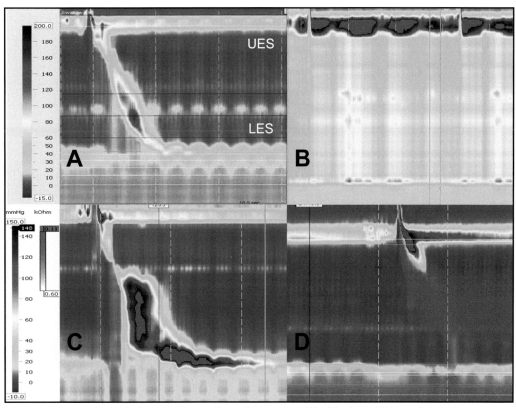

Figure 1-3. Representative high-resolution esophageal manometry (HRM) findings. (A) Normal peristaltic sequence. The upper esophageal sphincter (UES) and lower esophageal sphincter (LES) are seen as bands of pressure anchoring the topographic contour plot, called the "Clouse plot" in honor of Ray Clouse who pioneered HRM. Pressure in both sphincters dissipates, just preceding the contraction sequence, demonstrating adequate sphincter relaxation. (B) Achalasia. There is no esophageal-body peristalsis, with pan-esophageal compartmentalization of pressure and a nonrelaxing LES. (C) Esophageal spasm. The peristaltic sequence arrives prematurely at the distal esophagus, with fast contraction front velocity, seen as a vertical esophageal-body contraction sequence. Note that the LES relaxes preceding the sequence. (D) Aperistalsis. There is no esophageal body contraction, but the LES relaxes, so this is not achalasia. In this study, the bolus is visualized as purple contour that is seen to remain in the esophageal body. This example of impaired bolus transit is best seen with impedance HRM.

esophagitis as a cause for esophageal dysphagia has made upper endoscopy with biopsies a vital component of workup (see Figure 1-2); eosinophilic esophagitis is managed with topical steroid therapy, PPIs, and food elimination when trigger foods are identified; some advocate the six-food elimination diet as a therapeutic option, with gradual reintroduction of certain foods once symptom improvement is achieved.[10,11] If there is evidence of esophageal outflow obstruction from a structural obstructive process, such as an inoperable tumor, an endoscopic stent may be placed. For patients with severe obstructive lesions not amenable to endoscopic or surgical therapy, a gastrostomy or enterostomy tube can bypass the esophagus for enteral feeding. Infectious esophagitis is treated with antibiotics, acyclovir, or Nystatin, depending on the type of infection. Achalasia spectrum disorders (Figure 1-3) are managed endoscopically or surgically by disruption of the LES (Heller myotomy, pneumatic dilation, or perioral endoscopic myotomy); temporary benefit can be achieved by injecting botulinum toxin into the LES.[12] Dysphagia, from esophageal-body spastic disorders (see Figure 1-3) may improve with smooth muscle relaxants, such as calcium channel blockers, nitrates, and, rarely, botulinum toxin injection.[9]

TABLE 1-3 MECHANISMS CONTRIBUTING TO HEARTBURN AND CHEST PAIN OF ESOPHAGEAL ORIGIN	
Gastroesophageal reflux disease	Infectious esophagits
Eosinophilic esophagitis	Corrosive esophagitis (including pill esophagitis)
Esophageal motor disorders	Esophageal hypersensitivity
Functional symptoms	

HEARTBURN

Definition

Heartburn (pyrosis) is a burning feeling arising from the stomach and radiating to the retrosternal area, neck, and sometimes the back and arms. Heartburn is a typical symptom of gastroesophageal reflux disease (GERD) and may be associated with regurgitation, the effortless appearance of fluid in the mouth—either a bitter, acidic material or a salty fluid. In the setting of GERD, heartburn may be part of erosive GERD, which is readily treated with acid suppressive agents, many of which are available over the counter; therefore, nonerosive GERD is increasingly recognized as a mechanism for heartburn (Table 1-3). Certain foods, such as chocolate, foods high in fat, sugars, and onions, result in a lowering of LES tone, which may further worsen heartburn. Other triggers reported by patients include citrus juices, coffee, alcohol, and certain medications that reduce LES tone and esophageal peristalsis (eg, theophylline, calcium channel blockers). Activities that increase intra-abdominal pressure, such as bending over or lifting heavy objects, can also potentiate heartburn.[13]

Although GERD is the most common etiology of heartburn, this symptom can also occur from increased esophageal perception of physiological events, either chemical or mechanical (acid sensitivity), and from a functional process (functional heartburn). Other non-GERD mechanisms for esophageal mucosal inflammation, including infectious esophagitis, eosinophilic esophagitis, and caustic ingestions, can also result in heartburn (see Table 1-3).[13,14]

Pathophysiology

The most important pathophysiologic process involved in GERD-related heartburn is inappropriate or transient LES relaxation (TLESR), which allows reflux of gastric contents into the esophagus.[14] While even healthy individuals have TLESRs as a mechanism to vent gastric air, patients with GERD may have significantly reduced compliance at the EGJ such that TLESRs allow liquid content to escape into the esophagus; patients may also have increased frequency of TLESRs compared to healthy individuals.[15] A smaller proportion of the GERD population demonstrates low LES resting pressures (hypotensive LES). Structural disruption of the EGJ, where the LES has moved proximal to the level of the diaphragmatic crura (hiatus hernia), can further augment these LES physiologic alterations that promote reflux. The "acid pocket," an area of acidic supernatant residing at or close to the EGJ, has been recognized as a contributor to reflux, especially during TLESRs or in settings with structural disruption of the EGJ. Esophageal clearance of refluxed material may be compromised if esophageal body peristalsis is weak or hypomotile, resulting in prolonged esophageal acid exposure. Mucosal acidification following reflux events is partly neutralized by salivary bicarbonate following bolus clearance; this may be impaired in patients with reduced salivation, due to Sjogren syndrome, radiation to the head and neck, anticholinergic medications, and smoking.[16] Although the reflux of gastric acid commonly triggers heartburn, this symptom may be initiated by other processes, such as by esophageal balloon distention, reflux of bile salts, esophageal mucosal inflammation from nonreflux etiologies, and esophageal motor disturbances; it can be reproduced in the laboratory by esophageal acid infusion (Bernstein test) and esophageal balloon distention (thereby assessing esophageal hypersensitivity).[17]

Functional heartburn is characterized by reflux-related symptoms in the absence of esophagitis at endoscopy, normal esophageal acid exposure during esophageal pH monitoring, and unsatisfactory response to proton pump therapy.[18] The pathophysiology of this entity is believed to be related to disturbed esophageal perception, potentiated by psychological factors such as anxiety, panic disorder, and depression.[19]

The sensation of heartburn may be related to stimulation of mucosal chemoreceptors in the esophagus, which can become sensitive to acid following repeated acid exposure in reflux-associated heartburn.[20] However, it is unclear how discrete episodes of acid reflux trigger the symptomatic state that eventually leads to a diagnosis of GERD, since only 20% of discrete reflux episodes correlate with symptoms on esophageal pH monitoring. Moreover, as many as one-third of patients with Barrett esophagus (intestinal metaplasia in the distal esophagus exposed to prolonged acid exposure in predisposed individuals) are hyposensitive to acid. This suggests that the production of symptoms must involve more than contact of the esophagus with acid. Other factors that may influence the production of symptomatic heartburn include the acid clearance mechanism, salivary bicarbonate concentration, volume and extent of refluxed acid, interaction of pepsin with acid, and esophageal sensitivity.[14,16,17]

Although heartburn is commonly associated with GERD, gallbladder disease, peptic ulcer disease, and delayed gastric emptying may also generate symptoms that could mimic GERD.[16]

Evaluation and Diagnostic Testing

A good history is paramount in the initial evaluation of heartburn. It is now well recognized that the initial diagnostic and therapeutic approach to heartburn consists of empiric treatment with acid suppressive medications such as PPIs, the so-called PPI test (Figure 1-4). Improvement of heartburn following PPI therapy has a high sensitivity and predictive value for GERD as a mechanism for heartburn. In the absence of alarm symptoms (dysphagia or odynophagia, weight loss, prolonged symptoms, new-onset symptoms in patients older than 45 years, anemia and blood loss, family history of esophageal cancer, atypical reflux symptoms), symptomatic management can continue without the need for invasive testing in the short term (see Figure 1-4).

If there is no resolution of symptoms following a trial of PPI, or if there are alarm features, diagnostic evaluation starts with upper endoscopy (Table 1-4). The endoscopy is designed to evaluate alternative mechanisms of symptom generation (such as pill esophagitis, infectious esophagitis, eosinophilic esophagitis, or motor disorders) and to evaluate for complications of reflux disease, such as esophageal ulceration, stricture formation, Barrett's esophagus, and even esophageal adenocarcinoma. Practice guidelines recommend endoscopy to screen for Barrett's esophagus in high-risk patients and those with a long-standing history of GERD.[21] Endoscopy may also demonstrate findings of an alternative mechanism for symptoms, including eosinophilic esophagitis, infectious esophagitis, pill esophagitis, and other nonreflux disorders in the esophagus (see Figure 1-2).

Barium studies do not have a role in the diagnosis of reflux disease, since the presence or absence of TLESRs during the study will influence the results of the barium study, regardless of whether the patient has reflux disease (TLESRs can occur in normal individuals as well as GERD

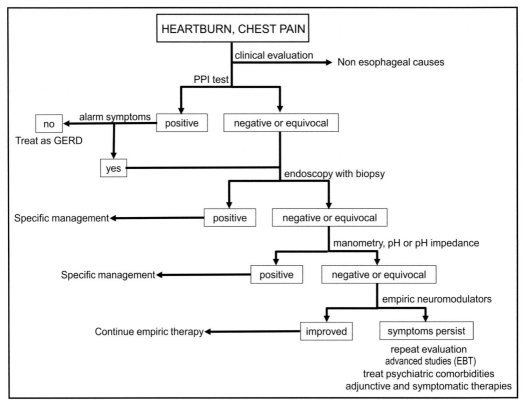

Figure 1-4. Algorithm for the evaluation of heartburn and chest pain. The approach starts with careful clinical history and physical examination to determine whether symptoms are of esophageal or nonesophageal origin. A proton pump inhibitor (PPI) test has clinical value in determining a reflux etiology if symptoms improve; the presence of alarm symptoms or a negative PPI test prompts endoscopy. If endoscopy (with biopsies to evaluate for eosinophilic esophagitis) is unrevealing, ambulatory pH or pH-impedance monitoring off therapy may allow further definition of a reflux-based mechanism for pain; the concurrent manometry study performed to assist pH probe placement may demonstrate a motor mechanism for symptoms. If specific diagnoses are made, appropriate management is initiated. In the absence of reflux or motor mechanisms for symptoms, empiric neuromodulator therapy can be considered. If symptoms persist further, repeat evaluation or advanced studies described in Table 1-4 can be considered. Psychiatric comorbidities need therapeutic attention, as these can propagate esophageal symptoms; adjunctive therapies such as acupuncture, cognitive and behavioral therapy, and hypnosis could be of value at this stage.

patients). Barium studies, however, provide accurate anatomic information and are frequently utilized in assessing anatomic relationships at the EGJ, especially prior to and following antireflux surgery. Barium studies have higher sensitivity for diagnosis of strictures (especially subtle strictures) and motor disorders compared to endoscopy.

Further characterization of esophageal acid and reflux exposure is provided by ambulatory pH and pH-impedance monitoring (see Figure 1-4). The additional benefit of impedance monitoring is that all types of reflux events—acidic, weakly acidic, liquid, and gaseous—can be identified (Figure 1-5). pH and pH-impedance monitoring are utilized most often in quantifying esophageal acid exposure, in correlating symptoms to reflux events, and in evaluating persisting symptoms despite adequate management of reflux disease (see Table 1-4). Quantification of acid exposure is frequently performed prior to antireflux surgery, when ambulatory pH or pH monitoring is performed off antisecretory therapy. Correlating symptoms to reflux events also requires testing when off antisecretory therapy. When symptoms persist despite adequate reflux management, prior evidence for reflux disease determines whether testing is performed on or off antisecretory therapy. If prior evidence for GERD is marginal or absent, it is best to study patients off antisecretory therapy. On the other hand, if there is robust prior evidence for GERD, pH-impedance

TABLE 1-4

TESTS USED FOR THE EVALUATION OF HEARTBURN AND CHEST PAIN OF ESOPHAGEAL ORIGIN

CLINICAL TESTS	TESTS UTILIZED IN RESEARCH
Proton pump inhibitor test	Electron microscopy of biopsies (especially evaluation for dilated intercellular spaces)
Upper endoscopy with biopsies to evaluate for eosinophilic esophagitis	Acid perfusion (Bernstein test)
Esophageal pH and pH-impedance monitoring	Esophageal functional luminal imaging probe
Esophageal manometry	High-frequency ultrasound
Baloon distension	Esophageal-evoked potentials
Endoscopic ultrasound	Neuroimaging, including functional magnetic resonance imaging
Barium swallow (less useful)	
Psychological evaluation	

monitoring on maximal antireflux therapy will help establish whether therapy is adequate and whether symptoms can be related to incompletely treated reflux. In addition to catheter-based pH and pH impedance, wireless pH monitoring is now possible for 48 to 96 hours using a pH probe attached to the esophageal mucosa that can communicate with a recorder that the patient wears on their belt (see Figure 1-5). Prolonged pH recording may have value in clarifying the presence or absence of abnormal acid exposure and/or symptom reflux correlation in patients with infrequent symptoms or unclear clinical evidence for GERD.[21-23]

Esophageal manometry does not enhance the initial evaluation of heartburn. However, manometry is utilized in determining the location of the LES for placement of pH and pH probes. It is also useful in excluding motor disorders that can mimic reflux symptoms and in assessing esophageal peristaltic performance, which can have implications on whether a standard fundoplication is possible.[8,9] Manometry with concurrent stationary impedance has value in diagnosing other, less common conditions that can mimic reflux disease, such as rumination syndrome, supragastric belching, and aerophagy.[24]

Management

The mainstay of management of reflux-related heartburn is antisecretory therapy that reduces gastric acid production, hence reducing the noxious chemical trigger from gastric acid in causing heartburn. Two classes of antisecretory medications are in common use: histamine-2 receptor antagonists (H2RAs) (eg, cimetidine, ranitidine, famotidine) and PPIs (eg, omeprazole, lansoprazole, rabeprazole, pantoprazole, esomeprazole, dexlansoprazole). These agents, used in once-a-day to twice-a-day dosing, are extremely effective in treating reflux-related heartburn in the vast majority of patients. PPIs need to be administered 30 to 45 minutes prior to a meal, as these agents deactivate proton pumps that are activated by a meal; they are typically administered before the first meal of the day when used as once-daily doses. While treatment typically starts with a PPI, this can be stepped down to an H2RA in patients with symptom resolution and uncomplicated reflux disease, in the absence of erosive esophagitis or Barrett's esophagus. When erosive esophagitis is present, over 80% of patients will demonstrate healing of esophagitis using a PPI; these

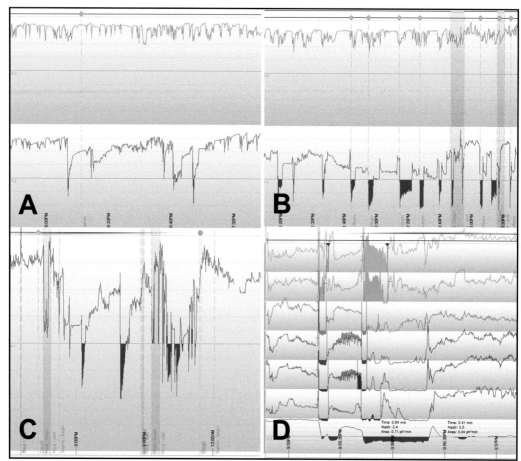

Figure 1-5. Ambulatory pH and pH-impedance tracings. (A) A two-channel pH study demonstrating infrequent reflux events in the distal channel with pH drops below a threshold of 4.0. (B) A two-channel pH study demonstrating frequent reflux events. The cumulative duration of pH < 4.0 is calculated as percentage time over the course of a day, termed the acid exposure time (AET). (C) Single-channel pH study using a wireless pH probe, demonstrating reflux events. A careful food diary is needed to determine if pH drops are caused by reflux events or ingested food. (D) A pH-impedance study demonstrating prolonged reflux events in the pH channel (last channel, in red) and impedance drops in the impedance channels. Note that the duration of impedance drop is far less than the pH drop, reflecting the fact that the bulk of reflux clearance may be prompt, but mucosal acidification can persist longer.

agents are maintained for long-term control of GERD. In patients with well-documented GERD, antireflux surgery is an option, with long-term results that resemble that from PPI therapy.[24]

For infrequent symptoms, neutralization of acid may be adequate with antacids containing magnesium hydroxide, calcium carbonate, or aluminum hydroxide. Nonpharmacologic measures, including avoiding large meals, avoiding lying down within 2 to 3 hours of a meal, avoiding food triggers, weight loss in the obese, and avoiding smoking and excessive alcohol intake, may complement medical management. Baclofen, a gamma-amino butyric acid B receptor agonist, has been demonstrated to reduce reflux events by decreasing TLESRs and can provide adjunctive benefit in patients with persisting reflux despite PPI therapy.[24]

Nonreflux etiologies of heartburn are treated depending on the etiology identified on clinical evaluation. Complications of reflux disease may also require management when encountered. Eosinophilic esophagitis, infectious esophagitis, pill esophagitis, and caustic esophagitis require specific management; most of these may benefit from additional acid suppression and topical antacids, sometimes combined with topical analgesics such as lidocaine elixir.

CHEST PAIN OF ESOPHAGEAL ORIGIN

Definition

Chest pain of esophageal origin is diagnosed in patients with retrosternal pain wherein cardiac disease has been ruled out; nonesophageal etiologies in the chest wall and other thoracic organs are also excluded when appropriate. The most common esophageal cause for chest pain is reflux disease; other causes include eosinophilic esophagitis, esophageal motor disorders, and esophageal visceral hypersensitivity (see Table 1-3). Heartburn may be reported as chest pain by some patients. Chest pain generates a lot of concern and can lead to emergency department visits and health care utilization. Demonstrating an esophageal source for the pain may help reduce health care utilization and lessen anxiety.[25] There is a strong association between esophageal chest pain and affective disorders, including anxiety, panic disorder, depression, and somatization.

Esophageal chest pain is characterized by a burning or squeezing sensation in the substernal region that may radiate to the neck, back, or jaws. It may last for minutes to hours, and can be severe enough to awaken the patient from sleep. When caused by reflux, it often abates spontaneously or with the use of antacids and may be accompanied by other typical reflux symptoms. Based on history alone, it is difficult to differentiate cardiac chest pain from pain of esophageal origin. In addition, relief of chest pain with nitroglycerin is not specific to cardiac chest pain and may be seen with chest pain of esophageal origin.

Pathophysiology

The mechanisms involved in the production of esophageal chest pain are not well elucidated but may involve stimulation of esophageal chemoreceptors (by acid, pepsin, or bile), mechanoreceptors (by distention or spasm), and thermoreceptors (by temperature changes, especially cold). For instance, ingestion of cold liquids can result in reduced peristalsis and distention of the esophagus, with resultant chest pain due to the luminal distention.[24,25]

Furthermore, altered pain perception may contribute to an individual's reaction to a noxious stimulus, which could explain why anxiolytics and antidepressants may improve esophageal chest pain.[20]

Gastroesophageal reflux produces pain through stimulation of esophageal chemoreceptors by acid. Two candidate receptors have been suggested to mediate acid sensitivity in the esophagus: the vanilloid receptor 1 (TRPV1) and the acid-sensing ion channels (ASIC). Upregulation of TRPV1 has been proposed to induce acid hypersensitivity in patients with esophageal chest pain.[14] Furthermore, motor abnormalities, such as exaggerated contractions and even spasm, can be induced by acid perfusion into the esophagus, correlating with concurrent chest pain. The degree of pain induced correlated to the amplitude and duration of esophageal contractions in these studies. Although patients with chest pain of esophageal origin have an increased frequency of esophageal contractions when compared to the control population, the mechanism by which these contractions result in pain is not clearly known.[20] Studies using high-frequency ultrasound have demonstrated that longitudinal esophageal smooth muscle contraction could be one of the mechanisms involved, as sustained longitudinal muscle contraction has been identified as a correlate of chest pain using these methods (see Table 1-4).

While peripheral sensitization with noxious triggers such as reflux events are thought to be the primary process in chest pain of esophageal origin, central sensitization and altered cerebral processing of peripheral stimuli are thought to contribute, particularly by inducing secondary hyperalgesia in surrounding healthy tissue.[20] Emotions, stress, and cognitive and psychological comorbidities also contribute to symptom generation and propagation.[17]

Diagnostic Approach

The diagnostic approach to chest pain involves a detailed clinical history and physical examination, as well as the exclusion of cardiac etiologies of the chest pain with appropriate testing (eg, stress tests, coronary angiography, as indicated).

The recognition that chest pain of esophageal origin is most commonly due to GERD directs the diagnostic and therapeutic approach, which is similar to that described earlier for heartburn (see Figure 1-4). Evaluation with a PPI taken twice daily serves to both diagnose GERD and alleviate esophageal chest pain (see Table 1-3). Upper endoscopy serves to evaluate for mucosal etiologies, including eosinophilic esophagitis, reflux esophagitis, and infectious esophagitis (see Figure 1-2). Ambulatory pH monitoring (see Figure 1-5) is useful in evaluating not just esophageal acid exposure times, but also the association between reflux and chest pain episodes.[21,22] Esophageal manometry evaluates for a motility disorder; spastic motor disorders and achalasia spectrum disorders may be associated with chest pain (see Figure 1-3). Esophageal hypersensitivity and functional chest pain are often encountered in patients with affective disorders such as anxiety, depression, panic disorder, and somatization; therefore, psychological evaluation may be useful in refractory cases.

Management

While management is directed by results of investigative studies, antireflux therapy is the initial approach to management when no specific etiology is identified (see Figure 1-4). Acid suppression and antireflux surgery may be options in patients with well-documented GERD. Eosinophilic esophagitis, infectious esophagitis, and other esophageal mucosal processes are treated with specific management if encountered.

Esophageal hypersensitivity may overlap with GERD, in which instance pain modulators are added to the management regimen.[20] Tricyclic antidepressants, atypical analgesics, and contemporary antidepressants (eg, paroxetine, venlafaxine, duloxetine) may be of value in suppressing symptoms under these circumstances. Spastic motor disorders may be markers of esophageal visceral hypersensitivity; in some instances, vigor of esophageal contraction could directly contribute to chest pain, in which instance smooth muscle relaxants and botulinum toxin injection may help resolve symptoms. Theophylline, an adenosine receptor antagonist, has been demonstrated to help esophageal chest pain, but its use is limited by side effects. Nonpharmacologic approaches, including hypnotherapy, cognitive and behavioral therapy, biofeedback, and transcutaneous nerve stimulation, have been utilized with varying results. Acupuncture and johrei can provide benefit in refractory cases.[17,20,25]

Identification of a specific etiology for esophageal chest pain improves the likelihood of symptom improvement and reduces health care utilization.[25] Psychological approaches complement management; reassurance and judicious utilization of investigative approaches provide the highest likelihood of a good outcome.

CONCLUSION

A systematic approach to the diagnosis of the common causes of esophageal symptoms is helpful in informing the appropriate management of patients. Several diagnostic modalities are utilized in medical practice for the evaluation of esophageal symptoms of dysphagia, heartburn, and chest pain. Such modalities, in coordination with an understanding of the pathophysiology and etiologies of the symptoms, direct management of these commonly encountered esophageal symptoms.

REFERENCES

1. Cook IJ. Diagnostic evaluation of dysphagia. *Nature Clinical Practice Gastroenterology and Hepatology*. 2008;5: 393-403.

2. Kuo P, Holloway RH, Nguyen NQ. Current and future techniques in the evaluation of dysphagia. *J Gastroenterol Hepatol*. 2012;27:873-881.

3. Lindgren MD, Janzon L. Prevalence of swallowing complaints and clinical findings among 50-79 year old men and women in an urban population. *Dysphagia*. 1991;6:187-192.

4. Cook IJ, Kahrilas PJ. AGA technical review on management of oropharyngeal dysphagia. *Gastroenterology*. 1999;116:455-478.

5. Trate DM, Parkman HP, Fisher RS. Dysphagia evaluation, diagnosis, and treatment. *Gastroenterology*. 1996;23:417-432.

6. Cook IJ. Oropharyngeal dysphagia. *Gastroenterol Clin N Am*. 2009;38:411-443.

7. Spechler SJ. AGA technical review on treatment of patients with dysphagia caused by benign disorders of distal esophagus. *Gastroenterology*. 1999;117:233-254.

8. Gyawali CP, Bredenoord AJ, Conklin JL, et al. Evaluation of esophageal motor function in clinical practice. *Neurogastroenterol Motil*. 2013;25:99-133.

9. Roman S, Kahrilas PJ. Challenges in the swallowing mechanism: nonobstructive dysphagia in the era of high resolution manometry and impedance. *Gastroenterol Clin N Am*. 2011;40:823-835.

10. Dellon ES. Diagnosis and management of eosinophilic esophagitis. *Clin Gastroenterol Hepatol*. 2012;10(10): 1066-1078.

11. Dellon ES, Gonsalves N, Hirano I, Furuta GT, Liacouras CA, Katzka DA. ACG clinical guideline: evidenced based approach to the diagnosis and management of esophageal eosinophilia and eosinophilic esophagitis (EoE). *Am J Gastroenterol*. 2013;108(5):679-692.

12. Vaezi MF, Pandolfino JE, Vela MF. ACG clinical guideline: diagnosis and management of achalasia. *Am J Gastroenterol*. 2013;108(8):1238-1249.

13. Kahrilas PJ. Clinical practice. Gastroesophageal reflux disease. *N Engl J Med*. 2008;359:1700-1707.

14. Kandulski A, Malfertheiner P. Gastroesophageal reflux disease – from reflux episodes to mucosal inflammation. *Nat Rev Gastroenterol Hepatol*. 2012;9:15-22.

15. Schneider JH, Küper MA, Königsrainer A, Brücher BL. Transient lower esophageal sphincter relaxation and esophageal motor response. *J Surg Res*. 2010;159(2):714-719.

16. Boeckxstaens GE. Review article: the pathophysiology of gastro-esophageal reflux disease. *Aliment Pharmacol Ther*. 2007;26(2):149-160.

17. Gyawali CP. Esophageal hypersensitivity. *Gastroenterol Hepatol*. 2010;6:497-500.

18. Kumar AR, Katz PO. Functional esophageal disorders: a review of diagnosis and management. *Expert Rev Gastroenterol Hepatol*. 2013;7:453-461.

19. Zerbib F, Bruley des Varannes S, Simon M, Galmiche JP. Functional heartburn: definition and management strategies. *Curr Gastroenterol Rep*. 2012;14(3):181-188.

20. Remes-Troche JM. The hypersensitive esophagus: pathophysiology, evaluation and treatment options. *Curr Gastroenterol Rep*. 2010;12:417-426.

21. Richter JE, Pandolfino JE, Vela MF, et al. Utilization of wireless pH monitoring technologies: a summary of the Proceedings from the Esophageal Diagnostic Working Group. *Dis Esophagus*. 2013;26(8):755-765.

22. Pandolfino JE, Vela MF. Esophageal-reflux monitoring. *Gastrointest Endosc*. 2009;69(4):917-930.

23. Fass R, Sifrim D. Management of heartburn not responding to proton pump inhibitors. *Gut*. 2009;58(2):295-309.

24. Katz PO, Gerson LB, Vela MF. Guidelines for the diagnosis and management of gastroesophageal reflux disease. *Am J Gastroenterol*. 2013;108:308-328.

25. Coss-Adame E, Erdogan A, Rao SS. Treatment of esophageal (noncardiac) chest pain: a review. *Clin Gastroenterol Hepatol*. 2013;Aug 28 (Epub ahead of print).

2

Gastroesophageal Reflux Disease

Wojciech Blonski, MD, PhD and Joel E. Richter, MD, FACP, MACG

KEY POINTS

- Gastroesophageal reflux disease (GERD) is defined as a presence of troublesome symptoms and/or complications caused by retrograde movement of gastric contents into the esophagus. The most typical symptoms are heartburn and regurgitation.

- GERD can be separated into esophageal and extraesophageal syndromes. Esophageal GERD syndromes are further divided into symptomatic syndromes (typical reflux syndrome and reflux chest pain syndrome) and syndromes with esophageal injury (reflux esophagitis, reflux stricture, Barrett's esophagus, and esophageal adenocarcinoma). Extraesophageal GERD syndromes are divided into established associations (reflux cough syndrome, reflux laryngitis syndrome, reflux asthma syndrome, and reflux dental erosion syndrome) and proposed associations (pharyngitis, sinusitis, idiopathic pulmonary fibrosis, and recurrent otitis media).

- Patients with suspected GERD symptoms should be placed on proton pump inhibitors (PPIs) and therapy should be maximized before further diagnostic workup.

- The initial diagnostic test should be endoscopy, especially if there are alarming symptoms such as dysphagia, bleeding, or weight loss.

- The most sensitive test for GERD is esophageal reflux testing. As a diagnostic test, this should be done off PPIs, with the key parameters to measure being acid reflux and symptom correlation. If the diagnosis of GERD is confirmed but symptoms persist on PPIs, then pH-impedance testing to measure both acid and nonacid reflux is the preferred test.

- PPIs and antireflux surgery are comparable in maintaining long-term remission. Careful selection of patients for antireflux surgery is warranted.

Rao SSC, Parkman HP, McCallum RW, eds.
Handbook of Gastrointestinal Motility and Functional Disorders (pp 19-33).

DEFINITION

Until recently, the definition of GERD has varied among studies without any consensus agreement. This changed with the publication of the Montreal consensus report in 2006.[1] According to the new Montreal definition, GERD is the presence of troublesome (adversely affecting patient's well-being) symptoms and/or complications caused by retrograde movement of gastric contents into the esophagus.[3] Data from population-based studies showed that mild troublesome symptoms occur at least twice a week, while moderate to severe symptoms occur more than 1 day per week.[1]

Gastroesophageal reflux disease was separated into esophageal and extraesophageal syndromes (Figure 2-1).[1] Esophageal syndromes were further divided into symptomatic syndromes (typical reflux syndrome and reflux chest pain syndrome) and syndromes with esophageal injury (reflux esophagitis, reflux stricture, Barrett's esophagus and esophageal adenocarcinoma). Extraesophageal syndromes were divided into established associations (reflux cough syndrome, reflux laryngitis syndrome, reflux asthma syndrome, and reflux dental erosion syndrome) and proposed associations (pharyngitis, sinusitis, idiopathic pulmonary fibrosis, and recurrent otitis media).

The Montreal definition recognized that symptoms caused by GERD might be due to acidic, weakly acidic, or gaseous refluxate. The diagnosis of GERD could be made based on typical symptoms; evidence of gastric refluxate into the esophagus determined by esophageal pH monitoring or intraesophageal pH-impedance monitoring; or injuries caused by the refluxate to the esophageal mucosa demonstrated on endoscopy, histologic, or electron microscopy evaluation.

DIAGNOSIS

According to the Montreal definition of GERD, typical reflux syndrome can be diagnosed without any additional diagnostic testing.[3] However, recent data from the Diamond study found that troublesome symptom-based diagnosis of GERD has only moderate sensitivity and specificity for family practitioners (63% and 63%) and gastroenterologists (67% and 70%) when compared with reference tests for GERD, such as upper endoscopy or abnormal esophageal pH testing.[4] In this study, 203 patients had GERD and 105 patients did not have GERD.[4] Heartburn was considered the most troublesome symptom in 40% and 21% of patients, with and patients without GERD, respectively, and the second most troublesome symptom in 25% of patients with GERD and 14% of patients without GERD.[4] Dyspepsia was marked as the most troublesome symptom in 21% of patients with GERD and 23% of patients without GERD.[4] Of note, regurgitation was only identified as the most troublesome symptom in 9% of GERD patients and 5% of non-GERD patients and the second most troublesome symptom in 17% of GERD patients and 7% of non-GERD patients.[4]

Trial With Proton Pump Inhibitors

Patients presenting with GERD symptoms usually undergo a trial test with proton pump inhibitors (PPIs) given at a single dose before breakfast for 2 to 4 weeks. However, a meta-analysis of 15 studies comparing the clinical response to a 1- to 4-week course of normal or high-dose PPIs in 2793 patients with chronic GERD symptoms showed good pooled sensitivity of 78% (95% CI 66% to 86%), but poor specificity of 54% (95% CI 44% to 65%) when compared with 24-hour esophageal pH monitoring, which is used as the gold standard to diagnose GERD.[5] These data were further supported by a recent study analyzing data from the Diamond study that demonstrated limited ability of the PPI test (esomeprazole 40 mg daily for 2 weeks) to diagnose GERD

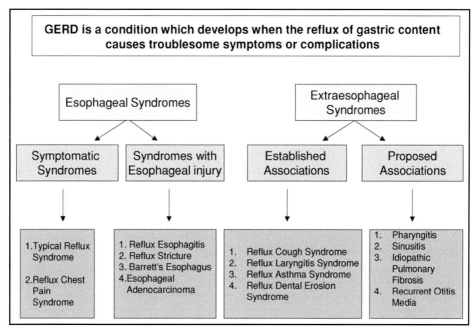

Figure 2-1. The overall definition of GERD and its constituent syndromes based on the Montreal consensus report. (Adapted with permission from Vakil N, van Zanten SV, Kahrilas P, et al. The Montreal definition and classification of gastroesophageal reflux disease: a global evidence-based consensus. *Am J Gastroenterol.* 2006;101:1900-1920.)

among 308 patients presenting with reflux symptoms with a positive response in 69% of patients with documented GERD and 51% of non-GERD patients.[4] On the other hand, a meta-analysis of 6 studies showed that high-dose PPI treatment up to 4 weeks duration was a cost-effective strategy with overall sensitivity of 80% (95% CI 64% to 83%) and specificity of 74% (95% CI 64% to 83%) in patients with noncardiac chest pain.[5] Despite these shortcomings, a PPI trial is recommended as the initial diagnostic test in patients with suspected GERD due to its simplicity, relatively cheap cost, and possibility of avoiding further expensive testing. In patients not responding to a single dose of PPIs, we recommend verifying drug compliance, then optimizing PPI therapy to twice daily (before breakfast and dinner) with symptom assessment after 4 to 8 weeks before considering additional testing.

Upper Endoscopy

Patients with persistent symptoms after a trial of twice-daily PPIs have "refractory GERD" and should undergo upper endoscopy as the next diagnostic test.[6] Upper endoscopy is also recommended as an early and first diagnostic step in those GERD patients who have alarming symptoms such as dysphagia, bleeding, anemia, weight loss, or recurrent vomiting.[6] Los Angeles (LA) classification of GERD with esophagitis has become the most universally accepted tool for grading erosive esophagitis.[7,8] Data from the large prospective European multicenter ProGERD study indicated that among 2721 patients with GERD symptoms at baseline before treatment, 45% had endoscopy-negative reflux disease, 38% had mild LA A/B esophagitis, 8% had more severe LA C/D esophagitis, and 9% had Barrett's esophagus.[9] After initial endoscopy, patients were treated for 2 to 8 weeks with esomeprazole and then followed by their primary care physicians. After 5 years of follow-up, the majority of patients either improved or had the same grade of esophagitis on follow-up endoscopy. Multivariate analysis suggested that family history of GERD (OR = 1.44, 95%CI 1.09 to 1.92) and lack of healing of esophagitis after initial treatment with PPI

(OR = 1.53, 95% CI 1.04 to 2.24) were the only baseline factors predicting progression to LA A/B or LA C/D esophagitis over 5 years. Progression to Barrett's esophagus was observed in 19.7% of patients with initial LA C/D esophagitis, 12.1% of LA A/B esophagitis, and 5.9% of endoscopy-negative reflux disease. Current guidelines recommend that patients with LA C/D esophagitis undergo follow-up upper endoscopy after a 2-month course of PPI to assess esophageal healing and rule out the presence of Barrett's esophagus. If Barrett's esophagus is not identified, then further screening endoscopies are not indicated.[6]

Esophageal Reflux Testing

The Esophageal Diagnostic Working Group has recently recommended that patients with suspected GERD failing PPIs and a lack of esophagitis on upper endoscopy should next undergo ambulatory esophageal pH testing off antacid therapy to confidently identify abnormal acid reflux.[10] This approach is preferred because esophageal pH monitoring done "on" PPIs given twice daily shows normal results in over 90% of patients with typical symptoms and nearly all patients with extraesophageal symptoms of GERD.[11] It is critical at this juncture to document abnormal acid reflux as the cause of symptoms and esophageal mucosal damage because this disease can be improved with aggressive PPI treatment or antireflux surgery. In patients without pathologic acid reflux off antisecretory therapy, the likelihood of clinically significant nonacid or bile reflux is low.[10] Those patients without pathologic acid reflux do not have GERD. They should undergo further evaluation for non-GERD causes of their symptoms, such as functional heartburn/chest pain; achalasia; eosinophilic esophagitis; gastroparesis; allergies; or diseases of the ear, nose, throat, and lungs not associated with acid reflux. A vigorous attempt should be made to discontinue PPI therapy, although one recent report found that 42% of patients continued PPI therapy despite negative results of pH testing.[12]

Traditionally, the standard test for evaluating esophageal pH was 24-hour ambulatory intra-esophageal pH monitoring.[13] In this test, the pH probe is passed transnasally, placed 5 cm above the lower esophageal sphincter (LES) (determined by esophageal manometry), and connected to a data recorder powered by batteries. The recorder collects pH values every 4 to 6 seconds for 24 hours. The patient is asked to record meals, time in recumbent position, and symptoms by pressing dedicated buttons. The most reproducible parameter of acid reflux disease is total time of esophageal pH < 4 exceeding 4% to 5.5%. The association between symptoms and acid reflux is assessed using the symptom index (SI) and the symptom association probability (SAP) expressed in percentages.[10]

Esophageal pH monitoring has 90% sensitivity and 85% to 100% specificity in patients with reflux esophagitis, but the test is rarely indicated in this setting.[14] However, in patients with normal esophageal mucosa, pH testing is only 60% sensitive and 85% to 90% specific. This disappointing sensitivity may be due to variability in reflux pattern from day to day and the tendency of the transnasal probe to be uncomfortable, limiting patients' daily activities and reducing the duration of the study.[10]

Due to these problems, the wireless ambulatory pH monitoring with the Bravo pH capsule (Given Imaging) has been recommended as the most desirable testing method for esophageal acid reflux.[10] The capsule is placed 6 cm above the squamocolumnar junction during upper endoscopy. Lack of the irritating transnasal catheter allows patients to have normal daily activities with sufficient time to monitor esophageal pH. The wireless capsule detaches and passes spontaneously within 2 weeks. The Esophageal Working Group recommends 48-hour monitoring of esophageal pH off PPIs for at least 7 days to minimize the potential for the negative effect of day-to-day variability in acid reflux and maximize symptom reflux correlation. The normative values of pathologic acid reflux during 48 hours were found to be similar to those for 24-hour assessment.[10]

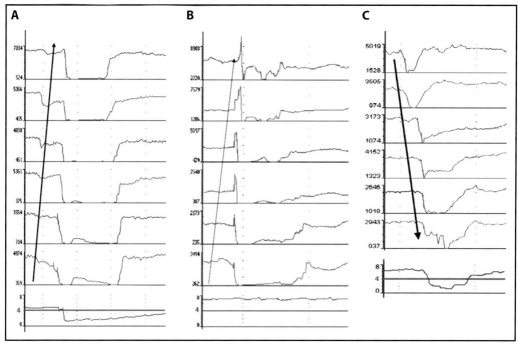

Figure 2-2. (A) An acid reflux episode detected by pH-impedance: retrograde bolus movement with accompanying drop in the distal esophageal pH to less than 4. (B) A nonacid reflux episode detected by pH-impedance: retrograde movement of the refluxate with accompanying distal esophageal pH greater than 4. (C) An acidic swallow identified by MII-pH: antegrade bolus movement with accompanying drop in the distal esophageal pH to less than 4.

Recently, a new technique of measuring gastroesophageal reflux was introduced: combined pH-impedance monitoring. Impedance has the ability to detect the retrograde movement of gastric contents into the esophagus independently from pH.[15] Combining impedance with pH monitoring detects both acid (pH < 4), weakly acidic (pH between 4 and 7), and nonacid (pH > 7) reflux episodes, whereas traditional pH monitoring allows only for the identification of acid reflux (Figure 2-2A and 2-2B). pH-impedance also automatically distinguishes between acid reflux events (Figure 2-2A) and swallowed acidic foods (Figure 2-3C). pH-impedance testing off antisecretory therapy is the most accurate method to identify acid reflux, but the transnasal catheter has the potential for more false-negative results for the reasons discussed.

pH-impedance performed on patients with persistent GERD symptoms despite PPI therapy finds that nearly 50% of patients tested on PPIs had a positive symptom index, with 37% of patients having positive symptom index for either weakly acid or nonacid reflux.[16] However, current treatment strategies for nonacid reflux (ie, baclofen, antireflux surgery) are limited and lack outcome data. The current recommendation by the Esophageal Working Group indicates that pH-impedance "on" PPI therapy is useful in adult patients with persistent heartburn and/or regurgitation, chronic cough, persistent belching, or rumination, provided the patients had either prior endoscopy showing erosive esophagitis or Barrett esophagus or a reflux-monitoring study done off antisecretory medications to document the presence of pathologic acid gastroesophageal reflux.[10] Only patients with documented symptoms related to weakly acidic or nonacid reflux with prior confirmation of pathologic acid gastroesophageal reflux should be considered for antireflux surgery.[10]

The proposed diagnostic approach to patients with symptoms suggestive of GERD is shown in Figure 2-3.[10]

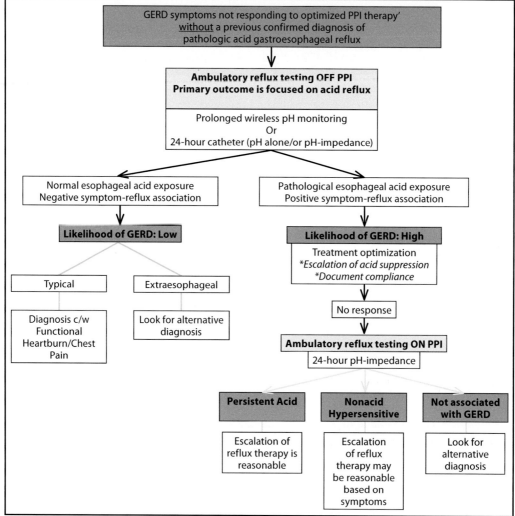

Figure 2-3. The approach to patients with GERD symptoms not responding to medical therapy developed by the Esophageal Diagnostic Working Group. (Adapted with permission from Richter JE, Pandolfino JE, Vela MF, et al. Utilization of wireless pH monitoring technologies: a summary of the proceedings from the Esophageal Diagnostic Working Group. *Dis Esophagus.* DOI:10.1111/j.142-2050.201201384.x Published August 7, 2012.) *The optimal proton pump inhibitor (PPI) dose threshold to define failure of acid suppression is unknown. Based on the data from Charbel et al., a dose that is either twice the Food and Drug Administration (FDA)–approved dose or a twice-daily dose of the FDA-indicated dose are the default regimens for defining PPI nonresponders.[11]

EPIDEMIOLOGY

Prevalence and Incidence

A recent systematic review of 28 population-based studies found geographic variations in the estimated prevalence of GERD, with 18.1% to 27.8% in North America (5 studies), 8.8% to 25.9% in Europe (8 studies), 8.7% to 33.1% in the Middle East (7 studies), 23.0% in South America (1 study), 11.6% in Australia (1 study), and 2.5% to 7.8% in East Asia (6 studies).[17] In the analyzed

TABLE 2-1

PREVALENCE OF REFLUX ESOPHAGITIS, HIATAL HERNIA, AND ENDOSCOPICALLY SUSPECTED ESOPHAGEAL METAPLASIA IN PROSPECTIVE POPULATION-BASED AND HEALTH-CHECK STUDIES[18]

STUDY		REFLUX ESOPHAGITIS	HIATAL HERNIA	ENDOSCOPICALLY SUSPECTED ESOPHAGEAL METAPLASIA
Population-based	Sweden	15.5%	23.9%	10.3%
	Italy	11.8%	43.0%	3.6%
	China	6.4%	0.7%	1.8%
Health-check	Japan	8.5%	19.5%	not reported
	Mainland China	4.3%	1.8%	1.0%
	Korea	3.4% to 7.9%	2.7% to 11.2%	3.4%
	Taiwan	9% to 24.6%	0.8% to 7.5%	0.0% to 0.3%

studies, GERD was diagnosed either by the Montreal definition, presence of heartburn, and/or regurgitation at least 1 day a week or by a clinician's assessment. In the same study they determined that the incidence of GERD per 1000 person years was 4.5 in the UK pediatric and adult population of approximately 3 million people aged 2 to 79 years, 0.84 in the UK pediatric population of approximately 2.3 million children and adolescents, and 5.4 in the US population sample obtained from Georgia Medicaid claims data of 163,000 people aged more than 27 years.

A recently published systematic review analyzed the data from 61,281 individuals from 3 general population studies (Sweden, Italy, and China) and 8 health-check studies from Asia regarding symptom-defined GERD (per Montreal definition) and esophageal endoscopic findings.[18] Health-check studies were performed among individuals undergoing routine health evaluations that included endoscopy. As shown in Table 2-1, large population-based studies have found the prevalence of reflux to be 15.5% in Sweden, 11.8% in Italy, and 6.4% in China. Asian health-check studies from Japan, China, and Korea reported a lower prevalence of reflux esophagitis (3.4% to 8.5%), whereas 4 Taiwanese studies showed esophagitis prevalence rates between 9% and 24.6%, comparable with values from the Italian and Swedish population studies. Of note, among patients without reflux symptoms, the prevalence of reflux esophagitis was 12.1% (Sweden), 8.6% (Italy), and 6.1% (China), whereas in Asian health-check studies, it ranged between 1.6% and 22.8%. Finally, the prevalence of endoscopically suspected esophageal metaplasia was 10.3% (Sweden), 3.6% (Italy), and 1.8% (China) in population-based studies and 0.0% to 3.4% in Asian health-check studies.[24] Of note, the prevalence of endoscopically suspected esophageal metaplasia was 9.4% (Sweden), 2.8% (Italy), and 1.8% (China) among asymptomatic patients undergoing endoscopy.[18] The available data suggest that a considerable subset of patients without reflux symptoms have reflux esophagitis (1.6% to 22.8%) or endoscopically suspected esophageal metaplasia (1.8% to 9.4%).

Risk Factors

According to recent systematic reviews, several genetic, demographic, behavioral, and comorbid factors may have significant positive or negative associations with GERD (Table 2-2).[17] It should be noted that factors reported in population-based studies were variable and the results sometimes conflicting. However, among these are 2 key risk factors of GERD: obesity and *Helicobacter pylori* infection. *H pylori* infection was not assessed in the studies included in the recent systematic reviews due to the fact that questionnaire-based surveys did not obtain this information. Nevertheless, most experts agree that the GERD epidemic is the result of increasing obesity, especially abdominal fat, and healthier stomachs as the indirect result of *H pylori* eradication.

TREATMENT

Lifestyle Modifications and Over-the-Counter Medications

Although lifestyle and dietary modifications are recommended in the treatment of GERD, an evidence-based review of 16 clinical trials assessing the impact of lifestyle modifications on GERD by improving symptoms, esophageal pH, or LES pressure found that only elevation of the head of the bed, left lateral decubitus position, and weight loss improved distal esophageal pH, with weight loss also improving GERD symptoms.[19] Data from the Nurses' Health Study suggest that a 3.5 reduction in body mass index (BMI) is associated with a 40% decrease in frequent reflux symptoms when compared to no change on BMI.[20]

Patients with GERD symptoms usually start treating themselves with over-the-counter (OTC) antacids, alginates, or H2 receptor antagonists. Over-the-counter PPIs are recommended for 2 weeks, but wide availability means that they are often used chronically. However, the presence of severe, frequent, or troublesome GERD symptoms or a long duration of symptoms should prompt evaluation by a physician and subsequent prescribing of long-term PPI therapy.[21]

Proton Pump Inhibitors

PPIs are the mainstay of GERD therapy. PPIs inhibit the H+K+ATPase pump, which is the final common pathway of secretion of gastric acid. PPIs maintain intragastric pH > 4 for between 15 and 21 hours, as compared to H2 receptor antagonists, which maintain it for only 8 hours daily.

Esophagitis

A Cochrane review of 134 randomized controlled trials involving 35,978 patients with esophagitis determined that treatment with PPI was superior to placebo (RR = 0.22; 95%CI 0.15 to −0.31 and number needed to treat [NNT] = 1.7; 95% CI 1.5 to 2.1), H2 receptor antagonists (pooled RR from 26 trials = 0.51, 95% CI 0.44 to −0.59), or prokinetics (RR from 1 trial = 0.38; 95% CI 0.22 to 0.66) in healing esophagitis at 4 to 8 weeks.[22] Maintenance treatment with PPI (24 to 52 weeks) was superior to H2 receptor antagonists in preventing recurrence of esophagitis (RR = 0.36; 95%CI 0.28 to 0.46 and NNT = 2.5; 95% CI 2.0 to 3.4) based on pooled data from 10 randomized controlled trials of 1583 patients.[23] PPIs were also more efficacious than H2 receptor antagonists given for 26 to 52 weeks in maintaining symptom-free (defined by absence of heartburn or low global symptom reflux score) remission (RR = 0.48; 95% CI 0.39 to 0.60 and NNT = 4.3; 95% CI 3.4 to 5.9) when data from 5 trials of 797 patients were pooled.[25] Data from 15,316 patients strongly suggest that the new-generation omeprazole, esomeprazole (40 mg in the morning), had a relative increase in probability of healing esophagitis of 10% at week 4 and 5% at week 8 and a

TABLE 2-2
RISK AND PROTECTIVE FACTORS OF GERD IN POPULATION STUDIES BASED ON MULTIVARIATE LOGISTIC REGRESSION ANALYSES[17]

	ODDS RATIO	95% CI
Low-Risk Factors		
Age per year	1.0	1.02 to 1.03
BMI per unit increase	1.1	1.09 to 1.13
Current or past smoker	1.3	1.10 to 1.54
Corticosteroids (oral or inhaled)	1.5	1.2 to 1.9
β2-adrenergic receptor agonist use	1.5	1.2 to 1.9
Use of anticholinergic medications	1.5	1.12 to 2.05
Past smoker vs never smoker	1.6	1.1 to 2.3
Congenital malformations	1.7	1.4 to 2.1
BMI > 30 vs $\leqq$ 30 (kg/m^2)	1.8	1.03 to 3.12
Current smoker vs never smoker	1.8	1.32 to 2.51
Alcohol (at least 7 drinks weekly) vs. none	1.9	1.1 to 3.3
Female sex	2.0	1.50 to 2.61
BMI 27 to 30 vs $\leqq$ 24 (kg/m^2)	2	1.2 to 3.3
Medium-Risk Factors		
Current smoker	2.5	1.07 to 5.70
BMI > 30 vs $\leqq$ 24 (kg/m^2)	2.8	1.7 to 4.5
Neurological disabilities	3.4	2.5 to 4.7
Nonsteroidal anti-inflammatory drug use 1 to 5 tablets weekly vs none	4.2	1.66 to 10.74
Congenital esophageal disorders	4.3	1.3 to 14.1
High-Risk Factors		
Hiatus hernia	7.4	2.7 to 20.3
Reported poor vs very good health status	20.1	10.33 to 39.13
Protective factors		
Oral contraceptives	0.76	0.63 to 0.93
Oral acne medications	0.4	0.2 to 0.9
Age 18 to 29 yrs vs 30 to 39 yrs	0.67	0.46 to 0.97
At least weekly but less than daily exercise vs daily exercise	0.68	0.49 to 0.94

relative increase of 8% at week 4 in probability of symptom relief in patients with erosive esophagitis compared to omeprazole 20 mg, lansoprazole 30 mg, and pantoprazole 40 mg.[24] Esomeprazole demonstrated the greatest therapeutic advantage in patients with severe disease (LA C and D) with a respective NNT of 14 and 8, whereas minimal benefit was found in patients with mild disease (LA A and B) with a respective NNT of 50 and 33.

Endoscopy-Negative Reflux Disease

Until recently, it was widely believed that PPIs were less effective in patients with nonerosive reflux disease when compared to erosive esophagitis. In one large systematic review, the therapeutic gain of PPI therapy over placebo for symptom relief was more than 75% higher among patients with erosive esophagitis (48%) than for patients with nonerosive reflux disease (27%).[25] However, a recent meta-analysis of randomized clinical trials challenged this concept, finding that 4-week therapy with PPIs was equally effective in complete relief of heartburn in nonerosive reflux disease confirmed by both negative upper endoscopy and abnormal pH test (pooled estimate from 2 trials of 0.73; 95% CI 0.69 to 0.74) and reflux esophagitis (pooled estimate from 32 trials of 0.72; 95% CI 0.69 to 0.74).[26] Treatment with PPIs was not as effective in patients with empirically treated heartburn (pooled estimate from 8 trials of 0.50, 95%CI 0.43 to 0.57) and in those with negative upper endoscopy but without pH testing (pooled estimate from 12 trials of 0.49, 95% CI 0.44 to 0.55). These findings underline the importance of appropriate esophageal functional testing; otherwise, it is impossible to distinguish between endoscopy-negative reflux disease, functional heartburn, or functional dyspepsia.[28]

Current guidelines by the American Gastroenterology Association support an increase in PPI dosing from once daily to twice daily in patients without symptom relief.[27] However, the new-generation PPI, dexlansoprazole modified release (MR), a derivative of lansoprazole with dual delayed-release technology, was shown in an open-label study to control heartburn in 88% of patients stepped down from twice-daily PPIs (lansoprazole, esomeprazole, pantoprazole, omeprazole, rabeprazole) to dexlansoprazole MR 30 mg daily for 6 weeks.[22] Therefore, patients who achieve relief of their heartburn on PPIs twice daily may be considered for once-daily therapy with dexlansoprazole to reduce costs, improve compliance, and reduce risk for side effects of high-dose PPIs. However, placebo-controlled trials are needed to validate these findings from an open-label study.

Extraesophageal Gastroesophageal Reflux Disease

There is variable efficacy of PPIs in treating patients with extraesophageal symptoms of GERD. A recent meta-analysis of 6 randomized controlled trials indicated that patients presenting with unexplained chest pain and abnormal esophageal pH testing and/or esophagitis were more than four-fold likely to respond to PPI treatment than placebo (RR = 4.3, 95% CI 2.8 to 6.7), whereas those with unexplained chest pain but without objective evidence of GERD were less likely to respond than placebo-treated patients (RR = 0.4; 95% CI 0.3 to 0.7).[29] Based on available data from systematic reviews, there is no evidence of predictable PPI efficacy in patients presenting with asthma,[30] cough,[31] hoarseness,[32] or laryngopharyngeal symptoms.[33] This observation is likely due to the complex multifactorial etiologies of these extraesophageal complaints.

Reflux Inhibitors

The efficacy of PPIs decreases in a stepwise fashion from esophagitis, heartburn, regurgitation, and chest pain to minimal predictive improvement in patients with cough, asthma, hoarseness, or laryngopharyngeal symptoms.[34] Therefore, an alternative therapeutic approach to GERD has been advocated by targeting and partially inhibiting TLESRs. Various inhibitors of TLESRs have been tested in GERD patients, such as baclofen, lesogaberan, and arbaclofen, with modest symptom improvement up to 26% as the result of decreasing all forms of gastroesophageal reflux.[34] Another TLESRs inhibitor, mGluR5-negative allosteric modulator (ADX10059), given as monotherapy,

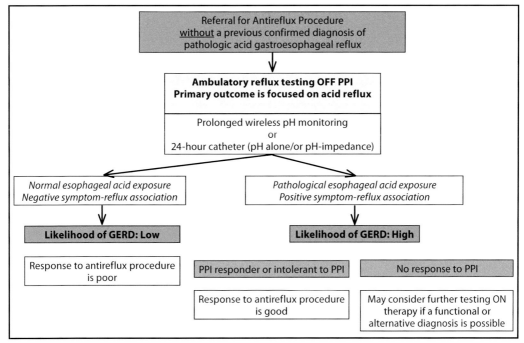

Figure 2-4. The approach to patients referred for antireflux procedures without a previous confirmed diagnosis of GERD, based on recommendations from the Esophageal Diagnostic Working Group. (Adapted with permission from Richter JE. Diagnostic tests for gastroesophageal reflux disease. *Am J Med Sci*. 2003;326:300-308.)

showed a significant increase in reflux symptom relief, but when given as an add-on therapy to PPIs it did not show substantial benefit. Overall, these new agents are not likely to exceed the effect of PPIs in treating GERD, but may have clinical utility among patients with persistent regurgitation or burping despite PPI therapy. At this time, all development programs for reflux inhibitors have been discontinued.[34]

Surgery

Antireflux surgery consists of the following steps: 1) reduction of the hiatal hernia back into the abdomen, 2) increasing the length of the LES within the abdomen, 3) closure of the gap in the crural diaphragm, and 4) wrapping the fundus of the stomach anteriorly or posteriorly around the esophagus.[35] Total (3600) Nissen fundoplication is the most popular procedure, whereas partial Toupet fundoplication is used in patients with aperistalsis or ineffective esophageal motility.[35]

Recent guidelines by the Society of American Gastrointestinal and Endoscopic Surgeons (SAGES) recommend that surgical therapy be considered if GERD patients have failed medical management, defined as inadequate control of symptoms; severe regurgitation on PPIs or side effects of PPIs; prefer surgery due to quality-of-life measures (ie, lifelong duration of PPIs or the cost of PPIs); developed GERD complications such as peptic stricture or Barrett's esophagus; or having extraesophageal manifestations of GERD such as asthma, hoarseness, cough, or chest pain.[36]

According to the newest recommendations issued by the Esophageal Diagnostic Advisory Panel, it is critical to evaluate the presence and severity of GERD with objective testing prior to antireflux surgery (Figure 2-4).[37] Preoperative workup should include upper endoscopy, barium esophagram, esophageal manometry, and pH testing. Patients with long-segment Barrett's esophagus of at least 3 cm do not need pH testing; however, those with short-segment Barrett's and mild esophagitis (LA A/B) require pH confirmation of abnormal distal esophageal acid exposure.

Esophageal pH testing should be performed off PPIs for 7 days or off H2 receptor antagonists for 3 days. Of note, this group recommended that positive SI or SAP alone is not a sufficient indication for antireflux surgery. All patients should undergo esophageal manometry to exclude achalasia and to tailor antireflux surgery, since weak esophageal peristalsis is associated with less dysphagia after partial rather than 3600 Nissen fundoplication. Patients with significant nausea, bloating, and food retention in the stomach after overnight fasting should have a 4-hour gastric emptying study.

Laparoscopic fundoplication is preferred over the open method due to shorter hospital stay (3 to 5 days), less abdominal pain, and fewer complications; however, it is a longer procedure and may have a higher reoperation rate. The partial fundoplication (Toupet) has lower rates of post-operative dysphagia and reoperations and comparable efficacy and patient satisfaction in controlling reflux symptoms up to 5 years after the procedure when compared with total fundoplication. However, recent SAGES guidelines do not support a tailored approach to fundoplication based upon esophageal motility unless there is aperistalsis.[36] Morbidly obese patients should undergo gastric bypass surgery rather than antireflux surgery due to higher failure rates of fundoplication in this patient population. Poor compliance with PPIs or poor response to PPIs prior to surgery is associated with poorer outcomes after surgery.[36] Fundoplication for suspected extraesophageal symptoms of GERD consistently has lower success rates when compared to patients with typical GERD symptoms.

Antireflux surgery is associated with several medical and surgical complications, including a 0% to 1% mortality rate (Table 2-3).[38] Failures after surgery usually occur within the first 2 years after surgery and include herniation of the fundoplication into the chest, slipped fundoplication, tight fundoplication, paraesophageal hernia, and malposition of fundoplication. To avoid potential pitfalls, a strict cooperation between gastroenterologist and surgeon is recommended.[38] The overall results of medical and surgical therapies for GERD seem comparable. Recent data from the LOTUS randomized clinical trial of 554 GERD patients support this point.[39] The majority of patients maintained 5-year remission of GERD after either laparoscopic antireflux surgery or treatment with esomeprazole, but estimated remission rates were higher in medically treated patients than in surgically treated patients (92% vs 85%, p = 0.048).

Lower Esophageal Sphincter Augmentation Device

A new treatment modality for GERD has emerged recently: an LES augmentation device (LINX Reflux Management System, Torax Medical, Inc). This device consists of interlinked titanium beads containing a magnetic core that are connected with each other by titanium wires. It is placed laparoscopically around the gastroesophageal junction in a simple operation that does not disrupt the hiatal structure. The U.S. Food and Drug Administration (FDA) approved LINX for patients with documented GERD by abnormal pH testing, with or without small hiatal hernia, who are symptomatic despite maximum medical therapy. It offers an alternative for patients reluctant to undergo traditional antireflux surgery because of possible complications and failure rates. This was confirmed by a recently published study on 100 consecutive patients with GERD who had the esophageal device implanted.[40] After 1 year, 64% of patients achieved at least a 50% reduction in distal esophageal acid exposure, 93% reduced their PPI use by at least 50%, and 92% had at least 50% improvement in their quality of life. Complete discontinuation of PPIs was observed in 86%, 87%, and 87% of patients after 1, 2, and 3 years, respectively. There was also a significant reduction in the proportion of patients complaining of moderate to severe regurgitation. Of note, dysphagia was the most frequently observed adverse event, occurring in 68% of patients after implantation. Persistent dysphagia was observed in 11% of patients after 1 year, 5% after 2 years, and 4% after 3 years. There were 3 patients who required device removal due to severe dysphagia.

Table 2-3 PREVALENCE OF MEDICAL AND SURGICAL COMPLICATIONS OF ANTIREFLUX SURGERY	
Mortality (< 30 days)	0% to 1%
Postoperative morbidity	8% to 17%
Open conversion rate	0% to 24%
Early postoperative complications	
Bowel perforation	0% to 4%
Bleeding and splenic injury	< 1%
Severe postoperative nausea and vomiting	2% to 5%
Late postoperative complications	
Gas-bloat syndrome	1% to 85%
Dysphagia	
Early	10% to 50%
Late	3% to 24%
Diarrhea	18% to 33%
Recurrent heartburn	10% to 62%
Need for revisional surgery	
Laparoscopic Nissen fundoplication	0% to 15%
Laparoscopic Toupet fundoplication	4% to 10%

Endoluminal Treatment

Endoluminal treatments of GERD have had a sordid history, with several being removed from the market in the early 2000s due to ineffectiveness, complications, and even deaths. Guidelines by the American Gastroenterology Association from 2007 clearly indicate that none of the endoluminal antireflux devices available at that time—radiofrequency energy (Stretta), endoscopic injection techniques (Enteryx, Gatekeeper), endoscopic suturing (EndoCinch, endoscopic suturing device), and endoscopic full-thickness plication—met criteria of being effective, easy to apply, and safe.[41] Furthermore, there was a lack of long-term follow-up data beyond 1 to 2 years on a large number of patients to assess safety and efficacy of endoluminal treatment; thus, endoscopic therapy for GERD was not recommended except as part of clinical trials.

However, current SAGES guidelines from 2013 recommend that the Stretta procedure be considered in adult GERD patients with typical symptoms and partial or complete response to PPI therapy who do not want laparoscopic fundoplication.[44] In this endoscopic procedure, radiofrequency energy is delivered to the gastroesophageal area, thus remodeling the musculature of the LES and gastric cardia, resulting in reductions in TLESRs and restoration of the natural barrier function of the LES. This method is not recommended in patients with severe esophagitis, a hiatus hernia longer than 2 cm, long-segment Barrett's esophagus, or dysphagia. Furthermore, a recent meta-analysis of the 4 randomized Stretta studies found no efficacy relevant to relief of symptoms, decrease in use of PPIs, increase in LES pressure or decrease in esophageal pH values.[45] The use of another currently available endoluminal method, an EsophyX device (EndoGastric Solutions, Inc) creating an incisionless fundoplication was not recommended due to lack of long-term data. Further studies are required to define optimal techniques and the most appropriate patient selection criteria and to further evaluate device and technique safety.

CONCLUSION

GERD is defined as a presence of troublesome symptoms and/or complications caused by retrograde movement of gastric contents into the esophagus. The most typical symptoms are heartburn and regurgitation. It is a common disease, with increasing prevalence in Western countries, with the major risk factors being obesity and eradication of *H pylori*. All patients with suspected GERD symptoms should be placed on PPIs and therapy should be maximized before further diagnostic workup. The most sensitive test for GERD is esophageal pH monitoring. PPIs are slightly superior to antireflux surgery in maintaining long-term remission. Careful selection of patients for antireflux surgery is warranted. A viable alternative for antireflux surgery may be an LES augmentation device.

REFERENCES

1. Vakil N, van Zanten SV, Kahrilas P, et al. The Montreal definition and classification of gastroesophageal reflux disease: a global evidence-based consensus. *Am J Gastroenterol.* 2006;101:1900-1920.
2. Dent J, Vakil N, Jones R, et al. Accuracy of the diagnosis of GORD by questionnaire, physicians and a trial of proton pump inhibitor treatment: the Diamond Study. *Gut.* 2010;59:714-721.
3. Numans ME, Lau J, de Wit NJ, et al. Short-term treatment with proton-pump inhibitors as a test for gastroesophageal reflux disease: a meta-analysis of diagnostic test characteristics. *Ann Inter Med.* 2004;140:518-527.
4. Bytzer P, Jones R, Vakil N, et al. Limited ability of the proton-pump inhibitor test to identify patients with gastroesophageal reflux disease. *Clin Gastroenterol Hepatol.* 2012;10:1360-1366.
5. Wang WH, Huang JQ, Zheng GF, et al. Is proton pump inhibitor testing an effective approach to diagnose gastroesophageal reflux disease in patients with noncardiac chest pain?: A meta-analysis. *Arch Intern Med.* 2005;165:1222-1228.
6. Shaheen NJ, Weinberg DS, Denberg TD, et al. Upper endoscopy for gastroesophageal reflux disease: best practice advice from the clinical guidelines committee of the American College of Physicians. *Ann Intern Med.* 2012;157:808-816.
7. Lundell LR, Dent J, Bennett JR, et al. Endoscopic assessment of oesophagitis: clinical and functional correlates and further validation of the Los Angeles classification. *Gut.* 1999;45:172-1780.
8. Richter JE. The many manifestations of gastroesophageal reflux disease: presentation, evaluation, and treatment. *Gastroenterol Clin North Am.* 2007;36:577-599, viii-ix.
9. Malfertheiner P, Nocon M, Vieth M, et al. Evolution of gastro-oesophageal reflux disease over 5 years under routine medical care: the ProGERD study. *Alimentary Pharmacol Ther.* 2012;35:154-164.
10. Richter JE, Pandolfino JE, Vela MF, et al. Utilization of wireless pH monitoring technologies: a summary of the proceedings from the Esophageal Diagnostic Working Group. *Dis Esophagus.* DOI:10.1111/j.1442-2050.2012.01384.x. Published August 7, 2012.
11. Charbel S, Khandwala F, Vaezi MF. The role of esophageal pH monitoring in symptomatic patients on PPI therapy. *Am J Gastroenterol.* 2005;100:283-289.
12. Gawron AJ, Rothe J, Fought AJ, et al. Many patients continue using proton pump inhibitors after negative results from tests for reflux disease. *Clin Gastroenterol Hepatol.* 2012;10:620-625.
13. Richter JE. Diagnostic tests for gastroesophageal reflux disease. *Am J Med Sci.* 2003;326:300-308.
14. Kahrilas PJ, Quigley EM. Clinical esophageal pH recording: a technical review for practice guideline development. *Gastroenterology.* 1996;110:1982-1996.

15. Tutuian R, Vela MF, Shay SS, et al. Multichannel intraluminal impedance in esophageal function testing and gastroesophageal reflux monitoring. *J Clin Gastroenterol*. 2003;37:206-215.
16. Mainie I, Tutuian R, Shay S, et al. Acid and non-acid reflux in patients with persistent symptoms despite acid suppressive therapy: a multicentre study using combined ambulatory impedance-pH monitoring. *Gut*. 2006;55:1398-1402.
17. El-Serag HB, Sweet S, Winchester CC, et al. Update on the epidemiology of gastro-oesophageal reflux disease: a systematic review. *Gut*. DOI:10.1136/gutjnl-2012-304269. Published July 13, 2013.
18. Dent J, Becher A, Sung J, et al. Systematic review: patterns of reflux-induced symptoms and esophageal endoscopic findings in large-scale surveys. *Clin Gastroenterol Hepatol*. 2012;10:863-873 e3.
19. Kaltenbach T, Crockett S, Gerson LB. Are lifestyle measures effective in patients with gastroesophageal reflux disease? An evidence-based approach. *Arch Intern Med*. 2006;166:965-971.
20. Jacobson BC, Somers SC, Fuchs CS, et al. Body-mass index and symptoms of gastroesophageal reflux in women. *New Engl J Med*. 2006;354:2340-2348.
21. Haag S, Andrews JM, Katelaris PH, et al. Management of reflux symptoms with over-the-counter proton pump inhibitors: issues and proposed guidelines. *Digestion*. 2009;80:226-234.
22. Khan M, Santana J, Donnellan C, et al. Medical treatments in the short term management of reflux oesophagitis. The Cochrane database of systematic reviews 2007:CD003244.
23. Donnellan C, Sharma N, Preston C, et al. Medical treatments for the maintenance therapy of reflux oesophagitis and endoscopic negative reflux disease. The Cochrane Database of systematic reviews. 2005:CD003245.
24. Gralnek IM, Dulai GS, Fennerty MB, et al. Esomeprazole versus other proton pump inhibitors in erosive esophagitis: a meta-analysis of randomized clinical trials. *Clin Gastroenterol Hepatol*. 2006;4:1452-1458.
25. Dean BB, Gano AD Jr, Knight K, et al. Effectiveness of proton pump inhibitors in nonerosive reflux disease. *Clin Gastroenterol Hepatol*. 2004;2:656-664.
26. Weijenborg PW, Cremonini F, Smout AJ, et al. PPI therapy is equally effective in well-defined non-erosive reflux disease and in reflux esophagitis: a meta-analysis. *Neurogastroenterol Motil*. 2012;24:747-757, e350.
27. Kahrilas PJ, Shaheen NJ, Vaezi MF. American Gastroenterological Association Institute technical review on the management of gastroesophageal reflux disease. *Gastroenterology*. 2008;135:1392-1413, 413 e1-5.
28. Fass R, Inadomi J, Han C, et al. Maintenance of heartburn relief after step-down from twice-daily proton pump inhibitor to once-daily dexlansoprazole modified release. *Clin Gastroenterol Hepatol*. 2012;10:247-253.
29. Kahrilas PJ, Hughes N, Howden CW. Response of unexplained chest pain to proton pump inhibitor treatment in patients with and without objective evidence of gastro-oesophageal reflux disease. *Gut*. 2011;60:1473-1478.
30. Gibson PG, Henry RL, Coughlan JL. Gastro-oesophageal reflux treatment for asthma in adults and children. *Cochrane Database Syst Rev*. 2003:CD001496.
31. Chang AB, Lasserson TJ, Gaffney J, et al. Gastro-oesophageal reflux treatment for prolonged non-specific cough in children and adults. *Cochrane Database Syst Rev*. 2011:CD004823.
32. Hopkins C, Yousaf U, Pedersen M. Acid reflux treatment for hoarseness. *Cochrane Database Syst Rev*. 2006:CD005054.
33. Gatta L, Vaira D, Sorrenti G, et al. Meta-analysis: the efficacy of proton pump inhibitors for laryngeal symptoms attributed to gastro-oesophageal reflux disease. *Alimentary Pharmacol Ther*. 2007;25:385-392.
34. Kahrilas PJ, Boeckxstaens G. Failure of reflux inhibitors in clinical trials: bad drugs or wrong patients? *Gut*. 2012;61:1501-1509.
35. Broeders JA, Roks DJ, Ahmed Ali U, et al. Laparoscopic anterior 180-degree versus Nissen fundoplication for gastroesophageal reflux disease: systematic review and meta-analysis of randomized clinical trials. *Ann Surg*. 2013;257:850-859.
36. Stefanidis D, Hope WW, Kohn GP, et al. Guidelines for surgical treatment of gastroesophageal reflux disease. *Surg Endosc*. 2010;24:2647-2669.
37. Jobe BA, Richter JE, Hoppo T, et al. Preoperative diagnostic workup before antireflux surgery: an evidence and experience-based consensus of the Esophageal Diagnostic Advisory Panel. *J Am Coll Surg*. 2013;217:586-597.
38. Richter JE. Gastroesophageal reflux disease treatment: side effects and complications of fundoplication. *Clin Gastroenterol Hepatol*. 2013;11:465-471; quiz e39.
39. Galmiche JP, Hatlebakk J, Atwood et al. Laparoscopic anti-reflux surgery vs. esomeprazole treatment for chronic GERD. The LOTUS randomized clinical trial. *JAMA*. 2011;305:1969-1977.
40. Ganz RA, Peters JH, Horgan S, et al. Esophageal sphincter device for gastroesophageal reflux disease. *New Engl J Med*. 2013;368:719-727.
41. Falk GW, Fennerty MB, Rothstein RI. AGA Institute medical position statement on the use of endoscopic therapy for gastroesophageal reflux disease. *Gastroenterology*. 2006;131:1313-1314.
42. Auyang ED, Carter P, Rauth T, et al. SAGES clinical spotlight review: endoluminal treatments for gastroesophageal reflux disease (GERD). *Surg Endosc*. 2013;27:2658-2672.
43. Lipka S, Kumar A, Richter JE. No evidence for efficiency of radiofrequencing ablation for treatment of GERD: a systematic review and meta-analysis. *Clin Gastroenterol Hep*. 2015;In press.

3

Achalasia

Andrew J. Gawron, MD, PhD, MS and John E. Pandolfino, MD, MSCI

KEY POINTS

- Achalasia results from myenteric plexus inflammation with subsequent degeneration and dysfunction of inhibitory postganglionic neurons in the distal esophagus, including the LES.

- The diagnosis of achalasia is made by demonstrating impaired lower esophageal sphincter (LES) relaxation and absent peristalsis in the absence of esophageal obstruction near the LES.

- The minimum evaluation includes manometry to document the motor findings and appropriate imaging studies to rule out obstruction.

- Three distinct subtypes of achalasia were quantitatively defined using high-resolution esophageal manometry. There is prognostic value of the achalasia subtypes: 1) type II patients have the best prognosis with myotomy or pneumatic dilation; 2) the treatment response of type I patients is less robust (and reduced further as the degree of esophageal dilatation increases); and 3) type III patients have a worse prognosis, probably because the associated spasm is less likely to respond to therapies directed at the LES.

- Definitive therapy of achalasia is mechanical disruption of the LES via myotomy or pneumatic dilation. Medical therapy should be reserved for those patients deemed poor candidates for a procedure due to other comorbidities or patient preference. An emerging endoscopic surgical approach, POEM, may offer similar benefits as traditional myotomy.

DEFINITION

Achalasia, derived from the Greek *khalasias* (to loosen), means "failure of a ring muscle to relax," and the term has been adopted to specifically describe esophageal achalasia. Achalasia is characterized by impaired lower esophageal sphincter (LES) relaxation and aperistalsis in the distal esophagus. However, it is important to note that aperistalsis, also termed "absent peristalsis,"

Rao SSC, Parkman HP, McCallum RW, eds.
Handbook of Gastrointestinal Motility and Functional Disorders (pp 35-46).
© 2015 Taylor & Francis Group.

means that there is no progressively sequenced esophageal contraction; it does not imply the complete absence of intraluminal pressure. Consequently, absent peristalsis does not exclude the occurrence of spastic contractions or panesophageal pressurization. Understanding these patterns of pressurization is key to understanding the current classification scheme for achalasia and management of this disease.[1]

PATHOPHYSIOLOGY

Achalasia is associated with functional loss of myenteric plexus ganglion cells in the distal esophagus and LES.[2] The initiating factor for the neuronal degeneration is likely an autoimmune process triggered by an indolent viral infection (herpes, measles) in conjunction with a genetically susceptible host.[3] The inflammatory reaction is associated with a T-cell lymphocyte infiltrate, which leads to a slow destruction of ganglion cells. The distribution and end result of this plexitis is variable and may be modified by the host response or the etiologic stimulus. Data to support a genetic basis come from studies in twins and siblings, as well as its association with genetic diseases, such as Allgrove syndrome, Down syndrome, and Parkinson disease.[4-6] Achalasia can also be one of several manifestations of the widespread myenteric plexus destruction found in Chagas disease, a late consequence of infection with the parasite *Trypanosome cruzi*.[7]

The consequence of the myenteric plexus inflammation leading to achalasia is degeneration and dysfunction of inhibitory postganglionic neurons in the distal esophagus, including the LES. These neurons utilize nitric oxide and vasoactive intestinal peptide as neurotransmitters, and their dysfunction results in an imbalance between excitatory and inhibitory control of the sphincter and adjacent esophagus. Unopposed cholinergic stimulation can result in impairment of LES relaxation, hypercontractility of the distal esophagus (including the LES), and rapidly propagated contractions in the distal esophagus. However, there is variable expression of these abnormalities among individuals, with specific features dominating in some and not manifesting in others; only impaired deglutitive LES relaxation is universally required as a defining feature of achalasia.

DIAGNOSIS

The diagnosis of achalasia is made by demonstrating impaired LES relaxation and absent peristalsis in the absence of esophageal obstruction near the LES by a stricture, tumor, vascular structure, implanted device (eg, Lap-Band [Apollo Endosurgery, Inc]), or infiltrating process.[8] The minimum evaluation includes manometry to document the motor findings and appropriate imaging studies to rule out obstruction. However, the increasing sophistication of diagnostic methods has led to increasing recognition of variations in the physiological manifestations of achalasia and of alternative disease processes that can mimic the disease.

With regard to esophageal manometry, a major technological evolution has occurred during the past decade wherein conventional water-perfused or strain-gauge systems with a polygraph and line tracing output have been replaced by high-resolution manometry (HRM) systems outputting pressure data in esophageal pressure topography (EPT). Diagnostic criteria have been tightened[1] and relevant physiological subtypes identified, as shown in Figure 3-1.[9] Our corresponding diagnostic algorithm is shown in Figure 3-2. Particularly instrumental in establishing uniform diagnostic criteria for achalasia was the development of a new metric devised for EPT to quantify esophagogastric junction (EGJ) relaxation pressure: the integrated relaxation pressure (IRP). Measurement of the IRP utilizes an "electronic sleeve sensor" initially described by Staino and Clouse[10] as conceptually similar to a Dent sleeve that compensates for potential LES movement by tracking the sphincter within a specified zone. This avoids the artifact of pseudorelaxation

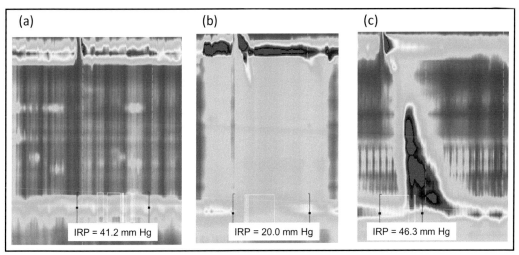

Figure 3-1. Subtypes of achalasia. (A) Type I is associated with absent peristalsis and no discernible esophageal contractility in the context of an elevated IRP. (B) Type II is associated with abnormal EGJ relaxation and panesophageal pressurization in excess of 30 mm Hg. (C) Type III achalasia is associated with premature (spastic) contractions and impaired EGJ relaxation.

(apparent sphincter relaxation caused by elevation of the sphincter above the sensor, displacing it into the stomach), which was a fatal flaw in the assessment of LES relaxation with nonsleeve conventional systems. The IRP is calculated from the electronic sleeve as the mean of 4 seconds of the lowest EGJ relaxation pressure after the pharyngeal contraction. The time scored can be continuous or noncontinuous, as when it is interrupted by a crural diaphragm contraction. The IRP provides a robust and accurate assessment of deglutitive EGJ relaxation and optimally discriminates defects of sphincter relaxation characteristic of achalasia.[11]

With the adoption of HRM with EPT, 3 distinct subtypes of achalasia were quantitatively defined using novel EPT metrics (see Figure 3-1).[9] There are now multiple publications supporting the prognostic value of these achalasia subtypes, consistently observing that 1) type II patients have the best prognosis with myotomy or pneumatic dilation; 2) the treatment response of type I patients is less robust (and reduced further as the degree of esophageal dilatation increases); and 3) type III patients have a worse prognosis, probably because the associated spasm is less likely to respond to therapies directed at the LES.[9,12-15] Emerging imaging modalities, such as combined HRM impedance manometry, have the potential to provide even more detailed information, including bolus retention parameters similar to timed barium esophagrams (Figure 3-3).

In addition, patients with impaired EGJ relaxation but some preserved peristalsis are now recognized as a distinct entity that can be a variant phenotype of achalasia. However, EGJ outflow obstruction can also be a manifestation of other disease entities, including eosinophilic esophagitis, LES hypertrophy, strictures, paraesophageal hernia, and pseudoachalasia due to tumor infiltration. An example of an EGJ outflow obstruction pattern is shown in Figure 3-4. In this case, the elevated IRP is due to a mechanical obstruction (prior fundoplication). This finding in patients without prior surgery always mandates careful imaging (often with biopsies) of the EGJ. We have also seen this pattern progress to achalasia (Figure 3-5), and patients should be followed on a regular basis.

The other requisite evaluation to establish a diagnosis of achalasia is of imaging studies to rule out obstruction in the region of the EGJ. In most instances, endoscopy will suffice. Endoscopy may also be helpful in determining the degree of esophageal dilatation, whether there is significant esophageal retention of food and fluid, and whether there is coexistent stasis or fungal esophagitis. A barium esophagram may suffice in this capacity in instances where there are equivocal manometric findings or when a manometry is not feasible because of severe dilatation and an

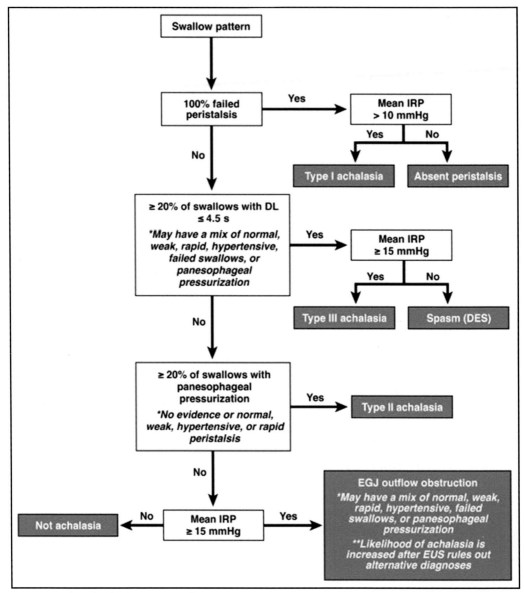

Figure 3-2. Algorithm for the diagnosis of achalasia.

inability to intubate the stomach with the manometry catheter. The esophagram can also quantify the efficacy of esophageal emptying when done as a "timed barium esophagram" protocol. When suspicion of pseudoachalasia is high, endoscopic ultrasound and/or computed tomography (CT) may be necessary.

EPIDEMIOLOGY

Achalasia remains a rare disease, and most patients are seen and treated at tertiary care centers, with an incident rate of about 1/100,000 cases per year. For example, in the entire country of Iceland over 51 years, 62 cases of achalasia were diagnosed (overall incidence 0.6/100,000/years and mean prevalence of 8.7 cases/100,000).[16] Gennaro et al[17] recently reported an incident rate in

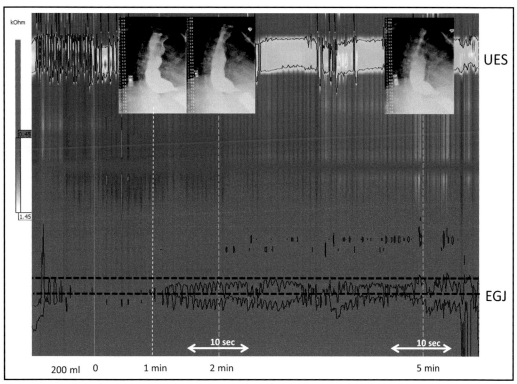

Figure 3-3. High-resolution impedance manometry of achalasia with corresponding barium esophagram. Note the impedance color contour (purple) showing similar sustained bolus retention as visualized in a concomitant barium esophagram at 1, 2, and 5 minutes.

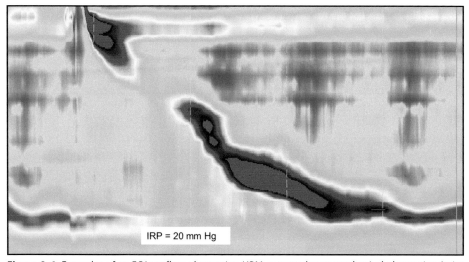

Figure 3-4. Examples of an EGJ outflow obstruction HRM pattern due to mechanical obstruction (prior fundoplication).

Italy of 1.59 cases/100,000/year (2001 to 2005).Research using the U.S.-based Clinical Outcomes Research Initiative (CORI) database of endoscopic procedures found that among 521,497 upper endoscopies performed from 2000 to 2008, 896 patients with achalasia were identified (0.2%).[18] There may be an increased risk with advanced age, but overall, achalasia affects both men and women of all races and ages fairly equally. More recent studies have suggested a higher incidence

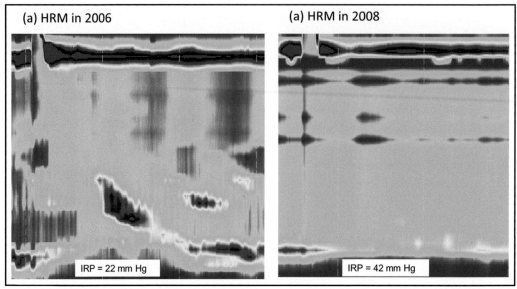

Figure 3-5. High-resolution manometry in a patient diagnosed with EGJ outflow obstruction in 2006 progressing to achalasia 2 years later (2008).

than much older studies (pre-1990); however, this likely reflects improvements in diagnostic testing and classification.

TREATMENT

Medical Treatment

Pharmacologic therapy with oral calcium channel blockers or nitrates causes a prompt reduction in LES pressure ranging from 0% to 50%, with mild benefit for dysphagia, but often has limiting side effects (headache, orthostatic hypotension, or edema). The use of calcium channel blockers or nitrates has not been shown to halt disease progression. Consequently, these products are poor long-term treatment options and should be reserved for patients who are judged to be poor candidates for myotomy or pneumatic dilation. Sublingual nifedipine in doses of 10 to 30 mg given 30 to 45 minutes before meals or sublingual isorbide dinitrate in doses of 5 to 10 mg given 15 minutes before meals may be useful as short-acting temporizing treatments.

5'-phosphodiesterase inhibitors, such as sildenafil, have also been utilized in achalasia and spastic disorders of the esophagus.[19] Sildenafil lowers EGJ pressure and attenuates distal esophageal contractions by blocking the enzyme that degrades cyclic guanosine monophosphate induced by nitric oxide. Hence, sildenafil is a viable alternative in patients not responding to or proving intolerant of calcium channel blockers or nitrates. The typical dose for sildenafil is from 25 to 50 mg with each meal. However, the current cost of sildenafil is much greater than that of nifedipine or isosorbide dinitrate, and patients are usually denied insurance coverage for the drug in this off-label indication. Furthermore, minimal long-term treatment data exist pertinent to using 5'-phosphodiesterase inhibitors in long-term achalasia treatment.

Botulinum Toxin

Botulinum toxin (Botox) injection into the muscle of the LES was proposed as an achalasia treatment based on its ability to block acetylcholine release from nerve endings by cleaving the

SNAP-25 protein, an essential component of that process. The standard approach is to inject 100 units of Botox with a sclerotherapy needle during endoscopy. Injections are done about 1 cm proximal to the squamocolumnar junction (SCJ) in 4 radially dispersed aliquots; this corresponds to the region of greatest tone within the LES. Using this technique, Pasricha et al[20] reported improved dysphagia in 66% of achalasics for 6 months. No increase in efficacy has been demonstrated with greater doses.[21] Physiologically, the effect of Botox is hard to demonstrate because it blocks only the nonmyogenic component of LES pressure. This effect is eventually reversed by axonal regeneration, and subsequent clinical series report minimal continued efficacy after 1 year.[20-23] On the positive side, Botox injection adds little time to endoscopy and is very safe, although it has been associated with chest pain after the injection, rare instances of mediastinitis, and allergic reactions to egg protein. On the negative side, most patients relapse and require retreatment within 12 months and repeated treatments have been shown to make subsequent Heller myotomy more challenging.[24] Botox injection has not been shown to attenuate the progressive esophageal dilatation, leaving these individuals prone to the long-term complications of achalasia. Consequently, Botox injection should rarely be utilized as a first-line therapy for achalasia, instead reserving it for poor surgical candidates and special circumstances.

Pneumatic Dilation

An achalasia dilator is a noncompliant, cylindrical balloon that is positioned across the LES and inflated with air using a handheld manometer. The only design currently available in the United States, the Rigiflex dilator (Boston Scientific), is positioned fluoroscopically over a guidewire and is available in 30-, 35-, and 40-mm diameters. Bougie and standard through-the-scope balloon dilators (maximal diameter of 20 mm) have no sustained efficacy in achalasia and should not be used. A cautious approach to dilation with the Rigiflex dilators is to initially use the 30-mm dilator and follow with a 35-mm dilator 2 to 4 weeks later if the initial dilation was insufficient. The reported efficacy of pneumatic dilation ranges from 32% to 98%.[25] Patients with a poor result or rapid recurrence of dysphagia are unlikely to respond to additional dilations, but subsequent response to myotomy is not influenced. The major complication of pneumatic dilation is esophageal perforation. Although the reported incidence of perforation from pneumatic dilation ranges from 0% to 16%, a recent systematic review on the topic concluded that when using the modern technique, the risk was less than 1%, comparable to the risk of unrecognized perforation during Heller myotomy.[26] Furthermore, most perforations are clinically obvious, "limited" perforations can be managed conservatively, and major perforations recognized and surgically repaired within 6 to 8 hours have outcomes comparable to patients undergoing elective Heller myotomy.

Pneumatic dilation should be performed by experienced physicians comfortable with the technique, and surgical back-up is requisite. The patient should have appropriate dietary instructions before the procedure so that there is minimal residual food in the esophagus during the procedure. The balloon dilator is completely deflated prior to both passage and withdrawal using a T-piece and large syringe to minimize trauma to the oropharynx. Pneumatic dilation requires concomitant endoscopy and fluoroscopy to place and visualize the guidewire and to verify appropriate balloon position. Our practice has been to use stiff spring-tip Savary guidewires rather than the flimsy wires provided by the manufacturer. The balloon size is chosen using a graded approach, starting with a 30-mm balloon and increasing to the 35-mm size if patients do not respond. We would not recommend using the 40-mm balloon because of data suggesting unacceptable perforation rates, preferring to refer patients failing 35-mm dilation for myotomy. Accurate placement of the balloon is crucial to the effectiveness of the procedure, and this must be verified fluoroscopically during the initial stages of balloon inflation. The inflation pressure of the balloon is not stipulated; full effacement of the sphincter on fluoroscopy is the endpoint of interest, which is usually associated with distention pressures of 8 to 15 psi. Patients should be observed in recovery for at least

2 hours with careful assessment for postprocedure pain. A gastrograffin/barium swallow study should be obtained if there is any worry of perforation. Patients should be explicitly advised to seek care emergently if they develop fever, shortness of breath, severe pain (especially if pleuritic), or subcutaneous emphysema.

Studies using pneumatic dilation as the initial treatment of achalasia have reported excellent long-term symptom control. However, one-third of patients will relapse in 4 to 6 years and may require repeat dilation. Response to therapy may be related to preprocedural clinical parameters, such as age (favorable if age > 45), gender (female > male),[27] esophageal diameter (inversely related to response), and achalasia type (type II better than I and III).[9,14] Although surgical myotomy has a greater response rate than a single pneumatic dilation, it appears that a strategy utilizing a series of dilations with the potential for repeat is comparable to surgery and a reasonable alternative to surgery. A recent randomized controlled trial (RCT) compared this type of graded strategy to surgical myotomy and found it to be noninferior in efficacy.[28]

Myotomy

The standard surgical approach to achalasia is a Heller myotomy, which divides the circular muscle fibers of the LES. This can be achieved by laparotomy, thoracotomy, thoracoscopy, or laparoscopy. Laparoscopy is currently the preferred approach due to its lower morbidity and comparable long-term outcome to that achieved with thoracotomy.[29] Laparoscopic Heller myotomy is superior to a single pneumatic dilation in terms of efficacy and durability, with reported efficacy rates in the 90% to 95% range.[25] However, the superiority of surgical myotomy over pneumatic dilation is less evident when compared to a graded approach to pneumatic dilation using repeat dilations as mandated by the clinical response.[28,29]

Similar to the case with pneumatic dilation, there is no standardized approach to Heller myotomy in terms of the specifics of the myotomy or the associated antireflux procedure. The most common recommendation is for a single anterior myotomy extending 2 cm onto the gastric cardia and about 7 cm in overall length. With respect to the antireflux repair, this can range from none to an anterior 180-degree fundoplasty (Dor) to a 270-degree partial fundoplication (Toupet). There is general agreement that a full 360-degree Nissen fundoplication is contraindicated. A recent RCT comparing the Dor procedure to Toupet fundoplication along with myotomy found no significant difference in abnormal pH testing between the 2 groups and similar dysphagia rates.[30] The current recommendation from the Society of American Gastrointestinal and Endoscopic Surgeons is that patients who undergo myotomy should have a fundoplication to prevent reflux without specifying which procedure.[31]

Per-Oral Endoscopic Myotomy

Although the current treatments for achalasia are extremely effective, both pneumatic dilation and laparoscopic myotomy are associated with a perforation risk of about 1%, and laparoscopic Heller myotomy still requires laparoscopy and surgical dissection of the EGJ. Consequently, there has been interest in developing a hybrid technique incorporating an endoscopic approach, but applying principles of natural orifice translumenal endoscopic surgery (NOTES) to perform a myotomy. This technique is termed *per-oral endoscopic myotomy*, or POEM, and was initially described by Pasricha et al[32] and subsequently developed by Inoue et al in Japan.[33] The procedure requires making a transverse mucosal incision in the midesophagus, entering it, and creating a submucosal tunnel all the way to the gastric cardia using a forward-viewing endoscope with a transparent distal cap and a triangular endoscopic submucosal dissection knife. Once the tunnel is complete, the endoscope is removed and its adequacy assessed by luminal inspection of the EGJ and proximal stomach (dye is instilled into the tunnel so that its path is visible intraluminally). The tunnel is then reentered and selective myotomy of the circular muscle accomplished

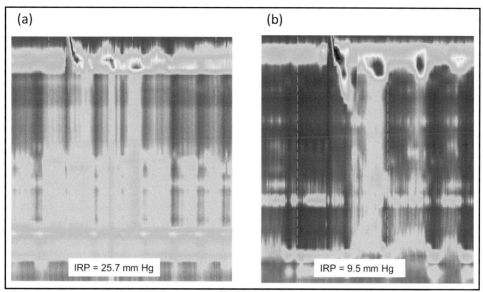

Figure 3-6. High-resolution manometry in type II achalasia (A) pre- and (B) post-POEM procedure.

with electrocautery tools for a minimum length of 6 cm up the esophagus and 2 cm distal to the SCJ onto the gastric cardia. The endoscope is then withdrawn, collapsing the tunnel, and endoclips are used to seal the entry incision. Initial reports of success rates of the POEM procedure in prospective cohorts of achalasia patients have been greater than 90%, comparable to those of laparoscopic Heller myotomy.[34-36] Data from a recent prospective, single-center study found that symptoms and postmyotomy IRPs were not different between patients with laparosocopic Heller myotomy or POEMs.[37] Our preliminary results comparing more than 30 POEM cases to laparoscopic Heller myotomy suggest comparable perioperative outcomes.[38] Figure 3-6 illustrates HRM in a patient with type II achalasia pre- and post-POEM procedure, demonstrating marked reduction in the IRP. There have been no randomized prospective comparison trials of POEM with either laparoscopic myotomy or pneumatic dilation. Hence, although POEM is clearly a promising technique for achalasia and related motility disorders, its relative efficacy compared to the well-studied alternatives of pneumatic dilation or laparoscopic Heller myotomy in terms of long-term dysphagia control, progression of esophageal dilatation, and postprocedure reflux remain to be established.

SUMMARY OF TREATMENT AND FOLLOW-UP

Patients who are deemed to be in good health should be counseled to pursue a definitive treatment capable of alleviating EGJ outflow obstruction such as myotomy (laparoscopic or endoscopic) or pneumatic dilation. Medical therapy with smooth muscle relaxants and/or botulinum toxin should be reserved for patients with substantial comorbidity making them poor surgical candidates, special circumstances in which a temporizing intervention is necessary, or rare instances where there is persistent uncertainty in the diagnosis of achalasia. Patients should have a postprocedure evaluation of effectiveness within the first 3 months after the intervention to assess adequacy of functional and symptom response. Patients with posttreatment symptoms should be evaluated based on the specific symptom, their pre-intervention anatomy and achalasia subtype. Patients with continued dysphagia, chest pain, and regurgitation after treatment should be evaluated to determine the effectiveness of the intervention in relieving EGJ outflow obstruction and improving esophageal emptying. Patients with significant bolus retention on timed barium esophagram or continued EGJ outflow obstruction defined by an IRP > 5 mm Hg on HRM should be considered treatment failures.

Patients who have failed pneumatic dilation may be referred for a repeat dilation with a larger balloon or myotomy. Patients who have undergone myotomy with an antireflux procedure should be evaluated for pseudoachalasia related to the fundoplication before repeat therapy is attempted. This can be assessed by performing manometry with amyl nitrite challenge to distinguish between an incomplete myotomy (EGJ relaxes with amyl nitrite) or a fixed obstruction related to the wrap (EGJ pressure does not change with amyl nitrite).[39] Patients with pseudoachalasia related to the fundoplication should also undergo endoscopy to determine whether the nature of the obstruction mandates surgical intervention (slipped fundoplication, paraesophageal hernia) versus an attempt at dilation (20 mm or pneumatic).

Patients with type III achalasia deserve special mention, because these patients can be difficult to manage. As currently defined, the key criterion for type III achalasia is 2 or more swallows with a premature contraction (distal latency < 4.5 seconds).[40] Based on the authors' experience, it is highly likely that the spastic contractions (and chest pain) will persist after pneumatic dilation or myotomy. Thus, these patients should be counseled accordingly and treatment with antispasmotics attempted.

CONCLUSIONS

Achalasia is the most well-defined esophageal motility disorder, but the presentation can be heterogeneous in terms of presenting symptoms and esophageal contractile patterns, which can result in a delayed or missed diagnosis. The commonality among all phenotypes is of EGJ outflow obstruction attributable to impaired LES relaxation, but the associated esophageal contractility can be of a completely flaccid esophagus, spasm, panesophageal pressurization, weak, or even normal peristalsis. Thus, the detection of achalasia requires vigilance and an understanding of the varied esophageal pressure topography phenotypes to confirm the diagnosis. This is clinically important because achalasia is unique among esophageal motility disorders in having specific effective therapies: disruption of the LES by either pneumatic dilation or myotomy (surgical or endoscopic). Once a diagnosis of achalasia is made, definitive therapy aimed at relieving EGJ outflow obstruction should be offered, assuming the patient is a good surgical candidate. With the recent advent of an improved diagnostic classification scheme and promising endoscopic therapy for achalasia, clinicians and patients have a range of options for effective treatments.

REFERENCES

1.   Bredenoord AJ, Fox M, Kahrilas PJ, et al. Chicago classification criteria of esophageal motility disorders defined in high resolution esophageal pressure topography. *Neurogastroenterol Motil.* 2012;24(Suppl 1):57-65.
2.   Goldblum JR, Whyte RI, Orringer MB, et al. Achalasia. A morphologic study of 42 resected specimens. *Am J Surg Pathol.* 1994;18:327-337.
3.   Boeckxstaens GE. Achalasia: virus-induced euthanasia of neurons? *Am J Gastroenterol.* 2008;103:1610-1612.
4.   Johnston BT, Colcher A, Li Q, et al. Repetitive proximal esophageal contractions: a new manometric finding and a possible further link between Parkinson's disease and achalasia. *Dysphagia.* 2001;16:186-189.
5.   Zárate N, Mearin F, Gil-Vernet JM, et al. Achalasia and Down's syndrome: coincidental association or something else? *Am J Gastroenterol.* 1999;94:1674-1677.
6.   Jung KW, Yoon IJ, Kim DH, et al. Genetic evaluation of ALADIN gene in early-onset achalasia and alacrima patients. *J Neurogastroenterol Motil.* 2011;17:169-173.
7.   Oliveira RB de, Rezende Filho J, Dantas RO, et al. The spectrum of esophageal motor disorders in Chagas disease. *Am J Gastroenterol.* 1995;90:1119-1124.

8. Pandolfino JE, Kahrilas PJ. American Gastroenterological Association medical position statement: clinical use of esophageal manometry. *Gastroenterol.* 2005;128:207-208.

9. Pandolfino JE, Kwiatek MA, Nealis T, et al. Achalasia: a new clinically relevant classification by high-resolution manometry. *Gastroenterol.* 2008;135:1526-1533.

10. Staiano A, Clouse RE. Detection of incomplete lower esophageal sphincter relaxation with conventional point-pressure sensors. *Am J Gastroenterol.* 2001;96:3258-3267.

11. Ghosh SK, Pandolfino JE, Rice J, et al. Impaired deglutitive EGJ relaxation in clinical esophageal manometry: a quantitative analysis of 400 patients and 75 controls. *Am J Physiol.* 2007;293:G878-G885.

12. Roman S, Zerbib F, Quenehervé L, et al. The Chicago classification for achalasia in a French multicentric cohort. *Dig Liver Dis.* 2012;44:976-980.

13. Salvador R, Costantini M, Zaninotto G, et al. The preoperative manometric pattern predicts the outcome of surgical treatment for esophageal achalasia. *J Gastrointest Surg.* 2010;14:1635-1645.

14. Pratap N, Reddy DN. Can achalasia subtyping by high-resolution manometry predict the therapeutic outcome of pneumatic balloon dilatation?: Author's reply. *J Neurogastroenterol Motil.* 2011;17:205.

15. Min M, Peng LH, Yang YS, et al. Characteristics of achalasia subtypes in untreated Chinese patients: a high-resolution manometry study. *J Dig Dis.* 2012;13:504-509.

16. Birgisson S, Richter JE. Achalasia in Iceland, 1952-2002: an epidemiologic study. *Dig Dis Sci.* 2007;52:1855-1860.

17. Gennaro N, Portale G, Gallo C, et al. Esophageal achalasia in the Veneto region: epidemiology and treatment. Epidemiology and treatment of achalasia. *J Gastrointest Surg.* 2011;15:423-428.

18. Enestvedt BK, Williams JL, Sonnenberg A. Epidemiology and practice patterns of achalasia in a large multi-centre database. *Aliment Pharmacol Ther.* 2011;33:1209-1214.

19. Bortolotti M, Mari C, Lopilato C, et al. Effects of sildenafil on esophageal motility of patients with idiopathic achalasia. *Gastroenterol.* 2000;118:253-257.

20. Pasricha PJ, Rai R, Ravich WJ, et al. Botulinum toxin for achalasia: long-term outcome and predictors of response. *Gastroenterol.* 1996;110:1410-1415.

21. Annese V, Bassotti G, Coccia G, et al. A multicentre randomised study of intrasphincteric botulinum toxin in patients with oesophageal achalasia. GISMAD Achalasia Study Group. *Gut.* 2000;46:597-600.

22. Vaezi MF, Richter JE, Wilcox CM, et al. Botulinum toxin versus pneumatic dilatation in the treatment of achalasia: a randomised trial. *Gut.* 1999;44:231-239.

23. Zaninotto G, Annese V, Costantini M, et al. Randomized controlled trial of botulinum toxin versus laparoscopic Heller myotomy for esophageal achalasia. *Ann Surg.* 2004;239:364-370.

24. Smith CD, Stival A, Howell DL, et al. Endoscopic therapy for achalasia before Heller myotomy results in worse outcomes than Heller myotomy alone. *Ann Surg.* 2006;243:579-584.

25. Spiess AE, Kahrilas PJ. Treating achalasia: from whalebone to laparoscope. *JAMA.* 1998;280:638-642.

26. Lynch KL, Pandolfino JE, Howden CW, et al. Major complications of pneumatic dilation and Heller myotomy for achalasia: single-center experience and systematic review of the literature. *Am J Gastroenterol.* 2012;107:1817-1825.

27. Farhoomand K, Connor JT, Richter JE, et al. Predictors of outcome of pneumatic dilation in achalasia. *Clin Gastroenterol Hepatol.* 2004;2:389-394.

28. Boeckxstaens GE, Annese V, Varannes SB des, et al. Pneumatic dilation versus laparoscopic Heller's myotomy for idiopathic achalasia. *N Engl J Med.* 2011;364:1807-1816.

29. Campos GM, Vittinghoff E, Rabl C, et al. Endoscopic and surgical treatments for achalasia: a systematic review and meta-analysis. *Ann Surg.* 2009;249:45-57.

30. Rawlings A, Soper NJ, Oelschlager B, et al. Laparoscopic Dor versus Toupet fundoplication following Heller myotomy for achalasia: results of a multicenter, prospective, randomized-controlled trial. *Surg Endosc.* 2012;26:18-26.

31. Stefanidis D, Richardson W, Farrell TM, et al. SAGES guidelines for the surgical treatment of esophageal achalasia. *Surg Endosc.* 2012;26:296-311.

32. Pasricha PJ, Hawari R, Ahmed I, et al. Submucosal endoscopic esophageal myotomy: a novel experimental approach for the treatment of achalasia. *Endoscopy.* 2007;39:761-764.

33. Inoue H, Minami H, Kobayashi Y, et al. Peroral endoscopic myotomy (POEM) for esophageal achalasia. *Endoscopy.* 2010;42:265-271.

34. Inoue H, Kudo S-E. [Per-oral endoscopic myotomy (POEM) for 43 consecutive cases of esophageal achalasia]. *Nihon Rinsho.* 2010;68:1749-1752.

35. Swanström LL, Rieder E, Dunst CM. A stepwise approach and early clinical experience in peroral endoscopic myotomy for the treatment of achalasia and esophageal motility disorders. *J Am Coll Surg.* 2011;213:751-756.

36. Renteln D von, Inoue H, Minami H, et al. Per-oral endoscopic myotomy for the treatment of achalasia: a prospective single center study. *Am J Gastroenterol.* 2012;107:411-417.

37. Bhayani NH, Kurian AA, Dunst CM, et al. A comparative study on comprehensive, objective outcomes of laparoscopic Heller myotomy with per-oral endoscopic myotomy (POEM) for achalasia. *Ann Surg.* 2013.

38. Hungness ES, Teitelbaum EN, Santos BF, et al. Comparison of perioperative outcomes between per-oral esophageal myotomy (POEM) and laparoscopic Heller myotomy. *J Gastrointest Surg.* 2013;17:228-235.

39. Dodds WJ, Stewart ET, Kishk SM, et al. Radiologic amyl nitrite test for distinguishing pseudoachalasia from idiopathic achalasia. *Am J Roentgenol.* 1986;146:21-23.
40. Pandolfino JE, Roman S, Carlson D, et al. Distal esophageal spasm in high-resolution esophageal pressure topography: defining clinical phenotypes. *Gastroenterol.* 2011;141:469-475.

Esophageal Spasm and Hypercontractile and Hypertensive Motility Disorders

Mark R. Fox, MD, MA, FRCP and Rami Sweis, MD, PhD, MRCP

KEY POINTS

- Dysphagia and chest pain may be due to esophageal spasm and related disorders; however, only a small proportion of patients with these symptoms have a major esophageal motility disorder on manometry.

- Esophageal spasm is characterized by premature (simultaneous) contractions related to impaired deglutitive inhibition (relaxation) of the esophagus on swallowing. Hypertensive contractions are caused by excessive excitation or response of the esophageal smooth muscle.

- High-resolution manometry with provocative challenge using solid foods that trigger esophageal dysmotility and symptoms can increase the sensitivity of physiological tests.

- Efficacy of established medical treatments such as smooth muscle relaxants and visceral analgesics is variable, and side effects may limit use. New treatments including sildenafil and botulinum toxin show promise.

- Empiric esophageal dilatation is not recommended. Surgical myotomy or POEM may be useful in well-characterized patients, but should be performed in specialist centers.

DEFINITION OF DISORDERS

Dysphagia and chest pain may be caused by esophageal dysfunction. Many patients who present with these symptoms have no evidence of "organic disorders" (eg, neoplasia, eosinophilia) or gastroesophageal reflux disease (GERD). In such cases, if symptoms are persistent, then the diagnosis of functional dysphagia or chest pain can be made. This classification includes esophageal motility disorders, and, in practice, patients and doctors often attribute symptoms to "esophageal spasm."

Rao SSC, Parkman HP, McCallum RW, eds.
Handbook of Gastrointestinal Motility and Functional Disorders (pp 47-61).
© 2015 Taylor & Francis Group.

However, symptom-based diagnosis is highly nonspecific and, on investigation, only a small proportion of cases are actually caused by abnormal esophageal function.

The "Chicago classification" of esophageal motility disorders for high-resolution manometry (HRM) defines esophageal spasm on the basis of premature contractions (short distal latency) with normal relaxation and opening of the esophagogastric junction (normal integrated relaxation pressure).[1] Hypertensive ("nutcracker") and hypercontractile ("jackhammer") esophagus are defined by the presence of high- or very high-pressure peristaltic contractions (elevated distal contractile index), respectively. High-resolution manometry has made it easier to differentiate these conditions from achalasia (eg, vigorous or "type III" achalasia) and outlet obstruction, which requires different therapy.

PATHOPHYSIOLOGY AND CAUSES OF SYMPTOMS

The causes of distal esophageal spasm (DES) and related disorders have not been identified; however, case reports of familial inheritance are exceptionally rare, and it is likely that environmental causes predominate.[2] Abnormal muscle contractions occur only in the mid-distal esophagus and are likely related to disturbed neuromuscular function (see later text). Endoscopic ultrasound imaging shows that such patients have a thicker muscularis propria and abnormal coordination between the longitudinal and circular muscle compared to healthy subjects.[3] Barium studies reveal that epiphrenic diverticulae are present in some cases. Interestingly, with few exceptions, surgical biopsies show that wall thickening is due to smooth muscle hypertrophy and not hyperplasia. Further, there is no neuropathy in the myenteric plexus as is present in achalasia. These findings indicate that muscle wall pathology may not be the primary cause of DES and related disorders, but rather may be the effect of poorly coordinated muscle function with increased resistance to bolus passage over time.

Normal esophageal motility and bolus transport depend on the dynamic, coordinated interplay of inhibition and excitation of the muscle wall. On swallowing, the pharyngeal swallow "pumps" fluid or food into the lumen. In the smooth muscle esophagus, inhibitory (relaxatory) and excitatory (contractile) motor neurons in the myenteric plexus are activated by preganglionic fibers that originate from the dorsal motor nucleus of the vagus (Figure 4-1). Inhibitory neurons release nitric oxide (NO), which relaxes the circular muscle layer to allow bolus passage. This "deglutitive relaxation" increases in duration from proximal to distal, which produces the normal peristaltic contraction. Subsequently, postganglionic excitatory neurons release acetylcholine (ACh) and other neurotransmitters (eg, serotonin [5-HT]), which mediate contraction of the muscle wall. This sequence of centrally coordinated events modulated by local reflexes activated by mechanical stimulation produces the esophageal contraction that clears the lumen of swallowed material.

Distal esophageal spasm and related conditions are caused either by impaired deglutitive inhibition or excessive excitation of the esophageal smooth muscle. Altered endogenous NO synthesis and/or degradation is involved in the pathogenesis of DES. NO synthase inhibitors decrease the duration of deglutitive inhibition, thereby reducing distal latency and increasing peristaltic velocity. Conversely, NO donors prolong the duration of deglutitive inhibition, thereby increasing distal latency and decreasing peristaltic velocity. In DES, deglutitive inhibition is reduced or absent when simultaneous contractions occur.[4] Further, NO donors can convert simultaneously into propagated contractions and improve dysphagia and chest pain.[2] Together, these studies provide strong evidence that endogenous NO is involved in the physiological regulation of esophageal motility and that loss of inhibitory control results in simultaneous and sometimes high-pressure contractions due to unopposed action of excitatory neurotransmitters.

In hypercontractile and hypertensive motility disorders, peristalsis is preserved but contractile pressure is elevated and repetitive contractions may occur. This pattern is consistent with

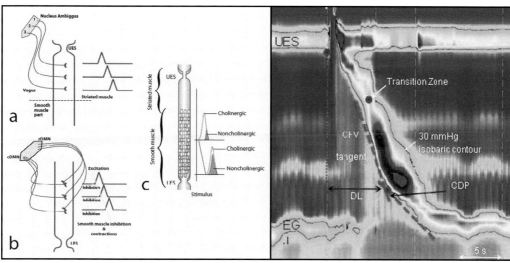

Figure 4-1. (A) Peristalsis in the proximal striated muscle esophagus is mediated by sequential excitation of lower motor neurons originating in the nucleus ambiguous via the vagus nerve. (B) On swallowing, there is rapid activation of short-latency inhibitory vagal fibers that relaxes the entire esophagus by releasing nitric oxide from the myenteric inhibitory neurons. There is a delayed activation of the cholinergic pathway in the long-latency vagal fibers. These cholinergic excitations only occur after the sequential termination of deglutitive inhibition. (C) The presence of an increasing number of inhibitory noncholinergic neurons (closed circles) and a decreasing number of excitatory cholinergic neurons (open circles) along the distal esophagus results in the gradual increase in duration of deglutitive inhibition and a coordinated peristaltic wave. (Reprinted with permission from Mashimo H and Goyal RK. <http://www.nature.com/gimo/contents/pt1/full/gimo3. html> [Accessed 27 June 2012] modified from Crist J, et al. *Proc Natl Acad Sci USA* 1984; 81(11):3595-3599 with permission). (D) Normal swallow on high-resolution manometry. The transition zone ("peristaltic break") represents the transition between the proximal striated (S1) and the mid-distal smooth muscle esophagus (S2 to S3). The contractile deceleration point (CDP) represents the inflection point in the contractile front propagation. It represents the transition from peristaltic contraction and clearance of the esophageal body to nonperistaltic clearance of the esophageal ampulla. Distal latency (DL) is the time from UES relaxation to the CDP and is a measurement of deglutitive relaxation. The distal contractile index (DCI; not shown) is an assessment of contractile vigor based on an integrated function of pressure, length, and duration of contraction.

preserved inhibitory but excessive excitatory stimulation. This view is supported by the finding of increased numbers of choline acetyltransferase-positive neurons in the myenteric plexus of affected patients.[5] Anticholinergic agents, such as atropine, reduce contractile pressures; however, its effects on esophageal physiology are complicated because presynaptic cholinergic nerves also promote the release of NO.[6] This may be the reason that anticholinergics do not reliably alleviate symptoms in patients with this form of dysmotility.

The cause of esophageal symptoms in patients with DES, hypercontractile, and hypertensive dysmotility is controversial. Distal esophageal spasm patients with predominant dysphagia tend to have a higher percentage of ineffective swallows with incomplete bolus transit compared to those with chest pain ($P < 0.05$). Conversely, those with predominant chest pain tend to have higher distal contractile pressure than those with dysphagia (amplitude 202 vs 118 mm Hg; $P < 0.05$). However, it is only when grossly elevated contractile pressures (> 260 mm Hg) occur that a direct causal association with chest pain can be demonstrated. Chest pain may also be associated with isolated spasm of the longitudinal muscle, as revealed by dramatic esophageal shortening detected by endoscopic ultrasound (EUS) or HRM.[3] Powerful contractions of the muscle wall may cause pain due to a massive increase in wall tension or, if prolonged, due to muscle wall ischaemia.[2] In addition, hypersensitivity to bolus escape (esophageal distension) and contractions (wall tension) may contribute to symptom generation. Recent studies have shown that visceral hypersensitivity and hyperresponsiveness to distension of the esophageal wall trigger typical symptoms in up to 75% patients with noncardiac, nonreflux chest pain.[7] This may be related to primary muscle dysfunction or to hypervigilance related to somatization and anxiety disorders that are more prevalent in patients with DES and nutcracker esophagus than healthy controls.[8]

EPIDEMIOLOGY AND NATURAL HISTORY

Dysphagia and noncardiac chest pain are common in the community, accounting for about 5% of all presentations to primary care physicians[9]; however, the underlying cause of these complaints is not known because only a fraction of affected patients are referred for physiologic investigations. In clinical series, 40% to 60% of patients with esophageal symptoms received a final diagnosis of GERD, with 10% to 30% diagnosed with any form of esophageal motor disorder and up to 50% receiving no definitive diagnosis.[10-13] Distal esophageal spasm is rare, found in 0.6% to 2.8% of patients referred with chest pain, 3.3% to 5.3% with dysphagia, and 4% to 4.5% if both symptoms are present. The prevalence of nutcracker esophagus (including hypertensive lower esophageal sphincter [LES]) is 6% to 48% in patients with chest pain and 3% to 6% in those with dysphagia, with more recent series providing lower estimates.[10,12]

There are no well-established associations between hypercontractile dysmotility and other clinical diseases. There are also no reliable data on the impact of gender or race on the prevalence of these conditions. Clinical series do suggest that nutcracker esophagus is somewhat more common in younger patients, whereas DES is more common in older patients. This could suggest disease progression over time; however, longitudinal studies do not support a systematic progression from nutcracker or DES to achalasia. The prognosis of these conditions is also uncertain. In a follow-up study of 72 patients with DES and related motility disorders, the majority reported an improvement in their symptoms over time, even though only 39% reported that medical treatment was beneficial. Overall, although these disorders cause persistent morbidity in some patients, it appears to run a benign course in others, with symptoms often subsiding spontaneously.

DIAGNOSIS

Patients with esophageal dysmotility often attend hospitals and even specialist clinics for years before receiving a definitive diagnosis. Typically, endoscopy and imaging studies are performed on multiple occasions; however, the patient is not referred for definitive tests. Thus, the utilization of health care resources is inefficient and unnecessary costs are incurred.

Certain presentations are more suggestive of dysmotility than reflux, angina, or musculoskeletal pain; however, patient presentation is nonspecific, and symptom-based diagnosis is not accurate.[14] This is illustrated by the finding that 38% to 75% of patients with achalasia also have symptoms of heartburn,[15,16] and the majority of patients with major motility disorders have received proton pump inhibitor (PPI) therapy to treat presumed GERD prior to diagnosis. Conversely, the description of dysphagia in achalasia can be vague, and the classic description of dysphagia to solids and liquids is reported by only 75% of patients.[17]

Initial Investigations

When suspected, cardiac chest pain must be excluded prior to other investigations; however, the presence of heart disease does not rule out other conditions, and patients who fail to respond well to anti-anginals should be investigated for esophageal disease. Laboratory tests rarely aid the diagnosis. Endoscopy with biopsy is indicated in all patients with dysphagia to identify neoplasia and mucosal disease (eg, reflux esophagitis, eosinophilia). Barium studies rarely provide useful information unless a classic corkscrew esophagus or an epiphrenic diverticulum is present or classic features of achalasia are seen. Computed tomography and EUS may detect thickening of the esophageal muscle wall (normally < 3 mm); however, this finding is not sensitive or specific for dysmotility.[18]

An empiric trial of high-dose acid suppression (eg, omeprazole 20 to 40 mg twice daily) is recommended before definitive tests, especially if chest pain predominates, because PPI treatment provides at least 50% improvement in up to 80% of patients with unexplained chest pain and GERD on 24-hour pH testing, but only 20% of those with no evidence of GERD.[19] A meta-analysis reported that a risk ratio for continued symptoms on PPI in this patient group was only 0.54 (95%CI: 0.41 to 0.71) representing a number-needed-to-treat of less than 3.[20] It is when PPIs do not provide adequate symptom relief that referral for physiologic studies is indicated.

Ambulatory Reflux Monitoring

GERD is a common cause of symptoms even in patients who fail to respond to PPIs. It is not known why some patients complain of heartburn and others of chest pain; however, ambulatory pH studies provide objective evidence of GERD in 40% to 60% of patients with noncardiac chest pain on the basis of pathologic acid exposure and/or a positive association between reflux events and chest pain.[10,12] Combined multichannel intraluminal impedance (MII) and pH studies increase sensitivity by detecting both acid and nonacid reflux and document failed esophageal clearance. This may be useful in this group because a high proportion may have heightened sensitivity, not only to acid reflux, but also to esophageal distention by nonacid "volume reflux" and bolus escape on swallowing. Patients with a proven association between acid reflux events and symptoms are more likely to respond to optimized antireflux therapy, including surgery, than those without such findings.[19] However, it is important to inspect the source data because pathological acid exposure is present in up to 20% of patients with achalasia and can be present in DES due to poor clearance rather than frequent reflux events. In addition, results can be confounded if fermentation of bacteria in food retained in the esophagus leads to lactic acid production.

Manometry

In diagnostic schemes such as the Chicago classification (Table 4-1), DES is characterized by the presence of simultaneous "spastic" contractions in the distal smooth muscle esophagus. Hypercontractile ("jackhammer") or hypertensive ("nutcracker") motility disorders require preservation of normal peristalsis with elevated contractile pressures. It is important to distinguish DES and related disorders from achalasia and outlet obstruction characterized by abnormal esophagogastric junction (EGJ) function because only the latter will respond to EGJ dilation or myotomy.

Using conventional manometry with 4 to 8 pressure sensors, it can be difficult to distinguish esophageal spasm in the distal esophagus from simultaneous "common cavity" pressure changes that occur throughout the lumen in achalasia and, occasionally, in obstruction.[21] High-resolution manometry increases the diagnostic sensitivity and specificity; in a series of 212 consecutive patients, conventional manometry missed one case of DES and misdiagnosed DES in 4 cases, which on HRM proved to be achalasia or aperistalsis.[22] The key criteria that improved diagnostic accuracy on HRM was the presence or absence of an increased esophagogastric pressure gradient (now integrated relaxation pressure).[23] High-resolution manometry was particularly useful in identifying achalasia patients with relatively low-pressure EGJ and in those with significant esophageal shortening (leads to "pseudorelaxation on conventional tests in achalasia patients").[21,23]

TABLE 4-1

HRM WORKING GROUP CHICAGO CLASSIFICATION OF ESOPHAGEAL MOTILITY DISORDERS V3.0

WITH NORMAL IRP/EGJ RELAXATION

Disorder	Criteria
Aperistalsis	Normal mean IRP, 100% swallows with absent peristalsis
Esophageal spasm	Normal mean IRP, > 20% premature contractions (DL < 4.5 s)
Hypercontractile peristalsis "jackhammer"	Normal mean IRP, normal DL > 4.5 s > 20% distal contractile integral (DCI) > 8000 mm Hg•s•cm
Hypertensive peristalsis "nutcracker"	Normal mean IRP, normal DL > 4.5 s Contractile pressure > 180 mm Hg or DCI > 5000 mm Hg•s•cm
Ineffective esophageal motility and frequent failed peristalsis	Normal mean IRP, normal DL > 4.5 s, > 50% failed or hypotensive (DCI < 450 mm Hg•s•cm) > 50% swallows with large breaks (> 5 cm in length) in the 20 mm Hg isobaric contour

WITH IMPAIRED IRP/EGJ RELAXATION

Disorder	Criteria
Achalasia	
Classic achalasia (type I)	Abnormal mean IRP/EGJ relaxation and aperistalsis
Achalasia with esophageal compression (type II)	Abnormal mean IRP/EGJ relaxation, aperistalsis, and panesophageal pressurization (IBP > 15 mm Hg) ≥ 20% swallows
Vigorous or spastic achalasia (type III)	Abnormal mean IRP/EGJ relaxation, aperistalsis, and premature contraction (ie, spasm) ≥ 20% of swallows
EGJ obstruction* *either structural obstruction or occasional achalasia variant	Abnormal mean IRP with instances of intact peristalsis or weak peristalsis such that criteria for achalasia not met

HRM: high resolution manometry; IRP: integrated relazation pressure; EGJ: esophagogastric junction; IBP: intrabolus pressure; DL: distal latency; DCI: distal contractile index (integrated pressure, duration and length of contraction wave).

Adapted from Kahrilas PJ, Brendenoord AJ, Fox M, et al. The Chicago classification of esophageal motility disorders, v3.0. *Neurogastroenterol Motil.* 2015;27(2):160-174.

In addition, HRM identifies achalasia subtypes in which spasm and prolonged contractions are limited to the mid- or lower-segment of the smooth muscle esophagus or restricted to the LES.

Version 3.0 of the Chicago classification (CC v3.0) defines spasm not by rapid "contractile front velocity" (CFV), but rather by short "distal contractile latency" (DL), which represents the duration

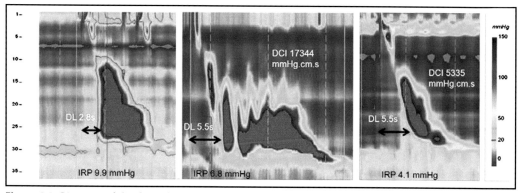

Figure 4-2. Diagnosis of distal esophageal spasm and related disorders by high-resolution manometry according to the Chicago classification. All peristaltic motility disorders have normal IRP (< 15 mm Hg)/EGJ function. (A) Distal esophageal spasm is characterized by premature contraction (DL < 4.5 s). (B) Hypercontractile "jackhammer" esophagus peristaltic contractions have normal DL, but contractile pressures are grossly elevated, often with repetitive contraction (DCI > 8000 mm Hg•cm•s). Hypertensive "nutcracker" esophagus has normal DL, but contractile pressures are elevated above normal (DCI 5000 to 8000 mm Hg•cm•s).

of deglutitive inhibition (see Figure 4-1).[24] This measurement is more objective and reproducible than CFV. Distal contractile latency is defined as the time from the start of upper sphincter relaxation to the contractile deceleration point (CDP), which is the point at which the esophageal contraction changes from a rapid, peristaltic "stripping" wave to a slower, nonperistaltic "emptying" phase.[24] A reduced DL (< 4.5 sec) defines a premature contraction, or spasm (Figure 4-2). The diagnosis of DES requires the presence of at least 20% premature contractions (DL < 4.5 sec) with normal EGJ relaxation. Using DL to define DES, the prevalence of DES is very low. In a study of 1070 HRM studies, only 24 (2.2%) exhibited a premature contraction (reduced DL), of which 18 (1.7%) had vigorous achalasia and only 6 (0.6%) had DES.[25] Swallows with normal EGJ relaxation and normal DL but with rapid CFV (> 9 cm/s) are "rapid contractions"; however, these are a normal variant and no longer included in CC v3.0.

Hypertensive ("nutcracker") and hypercontractile ("jackhammer") esophageal motility disorders are defined by the presence of normal EGJ relaxation and normal DL (see Figure 4-2). In hypertensive motility disorders, contractile pressures are abnormally high (distal contractile index [DCI] exceeds 5000 mm Hg•cm•s but lies below 8000 mm Hg•cm•s). This is above the upper end of the normal range; however, contractile pressure in this range can be found in healthy subjects, and this diagnosis is no longer included in CC v3.0. Notwithstanding this, nutcracker esophagus is more prevalent in patients with noncardiac chest pain than in healthy controls[26]; however, this association may be related to concurrent anxiety rather than esophageal pathology. Also, the use of opiates systematically increases contractile pressures. In hypercontractile motility pressures exceed a DCI of 8000 mm Hg•cm•s) with water swallos and often can include repetitive contractions (hence, "jackhammer" esophagus). This major motility disorder is never seen in health and is often, but not always, directly associated with chest pain.[27]

Despite advances in technology and classification, the clinical significance of high pressure contractions and of (intermittent or low pressure) esophageal spasm is not always certain. Combined manometry with impedance can document motility and bolus transport. This information can refine the diagnosis into cases with and without impaired esophageal function; however, this does not clarify the relationship between dysmotility and patient symptoms. More convincing evidence of a causal link is provided by a clear temporal association of dysmotility with symptoms in a real-life setting. Current protocols and diagnostic criteria are based on a series of small-volume swallows of fluid that rarely triggers symptoms even in patients with major motility disorders. Some centers include multiple water swallows, solid swallows, or provocative testing using acid

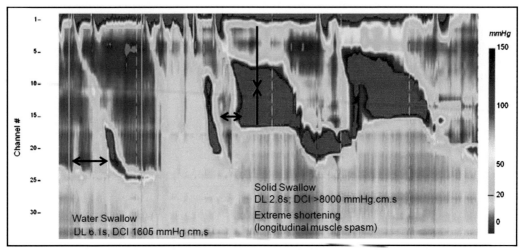

Channel #

mmHg
150
100
50
20
0

Water Swallow
DL 6.1s, DCI 1605 mmHg.cm.s

Solid Swallow
DL 2.8s; DCI >8000 mmHg.cm.s
Extreme shortening
(longitudinal muscle spasm)

Figure 4-3. Diagnosis of distal esophageal spasm by high-resolution manometry with test meal. Motility was normal and the patient symptom free during water swallows; however, on taking solids, spasm with high contractile pressure and esophageal shortening was observed. The patient reported typical chest pain. The use of physiological challenges that reproduce the situation in which the patient experiences symptoms can increase the sensitivity of tests.

perfusion, balloon distension, or edrophonium to increase study sensitivity; however, normal values have not been established and the clinical value of provocative testing remains controversial. More relevant is the ability to link esophageal dysmotility to spontaneous patient reports of symptoms, as is done routinely in ambulatory pH studies. Barham et al[28] reported findings of ambulatory manometry in 390 consecutive patients with suspected esophageal symptoms. Sixteen patients (4%) were found to have symptomatic dysmotility during ambulatory testing, of whom 14 had normal findings on stationary manometry. Conversely, the majority (53/55) of patients with asymptomatic spasm on stationary manometry had no symptomatic dysmotility during ambulatory studies.[28] This technique has not been adopted in clinical practice because interpretation of prolonged conventional manometry records, especially during meals, is challenging. An alternative for stationary HRM studies is to provide a test meal or specific foods that are suspected to trigger symptomatic dysmotility in patients with no diagnosis after water swallows. In a recent pilot study of patients with esophageal symptoms, manometric classification was altered in 67% and clinical diagnosis based on symptomatic dysmotility was altered in 39% of patients who underwent HRM with a standardized test meal (Figure 4-3).[29] These findings altered clinical management in several cases and, if this is repeated in larger clinical studies, it will likely alter the way manometry is performed.

How to Manage Esophageal Spasm and Related Conditions

The evidence base that informs the management of patients with nonachalasic hypercontractile disorders is not strong (Table 4-2). To recruit more than a handful of patients, studies have often enrolled heterogeneous patient groups, including motility disorders that may have quite distinct pathophysiology. As a result, most of what we know is based on retrospective data reviews and small, uncontrolled therapeutic trials.

Overall, the efficacy of medical treatments such as smooth muscle relaxants and visceral analgesics is variable and side effects may limit use. Only about half of the patients with spastic and hypertensive esophageal motor disorders find medical therapy to be of benefit. In this

TABLE 4-2

EVIDENCE BASE FOR MEDICAL THERAPY OF DISTAL ESOPHAGEAL SPASM AND HYPERCONTRACTILE DYSMOTILITY

MEDICATION	DOSE	ROUTE AND FREQUENCY	COST	EVIDENCE GRADE
Peppermint oil	1 capsule	oral prn or tid	$	C
Nifedipine MR	10-20 mg	oral prn or tid	$	B (1 RCT)
Diltiazem MR	60 mg	oral prn or tid	$	B (1 RCT)
Glyceryl trinitrate	300 mg	S/L prn or tid	$	C
Isosorbide dinitrate	10-40 μg	PO od or tid	$	C
Sildenafil	20 mg	Oral prn or tid	$$$	C
Trazodone	50 mg	Oral od qhs	$	B
Imipramine	25 mg	Oral od qhs	$	B
Clomipramine	25 mg	Oral od qhs	$	C
Botulinum toxin	50-200 IU	Endoscopic injection repeat ~6 months	$$$	B (1 RCT)
Esophageal dilation		Endoscopic balloon or bougie dilation		C
Esophageal myotomy		Surgery		C

prn: as required; tid: 3 times per day; S/L: under the tongue; po: by mouth; od: once daily; qhs: every night at bedtime; RCT: randomized controlled trial; $: cheap; $$: moderate; $$$: expensive.

situation, it is essential to explain the causes of symptoms, provide a clear "diagnosis," and reassure patients. This is an important initial step and is therapeutic in and of itself. In patients who require treatment, the primary aim is symptom control. This can often be achieved by empirical measures, such as (1) avoiding factors that trigger esophageal dysmotility by lifestyle intervention (eg, diet, stress reduction) and acid suppression; (2) promoting normal esophageal motility (eg, reducing contractile pressure, promoting peristaltic contractions); and/or (3) reducing esophageal sensitivity to dysmotility and bolus retention. Careful history, including an assessment of psychosocial factors, may highlight specific issues and direct intervention at this level.

Lifestyle Interventions

In general, patients with DES and related disorders find that soft foods and liquids trigger fewer symptoms because these reduce resistance to bolus passage and the stimulus to the esophagus. Certain patients report esophageal symptoms following ingestion of cold fluids or particular foods, and these should be avoided. It is also recommended that patients avoid caffeine and other procholinergic substances. There is little evidence that smoking or alcohol has direct effects on esophageal motility; however, any factor that increases acid reflux should be avoided.

Acid Suppressant Medications

A trial of high-dose PPIs should be considered in all patients; a link between acid reflux and dysmotility has been reported that may be due to stimulation of the esophagus by acid irritation or volume distension. Patients with pathological acid reflux on pH studies, and especially those with a positive symptom association, may respond to this therapy even in the presence of esophageal dysmotility.

Smooth Muscle Relaxants

A variety of medications that decrease contractile pressure (eg, anticholinergics, calcium channel blockers, and nitrate donors) have been applied in DES and related conditions; however, their effect that decrease contractile pressure, have been applied in DES and related conditions; however, their effect on chest pain and dysphagia is inconsistent and side effects are often limiting.

Calcium Channel Blockers

Calcium channel blockers reduce LES pressure and peristaltic amplitude within 20 to 30 minutes of oral ingestion. Nifedipine (20 mg) appears to have a greater effect than other calcium channel blockers.[30,31] Further, controlled trials have shown little or no overall benefit in symptom control for this class of medications, and the side effect profile (hypotension, bradycardia, pedal edema) impacts long-term tolerability even in those with a symptom response.

Nitrate Donors

It is well established that nitrate donors (eg, glyceryl trinitrate [GTN] spray, isosorbide dinitrate) reduce contractile amplitude and velocity, thus promoting normal peristalsis.[32] However, although clinical studies indicate that these effects can improve symptoms, side effects (dizziness and headaches) are often limiting.[32] Nitrate donors may be more effective in patients with no evidence of GERD.[33] Patients with good response to short-acting preparations seem to also do well on long-acting preparations, which may be better tolerated.

An alternative to nitrate donors could be phosphodiesterase type V inhibitors (eg, sildenafil), which inhibit the breakdown of NO in the synaptic cleft. This increases intracellular NO concentration and so induces smooth muscle relaxation. Sildenafil has been shown to reduce LES resting pressure, prolong the duration of LES relaxation, reduce contractile pressure, and normalize contraction duration.[34,35] Two case series have reported manometric improvement on sildenafil in patients with DES and related disorders (Figure 4-4).[34,36] Taken together, 5 of 7 patients with DES but none with achalasia had a symptomatic response to treatment that was maintained for several months.

Smooth muscle relaxants are available in short- and long-acting preparations. In patients who find them effective and tolerate the side effects, these medications can be given regularly or on demand, depending on symptom frequency. Sublingual GTN may be convenient in patients with intermittent chest pain or dysphagia. Long-acting phosphodiesterase type V inhibitors may be a useful medication for patients with frequent symptoms (special permission may be required to prescribe).

Botulinum Toxin

Botulinum toxin A causes muscle relaxation by inhibiting the release of ACh from neurons at the neuromuscular junction. Several studies, including one randomized controlled trial, have reported symptom relief in DES patients following endoscopic injection of botulinum toxin into the distal smooth muscle esophagus. Storr et al[37] injected a total of 100 IU botulinum toxin at multiple sites along the esophagus wall and into endoscopically visible contraction rings. At

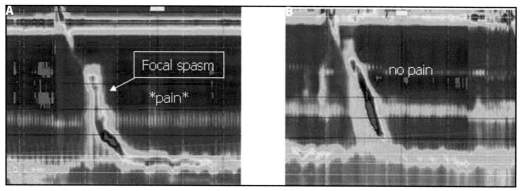

Figure 4-4. Distal esophageal spasm diagnosed in a 63-year-old woman with central chest pain on swallowing. (A) Baseline HRM after swallowing 5 mL of water showing esophageal spasm (short DL). This was associated with typical chest pain symptoms when eating bread. (B) Thirty minutes after administering 20 mg sildenafil, peristalsis was normal and symptoms were not reported even when challenged with bread swallows. (Reprinted with permission from Fox M, Sweis R, Wong T, Anggiansah A. Sildenafil relieves symptoms and normalizes motility in patients with oesophageal spasm: a report of two cases. *Neurogastroenterol Motil.* 2007;19(10):798-803.)

4 weeks, 8 of 9 patients reported almost complete symptom relief that was maintained at 6 months without further treatment. Subsequently, 4 patients required reinjection 8, 12, 15, or 24 months after the initial treatment with similarly good results. Miller et al[38] reported complete symptom relief in 14/29 (48%) DES patients treated with 100 IU of botulinum toxin at the LES, which lasted, on average, over 7 months. Vanuytsel et al[39] reported findings from a randomized, placebo-controlled, double-blind, partial crossover study in 22 patients with nonachalasia esophageal hypermotility disorders. Botulinum toxin (8 injections of 12.5 IU in each patient, 4 injections at and 5 cm above the EGJ) or sham injections were performed in a 4-week crossover design.[39] Active treatment significantly improved motility compared to placebo (Figure 4-5). Treatment also relieved dysphagia in about half the patients treated; however, no significant effects were seen for chest pain, regurgitation, or heartburn. To date, no serious adverse effects were reported even after repeated injection of botulinum toxin. Botulinum toxin is the only treatment with proven efficacy in patients with DES on manometry as opposed to patients with chest pain thought to be related to dysmotility. It is a valuable addition to the treatment options in patients with severe symptoms, especially dysphagia, when other treatments have failed. Endoscopic injection can be repeated when symptoms return, and extensive use in other conditions has revealed no evidence of long-term harm.

Pain Modulators

The benefits of tricyclic antidepressants, serotonin reuptake inhibitors, and other antide-pressants are well established in functional gastrointestinal (GI) disease, including in the treatment of noncardiac chest pain.[40-42] Although this group of drugs has no effect on esophageal function, it is thought to reduce symptoms due effects on visceral sensitivity. Central effects on anxiety and depression, which often coexist with chronic functional syndromes, may also be beneficial.

Initially, low doses are taken at nighttime to avoid daytime drowsiness. Patients must be encouraged to persist with treatment because, whereas side effects decrease after several days of treatment, beneficial effects may take 4 to 8 weeks to become apparent. If symptom relief is not adequate at this stage, doses can be increased at intervals until clinical improvement occurs, side effects become troublesome, or a full antidepressant dose is reached. After symptom remission is achieved, the optimal duration of treatment and the likelihood of symptom recurrence after with-drawal of these medications have not been defined. Patients with good treatment response can continue treatment indefinitely.

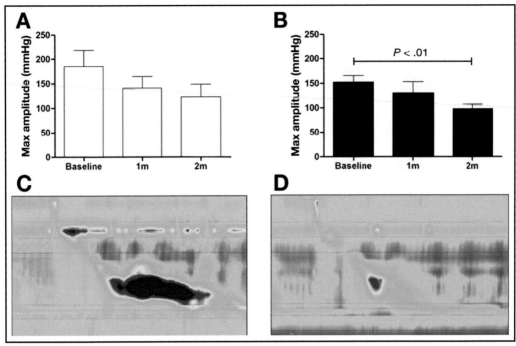

Figure 4-5. Maximal distal amplitude and symptoms before and after botulinum toxin (BTX) injection. (A) Maximal distal amplitude in patients at baseline, 1 month, and 2 months after BTX injection. (B) Dysphagia score in patients at baseline and 6 months after BTX or sham injection. Significant improvement was seen in patients after BTX but not sham injection. (C, D) Representative pictures of a patient with hypercontractile ("jackhammer") esophagus before and 1 month after BTX. (Reprinted with permission from Vanuytsel T, Bisschops R, Farre R, et al. Botulinum toxin reduces dysphagia in patients with nonachalasia primary esophageal motility disorders. *Clin Gastroenterol Hepatol.* 2013;11:1115-1121.)

Although amitriptyline and imipramine (both 10 to 25 mg at night) are commonly prescribed in noncardiac chest pain, the serotonin reuptake inhibitor trazodone is the most studied in patients with documented esophageal dysmotility. In a double-blind, placebo-controlled study, including patients with chest pain and DES or related disorders, trazodone (100 to 150 mg/d) improved overall symptoms to a greater degree than placebo without effects on manometric abnormalities.[40] In a subsequent study, trazodone was found to have superior clinical efficacy compared to isosorbide dinitrate in unselected patients with these conditions.[43]

The effects of psychological intervention on esophageal dysmotility and symptoms have not been assessed; however, in common with other functional GI diseases, patients may profit from cognitive behavioral or interpersonal therapies. Patients learn to cope with their symptoms by diverting attention away from GI sensations and addressing unhelpful thoughts and behavior related to the condition.

Bougienage and Pneumatic Dilation

In achalasia, dilation reduces outflow obstruction by disrupting the LES; however, the mechanism of action (if any) in DES patients is uncertain. Bougienage by a variety of rigid dilators (incremental to 18 mm) and pneumatic dilation (incremental to 30 mm) has been used in patients with DES not responding to pharmacological therapy. Case series suggest that up to half can have a good outcome, although there is an approximate 5% risk of perforation and/or bleeding.[44] There is also a risk of gastroesophageal reflux after the procedure. In one case series, 20 patients with

DES had pneumatic dilatations of whom 14 had a good response, 5 had a poor response, and 1 had perforation. Of those with poor response, 3 proceeded to full-length myotomy, 2 of whom had relief of symptoms.[45] No controlled trials have been performed, and it is possible that those who benefited from this approach had a diagnosis either of achalasia or outlet obstruction rather than DES that had been missed by conventional manometry.

Surgery

Surgical management of DES and related conditions is reserved for patients with severe symptoms that have failed to respond to medical and endoscopic therapies. Laparoscopic and thoracoscopic operative techniques are described. The procedure is based on esophagomyotomy, with the incision extending along the entire smooth muscle esophagus and 2 cm below the EGJ. Two methods are considered equally effective in avoiding postmyotomy reflux: a "short, floppy" wrap or a sphincter-sparing myotomy when LES function is preserved. There are no controlled studies; however, in one case series, outcomes after surgery were better than continued medical care.[46] Historically, the results are less good than those following esophagomyotomy for achalasia; however, recent surgical series report good long-term functional outcomes in 80% of cases of severe DES with extended myotomy and anterior fundoplication.[46] If patients continue to experience persistent or recurrent pain and dysphagia after surgery, then a total esophagectomy and cervical esophagogastrostomy may be required. Experts agree that these difficult operations should be performed only by specialist surgeons on carefully selected patients with evidence of esophageal dysfunction and a clear rationale to expect benefit from this procedure.

CONCLUSION

DES and hypercontractile esophageal motility disorders are rare diseases that typically present with chest pain and dysphagia. The etiology is related to abnormal neuromuscular function. The diagnosis is based on manometry. Distal esophageal spasm is characterized by the presence of premature (simultaneous) contractions, whereas other conditions, such as "jackhammer" and "nutcracker" esophagus are characterized by high-pressure contractions. The clinical significance of manometric abnormalities is greatly supported if symptoms accompany dysmotility. It is to be hoped that the introduction of the Chicago classification for HRM with a well-accepted definition of these disorders will facilitate recruitment of well-characterized patients to the multicenter studies that will be required to provide robust information about the management of these disorders.

Therapeutic options are limited; however, careful history and examination of the physiologic investigations may highlight specific pathology and guide effective therapy. Initial therapy with high-dose acid suppression is appropriate, as dysmotility may be triggered or symptoms aggravated by acid reflux. Initial pharmacotherapy involves smooth muscle relaxants such as calcium channel blockers or nitrate donors (eg, GTN); however, efficacy of these medications is variable and is often limited by side effects. Medications that reduce visceral sensitivity such as trazodone may be helpful in other cases, although they do not reduce dysmotility. Increasing evidence supports the clinical efficacy of botulinum toxin injected into the esophageal wall as second-line therapy. Endoscopic LES dilation and surgical myotomy of the distal esophagus are reserved for use in specialist centers.

There is growing interest in the use of POEM (per-oral endoscopic myotomy) as an alternative method to surgery whereby the circular muscles of the esophagus that are contributing to spasm can be manometrically identified and incised endoscopically in a targeted manner up to the proximal point of spasm in patients with refractory hypercontractility disorders.[47, 48]

REFERENCES

1. Pandolfino JE, Kwiatek MA, Nealis T, Bulsiewicz W, Post J, Kahrilas PJ. Achalasia: a new clinically relevant classification by high-resolution manometry. *Gastroenterology.* 2008;135(5):1526-1533.

2. Grubel C, Hiscock R, Hebbard G. Value of spatiotemporal representation of manometric data. *Clin Gastroenterol Hepatol.* 2008;6(5):525-530.

3. Mittal RK, Liu J, Puckett JL, et al. Sensory and motor function of the esophagus: lessons from ultrasound imaging. *Gastroenterology.* 2005;128(2):487-497.

4. Sifrim D, Janssens J, Vantrappen G. Failing deglutitive inhibition in primary esophageal motility disorders. *Gastroenterology.* 1994;106(4):875-882.

5. Kim HS, Park H, Lim JH, et al. Morphometric evaluation of oesophageal wall in patients with nutcracker oesophagus and ineffective oesophageal motility. *Neurogastroenterol Motil.* 2008;20(8):869-876.

6. Crist J, Gidda JS, Goyal RK. Intramural mechanism of esophageal peristalsis: roles of cholinergic and noncholinergic nerves. *Proc Natl Acad Sci USA.* 1984;81(11):3595-3599.

7. Nasr I, Attaluri A, Hashmi S, Gregersen H, Rao SS. Investigation of esophageal sensation and biomechanical properties in functional chest pain. *Neurogastroenterol Motil.* 2010;22(5):520-526, e116.

8. Song CW, Lee SJ, Jeen YT, et al. Inconsistent association of esophageal symptoms, psychometric abnormalities and dysmotility. *Am J Gastroenterol.* 2001;96(8):2312-2316.

9. Eslick GD, Coulshed DS, Talley NJ. Review article: the burden of illness of non-cardiac chest pain. *Aliment Pharmacol Ther.* 2002;16(7):1217-1223.

10. Katz PO, Dalton CB, Richter JE, Wu WC, Castell DO. Esophageal testing of patients with noncardiac chest pain or dysphagia. Results of three years' experience with 1161 patients. *Ann Intern Med.* 1987;106(4):593-597.

11. Dekel R, Pearson T, Wendel C, De Garmo P, Fennerty MB, Fass R. Assessment of oesophageal motor function in patients with dysphagia or chest pain: the Clinical Outcomes Research Initiative experience. *Aliment Pharmacol Ther.* 2003;18(11-12):1083-1089.

12. Xiao Y, Nicodeme F, Kahrilas PJ, Roman S, Lin Z, Pandolfino JE. Optimizing the swallow protocol of clinical high-resolution esophageal manometry studies. *Neurogastroenterol Motil.* 2012;24(10):e489-496.

13. O'Neill J, McMahon SB, Undem BJ. Chronic cough and pain: Janus faces in sensory neurobiology? *Pulmonary Pharmacol Ther.* 2013;26(5):476-485.

14. Herbella FA, Raz DJ, Nipomnick I, Patti MG. Primary versus secondary esophageal motility disorders: diagnosis and implications for treatment. *J Laparoendosc Adv Surg Tech A.* 2009;19(2):195-198.

15. Howard PJ, Maher L, Pryde A, Cameron EW, Heading RC. Five year prospective study of the incidence, clinical features, and diagnosis of achalasia in Edinburgh. *Gut.* 1992;33(8):1011-1015.

16. Ponce J, Ortiz V, Maroto N, Ponce M, Bustamante M, Garrigues V. High prevalence of heartburn and low acid sensitivity in patients with idiopathic achalasia. *Dig Dis Sci.* 2011;56(3):773-776.

17. Vela MF, Richter JE, Khandwala F, et al. The long-term efficacy of pneumatic dilatation and Heller myotomy for the treatment of achalasia. *Clin Gastroenterol Hepatol.* 2006;4(5):580-587.

18. Nino-Murcia M, Stark P, Triadafilopoulos G. Esophageal wall thickening: a CT finding in diffuse esophageal spasm. *J Comput Assist Tomogr.* 1997;21(2):318-321.

19. Wang WH, Huang JQ, Zheng GF, et al. Is proton pump inhibitor testing an effective approach to diagnose gastroesophageal reflux disease in patients with noncardiac chest pain?: a meta-analysis. *Arch Intern Med.* 2005;165(11):1222-1228.

20. Cremonini F, Wise J, Moayyedi P, Talley NJ. Diagnostic and therapeutic use of proton pump inhibitors in non-cardiac chest pain: a meta-analysis. *Am J Gastroenterol.* 2005;100(6):1226-1232.

21. Fox MR, Bredenoord AJ. Oesophageal high-resolution manometry: moving from research into clinical practice. *Gut.* 2008;57(3):405-423.

22. Clouse RE, Staiano A, Alrakawi A, Haroian L. Application of topographical methods to clinical esophageal manometry. *Am J Gastroenterol.* 2000;95(10):2720-2730.

23. Staiano A, Clouse RE. Detection of incomplete lower esophageal sphincter relaxation with conventional point-pressure sensors. *Am J Gastroenterol.* 2001;96(12):3258-3267.

24. Roman S, Lin Z, Pandolfino JE, Kahrilas PJ. Distal contraction latency: a measure of propagation velocity optimized for esophageal pressure topography studies. *Am J Gastroenterol.* 2011;106(3):443-451.

25. Pandolfino JE, Roman S, Carlson D, et al. Distal esophageal spasm in high-resolution esophageal pressure topography: defining clinical phenotypes. *Gastroenterology.* 2011;141(2):469-475.

26. Tutuian R, Mainie I, Agrawal A, Gideon RM, Katz PO, Castell DO. Symptom and function heterogenicity among patients with distal esophageal spasm: studies using combined impedance-manometry. *Am J Gastroenterol.* 2006;101(3):464-469.

27. Bredenoord AJ, Fox M, Kahrilas PJ, Pandolfino JE, Schwizer W, Smout AJ. Chicago classification criteria of esophageal motility disorders defined in high resolution esophageal pressure topography. *Neurogastroenterol Motil.* 2012;24(Suppl 1):57-65.

28. Barham CP, Gotley DC, Fowler A, Mills A, Alderson D. Diffuse oesophageal spasm: diagnosis by ambulatory 24 hour manometry. *Gut.* 1997;41(2):151-155.

29. Sweis R, Anggiansah A, Wong T, Brady G, Fox M. Assessment of esophageal dysfunction and symptoms during and after a standardized test meal: development and clinical validation of a new methodology utilizing high-resolution manometry. *Neurogastroenterol Motil.* 2014;26(2):215-228.

30. Richter JE, Spurling TJ, Cordova CM, Castell DO. Effects of oral calcium blocker, diltiazem, on esophageal contractions. Studies in volunteers and patients with nutcracker esophagus. *Dig Dis Sci.* 1984;29(7):649-656.

31. Konrad-Dalhoff I, Baunack AR, Ramsch KD, et al. Effect of the calcium antagonists nifedipine, nitrendipine, nimodipine and nisoldipine on oesophageal motility in man. *Eur J Clin Pharmacol.* 1991;41(4):313-316.

32. Konturek JW, Gillessen A, Domschke W. Diffuse esophageal spasm: a malfunction that involves nitric oxide? *Scand J Gastroenterol.* 1995;30(11):1041-1045.

33. Swamy N. Esophageal spasm: clinical and manometric response to nitroglycerine and long acting nitrites. *Gastroenterology.* 1977;72(1):23-27.

34. Eherer AJ, Schwetz I, Hammer HF, et al. Effect of sildenafil on oesophageal motor function in healthy subjects and patients with oesophageal motor disorders. *Gut.* 2002;50(6):758-764.

35. Bortolotti M, Pandolfo N, Giovannini M, Mari C, Miglioli M. Effect of sildenafil on hypertensive lower oesophageal sphincter. *Eur J Clin Invest.* 2002;32(9):682-685.

36. Sifrim D, Mittal R, Fass R, et al. Review article: acidity and volume of the refluxate in the genesis of gastro-oesophageal reflux disease symptoms. *Aliment Pharmacol Ther.* 2007;25(9):1003-1017.

37. Storr M, Allescher HD, Rosch T, Born P, Weigert N, Classen M. Treatment of symptomatic diffuse esophageal spasm by endoscopic injections of botulinum toxin: a prospective study with long-term follow-up. *Gastrointest Endosc.* 2001;54(6):754-759.

38. Miller LS, Pullela SV, Parkman HP, et al. Treatment of chest pain in patients with noncardiac, nonreflux, nonachalasia spastic esophageal motor disorders using botulinum toxin injection into the gastroesophageal junction. *Am J Gastroenterol.* 2002;97(7):1640-1646.

39. Vanuytsel T, Bisschps R, L H, al. e. A sham-controlled study of injection of botulinum toxin in non-achalasia esophageal motility disorder. *Gastroenterology.* 2009;136: p131.

40. Clouse RE, Lustman PJ, Eckert TC, Ferney DM, Griffith LS. Low-dose trazodone for symptomatic patients with esophageal contraction abnormalities. A double-blind, placebo-controlled trial. *Gastroenterology.* 1987;92(4):1027-1036.

41. Cannon RO, 3rd, Quyyumi AA, Mincemoyer R, et al. Imipramine in patients with chest pain despite normal coronary angiograms. *N Engl J Med.* 1994;330(20):1411-1417.

42. Broekaert D, Fischler B, Sifrim D, Janssens J, Tack J. Influence of citalopram, a selective serotonin reuptake inhibitor, on oesophageal hypersensitivity: a double-blind, placebo-controlled study. *Aliment Pharmacol Ther.* 2006;23(3):365-370.

43. Handa M, Mine K, Yamamoto H, et al. Antidepressant treatment of patients with diffuse esophageal spasm: a psychosomatic approach. *J Clin Gastroenterol.* 1999;28(3):228-232.

44. Nair LA, Reynolds JC, Parkman HP, et al. Complications during pneumatic dilation for achalasia or diffuse esophageal spasm. Analysis of risk factors, early clinical characteristics, and outcome. *Dig Dis Sci.* 1993;38(10):1893-1904.

45. Irving JD, Owen WJ, Linsell J, McCullagh M, Keightley A, Anggiansah A. Management of diffuse esophageal spasm with balloon dilatation. *Gastrointest Radiol.* 1992;17(3):189-192.

46. Patti MG, Pellegrini CA, Arcerito M, Tong J, Mulvihill SJ, Way LW. Comparison of medical and minimally invasive surgical therapy for primary esophageal motility disorders. *Arch Surg.* 1995;130(6):609-615.

47. von Renteln D, Fuchs KH, Fockens P. Peroral endoscopicmyotomy for the treatment of achalasia: an international prospective multicenter study. *Gastroenterology.* 2013;145:309-311.

48. Minami H, Isomoto H, Yamaguchi N, et al. Peroral endoscopic myotomy (POEM) for diffuse esophageal spasm. *Endoscopy.* 2014;46 Suppl 1 UCTN:E79-E81.

5

Cricopharyngeal Disorders

Kevin A. Ghassemi, MD and Jeffrey L. Conklin, MD

KEY POINTS

- Cricopharyngeal disorders, while of varying origin, lead to impaired bolus passage from the pharynx into the esophagus.

- Transfer dysphagia refers to swallowing difficulty arising from the oropharyngeal phase of swallowing. The result is impaired bolus movement from the oral cavity and pharynx into the esophagus.

- For most of the cricopharyngeal disorders, videofluoroscopic evaluation is the primary tool used in making the diagnosis. While esophageal manometry is not part of the diagnostic workup, it sometimes provides the first clue that dysphagia is the result of striated neuro-muscular disease.

- Treatment options depend on the underlying disorder. In the cases of a cricopharyngeal bar or cricopharyngeal achalasia, therapeutic choices include dilation, botulinum toxin injection, and cricopharyngeal myotomy. Videofluoroscopic swallow evaluation can help determine behavioral techniques that might improve swallowing function and identify consistencies of oral intake that reduce the risk of aspiration. Therapies for dysphagia due to stroke or following chemoradiotherapy include rehabilitative and compensatory techniques.

TRANSFER DYSPHAGIA

Definition

Transfer dysphagia refers to swallowing difficulty arising from the oropharyngeal phase of swallowing. The result is impaired bolus movement from the oral cavity and pharynx into the esophagus.

Rao SSC, Parkman HP, McCallum RW, eds.
Handbook of Gastrointestinal Motility and Functional Disorders (pp 63-75).

TABLE 5-1	
NEUROLOGIC AND MUSCULAR ETIOLOGIES OF TRANSFER DYSPHAGIA	
NEUROLOGIC	**MUSCULAR**
Stroke	Hereditary disorders
Parkinson's disease	Oculopharyngeal muscular dystrophy
Amyotrophic lateral sclerosis	Myotonic dystrophy
Multiple system atrophy	Duchenne muscular dystrophy
Progressive supranuclear palsy	Limb girdle muscular dystrophy
Multiple sclerosis	Oculopharyngodistal myopathy
Spinocerebellar ataxia	Nemaline rod myopathy
Friedreich ataxia	Mitochondrial myopathies
Ataxia telangiectasia	Acquired disorders
Myasthenia gravis	Polymyositis
Huntington's disease	Dermatomyositis
Wilson disease	Inclusion body myositis
Postpolio syndrome	Thyrotoxic myopathy
Guillain-Barré syndrome	

Pathophysiology

In general, transfer dysphagia results from disrupted neural control of the oropharyngeal musculature, a primary muscle disorder, or anatomical obstruction of the pharynx. The differential is exhaustive, and an extensive list of neuromuscular etiologies is found in Table 5-1. The more common and rare but well-recognized causes of oropharyngeal will be discussed here. Mechanical causes for transfer dysphagia, such as head and neck tumors and cervical osteophytes, will not be discussed. Cricopharyngeal bar and Zenker diverticulum will be discussed specifically later in this chapter.

Neurologic Diseases

Because the central pattern generator for swallowing is located in the medulla, damage to this region from a stroke often results in dysphagia. However, stroke might cause dysphagia by affecting other areas that provide input to the central pattern generator, including motor and somatosensory cortices, insula, basal ganglia, anterior cingulate gyrus, internal capsule, and connecting white matter pathways.[1] Parkinson disease (PD), which affects dopaminergic pathways, interferes with bolus transfer by causing hypokinesia and a reduced rate of spontaneous swallowing movements.[2] Amyotrophic lateral sclerosis (ALS), which affects upper and lower motor neurons, can cause spasticity of the bulbar musculature, atrophy and fasciculation of the tongue, and disruption of the respiratory-swallow coordination.[3] Myasthenia gravis, an autoimmune condition in which circulating antibodies block nicotinic acetylcholine receptors at the postsynaptic

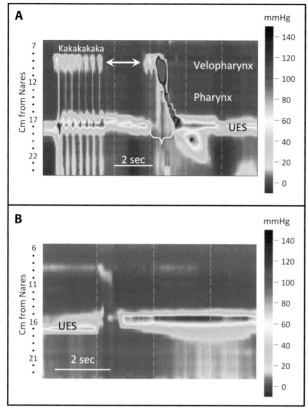

Figure 5-1. (A) High-resolution pressure topography of the pharynx and striated muscle esophagus from a normal individual, and (B) a patient with myasthenia gravis. Distance from the naries is to the left, time is along the x-axis, and pressure is depicted as color, with the association between pressure and color demonstrated by the color bar to the right. In panel A, vocalization by saying ka-ka-ka identifies where velopalatine (VP) closure occurs (white arrow pointing left). The white arrow pointing right indicates the location of VP closure during a swallow. At about the time of VP closure, the upper esophageal sphincter (UES) opens (bracket). Notice that pharyngeal pressure approximates pressure in the proximal esophagus during UES opening. Peristalsis produced by pharyngeal and tongue base contraction is seen as a diagonal band of high pressure (hot color) between the velopharynx and UES. The asterisk indicates peristalsis in the striated muscle esophagus. In the patient with myasthenia gravis (B), there is profound weakness of the pharyngeal musculature and striated muscle esophageal.

neuromuscular junction, leads to weakness and fatigue of facial, jaw, buccal, lingual, and pharyngeal muscles (Figure 5-1).[4]

Muscular Diseases

The common thread among the myopathies, whether acquired or genetic, is that they cause skeletal muscle weakness. Dysphagia can result from difficulty with mastication, bolus transfer, or cricopharyngeal dysfunction. Some of the best-known hereditary myopathies include oculopharyngeal muscular dystrophy (autosomal dominant), myotonic dystrophy (autosomal dominant), and Duchenne muscular dystrophy (X-linked). Primary inflammatory myopathies include polymyositis (PM), dermatomyositis (DM), and inclusion body myositis (IBM). In PM and IBM, cytotoxic T-cells infiltrate muscle fibers and lead to muscle fiber necrosis. Dermatomyositis is a microangiopathy caused by B- and T-lymphocytes that activate the complement cascade, which lyses endomysial capillaries, leading to muscle ischemia. Striated muscle myopathies frequently affect the striated muscle esophagus, and on some occasions, the smooth muscle esophagus as well.[5] Polymyositis and DM have been associated with infections, connective tissue diseases, and a variety of cancers.[6]

Chemotherapy and Radiation Treatment

Treatment of head and neck tumors with chemotherapy and/or radiation can impair bolus clearance from the oral cavity and pharynx. Mechanisms for this include mucositis, impaired pharyngeal sensation, peripheral neuropathy, fibrosis, and reduced muscle strength. The fibrosis in particular can affect pharyngeal constrictor motion, reduce laryngeal motion and compromise airway protection, and reduce upper esophageal sphincter (UES) opening. Radiation injury can occur soon after treatment or years later.[7]

Epidemiology

The prevalence/incidence of transfer dysphagia is high overall, but varies for specific etiologies. Stroke affects nearly 800,000 people a year in the United States. Almost 50% of stroke sufferers complain of dysphagia,[8] and videofluoroscopy identifies aspiration in up to 70%.[9] Over 80% of patients with PD complain of dysphagia.[10] The incidence of ALS is 2 in 100,000, with dysphagia being reported in almost 90% of patients experiencing bulbar involvement.[11] Myasthenia gravis affects 1 in 5000 people, and 40% will develop dysphagia at some point in the course of the disease.[12] Among patients with striated muscle myopathies, dysphagia has been reported in about 40% with a hereditary type and 30% with an acquired inflammatory myopathy.[13]

Diagnosis

Following a stroke, evaluation of dysphagia and assessment of aspiration risk should begin with a clinical swallowing examination performed by a speech pathologist. This will determine whether an instrumental evaluation is needed, identify potential management strategies, and indicate the appropriate diet. Cognitive screening helps to decide on the appropriate instrument for further evaluation. The videofluoroscopic swallow study assesses oral, pharyngeal, and esophageal phases of swallowing. A videoendoscopic assessment does not evaluate the oral phase, but because the apparatus is portable, it is preferred when the patient cannot be transported to radiology or is ventilator dependent.[14]

Videofluoroscopic swallow evaluation is the primary method for evaluating patients with a history suggestive of transfer dysphagia. It is used to help determine behavioral techniques that might improve swallowing function and identify consistencies of oral intake that reduce the risk of aspiration. With progressive neuromuscular disorders, however, one may forgo such diagnostic testing based on the expectation that dysphagia will develop and deglutitive function will continue to deteriorate.

Elevated levels of muscle enzymes, such as creatine kinase, and identification of inflammatory markers support the diagnosis of myopathy. Specific autoantibodies are often present with inflammatory myopathies: anti-Jo1 for PM/DM that is associated with interstitial lung disease, and anti-Mi-1 and 2 for DM.[15] Muscle biopsy is needed to confirm the diagnosis.

While esophageal manometry is not part of the diagnostic workup, it sometimes provides the first clue that dysphagia is the result of striated neuromuscular disease (see Figure 5-1).

Treatment

Therapies for dysphagia due to stroke or following chemoradiotherapy include rehabilitative and compensatory techniques. Rehabilitative exercises, such as the Shaker exercise and tongue-hold maneuver, are designed to improve UES opening and bolus clearance. Compensatory management, such as breath holding and bolus modification, focuses on temporarily eliminating symptoms to facilitate swallowing. Unfortunately, it does not alter deglutitive physiology or provide long-term benefit.[16]

While levodopa is the standard treatment for symptoms related to PD, it does not appear to be an effective treatment for PD-related dysphagia. Compensatory behavioral strategies, such as the chin tuck maneuver and using thickened liquids, might be helpful, and cricopharyngeal myotomy can help patients with cricopharyngeal dysfunction.[17] Pharyngeal muscle fatigue common to myasthenia gravis can be reduced by eating smaller but more frequent meals. Pharmacologic management of dysphagia associated with myasthenia can be difficult, as it is less efficacious for corticobulbar than other symptoms. The treatment of ALS is mainly palliative. Feeding tube placement should be considered early on, as placement once the patient becomes nutritionally compromised might be unsafe and inappropriate.

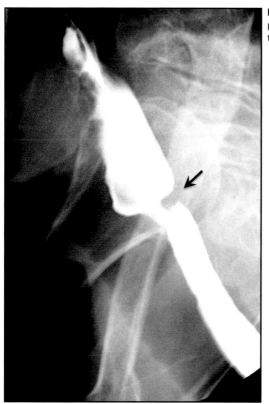

Figure 5-2. Cricopharyngeal bar. The arrow indicates the posterior indentation of the cricopharyngeus muscle on the cervical esophagus.

Dysphagia related to acquired inflammatory myopathies is best treated by immunosuppression. Noninflammatory myopathy-related dysphagia is initially managed with compensatory methods, including positioning and optimizing food textures. However, long-term enteral feeding is needed if the dysphagia progresses.

CRICOPHARYNGEAL ACHALASIA/BAR

Definition

The terms *cricopharyngeal achalasia* and *cricopharyngeal bar* are frequently used interchangeably, but they are distinct entities. A cricopharyngeal bar is a prominence of the cricopharyngeus muscle that is seen on lateral films during videofluoroscopy (Figure 5-2).[18] Cricopharyngeal achalasia may be best described as a condition in which the cricopharyngeus muscle is either incompletely inhibited or more activated during deglutition.[19]

Pathophysiology

The pathogenesis of a cricopharyngeal bar is not impaired UES relaxation, but rather, increased muscle stiffness that reduces UES opening during swallowing. Flow across the UES remains the same as in healthy individuals because there is an increase in intrabolus pressure in the pharynx above the UES.[20] Cricopharyngeal bar is characterized histopathologically as interstitial fibrosis seen in the setting of striated muscle fiber degeneration.[22]

TABLE 5-2 CONDITIONS ASSOCIATED WITH CRICOPHARYNGEAL ACHALASIA	
Central Nervous System Disorders	*Spinal or Neuromuscular Disorders*
Parkinson's disease	Multiple sclerosis
Alzheimer's disease	Myasthenia gravis
Stroke (cortical and lateral medullary)	Amyotrophic lateral sclerosis
Cancer (primary CNS or metastatic)	Trauma
Postpolio syndrome	Cerebral palsy
Multiple system atrophy	Myotonic dystrophy
Ataxia telangiectasia	Inclusion body myositis
CNS: central nervous system.	

The etiology of cricopharyngeal achalasia is unknown due mainly to its rarity, lack of a consensus definition, and difficulty performing an adequate investigation. However, given its association with a number of neuromuscular conditions, it might be due to deterioration of parts of neuronal circuitry in the medullary brainstem that makes up the central pattern generator for swallowing.[19] Due to a lack of a consensus definition, cricopharyngeal achalasia may be considered part of a more general group of disorders called UES dysfunction.

Epidemiology

Cricopharyngeal bars are reported in 5% to 19% of patients undergoing dynamic pharyngeal radiography. Although common, its clinical significance is controversial, since in most cases other etiologies for dysphagia are discovered.[20] It is more frequently seen in older patients. Cricopharyngeal achalasia is rare, but has been associated with several neuromuscular conditions (Table 5-2).

Diagnosis

The most common symptom for both conditions is dysphagia, and for solids more often than liquids. When severe, weight loss and/or dehydration might occur. In the case of cricopharyngeal bars, however, most of the time patients are asymptomatic. Patients should undergo evaluation by endoscopy, radiography, and manometry. Endoscopy is usually not helpful to establish the diagnosis of either condition, but is performed to rule out other potentially serious etiologies of dysphagia.

Fluoroscopy is the mainstay for diagnosing both disorders. A cricopharyngeal bar appears as an indentation seen in the posterior aspect of the esophagus between the C3 and C6 vertebral levels (see Figure 5-2).[18] Cricopharyngeal achalasia is characterized videofluoroscopically as a reduced opening of the pharyngoesophageal segment and bolus retention in the hypopharynx.

While not required to diagnose a cricopharyngeal bar, manometry often demonstrates an elevated intrabolus pressure above the UES that represents an obstruction to flow across the UES (Figure 5-3).[23] With cricopharyngeal achalasia, manometry might detect a decrease in the duration and degree of UES deglutitive relaxation, as well inappropriate contraction of the UES in its resting state.[19]

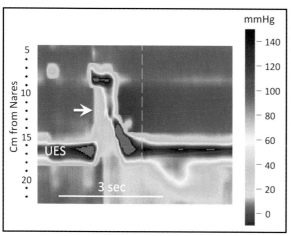

Figure 5-3. High-resolution pressure topography of the pharynx and striated muscle esophagus from a patient with a cricopharyngeal bar. Notice that there is an elevated intrabolus pressure in the pharynx (arrow).

Treatment

Treatment of a cricopharyngeal bar depends on symptoms; if the patient is asymptomatic, no therapy is necessary. The two options that have been reported in the literature are cricopharyngeal dilation and myotomy. Botulinum toxin injection has not been studied in cricopharyngeal bars specifically, but has in UES dysfunction.

There are a few studies reporting outcomes of cricopharyngeal dilation. In one of the largest studies, 31 patients undergoing Savary dilation (dilator size ranging from 45 to 60 Fr) during a period of 5 years were retrospectively evaluated.[24] About half of the patients did not experience recurrent dysphagia for at least 6 months following a single dilation. Only 2 did not respond to multiple dilations. Dilation-related adverse events were not reported. A smaller retrospective study evaluated 6 patients—5 who underwent Savary dilation and 1 who was dilated by a through-the-scope balloon. During a follow-up period of up to 27 months, 3 patients did not have recurrent dysphagia, and the other 3 had recurrent symptoms beginning at 6 to 22 months.[25] There were no postdilation adverse events.

Cricopharyngeal myotomy can normalize the UES opening dimensions and improve pharyngeal contraction. Most studies group cricopharyngeal disorders when evaluating the effect of myotomy. One study of 14 patients looked at manometric, fluoroscopic, and functional outcomes after endoscopic laser cricopharyngeal myotomy specifically for cricopharyngeal bar.[26] The mean functional outcome swallowing scale decreased from a baseline of 2.6 to 0.9, the mean cricopharyngeal cross-sectional opening increased from 32.8 to 123.5 mm^2, and the intrabolus pressure gradient across the cricopharyngeal region decreased by about 50%.

Treatment options for cricopharyngeal achalasia/UES dysfunction include botulinum toxin injection, dilation, and cricopharyngeal myotomy. Dilation performed similarly to that for a cricopharyngeal bar reduces resting UES pressure and improves cricopharyngeal opening.[27] Botulinum toxin injection usually is performed bilaterally, and varying doses have been described in the literature. The duration of benefit is around 3 to 4 months, and treatment can be repeated. While the risk of complications is low, the toxin can spread to laryngeal and pharyngeal muscles, which could exacerbate dysphagia or compromise the airway.[19,28] Cricopharyngeal myotomy is performed in a similar manner as that for a cricopharyngeal bar. It might be predisposed to esophagopharyngeal reflux and aspiration, but most studies suggest that the myotomy does not eliminate resting UES tone completely.[29]

ZENKER DIVERTICULUM

Definition

A Zenker diverticulum is a herniation through an area of weakness between the inferior constrictor and cricopharyngeus muscles. Histopathologically, the diverticulum consists of stratified squamous epithelial mucosa and submucosa and is often surrounded by fibrous tissue. Muscle fibers are absent; thus, it is more correctly considered a pseudodiverticulum.[30]

Pathophysiology

Zenker diverticula result from increased pressure in the hypopharynx leading to herniation through a defect in the muscular wall in a region known as Killian triangle, which is formed by the inferior pharyngeal constrictor and cricopharyngeus muscles. The primary underlying reason for increased hypopharyngeal pressure is stiffening of the cricopharyngeal muscle.[31] This stiffening is caused by cricopharyngeus muscle fiber degeneration and their replacement with fibroadipose tissue.[32] Other potential mechanisms, such as a hypertensive UES or uncoordinated UES contraction, have been proposed as the mechanism for increased hypopharyngeal pressure, but results are conflicting.[33]

Epidemiology

The annual incidence of Zenker diverticulum is estimated to be 2/100,000 people, although the true incidence might be higher, as most are asymptomatic or produce minimal symptoms. The prevalence in the general population is thought to be between 0.01% and 0.11%.[34] It is usually seen in the geriatric population, with a median age of presentation after the age of 60 years. It is found in males more commonly than females by a factor of 3:1, and it appears to occur more frequently in people of European descent, particularly Northern Europe.[35]

Diagnosis

Symptoms of Zenker diverticulum include dysphagia and regurgitation of undigested food, the degree of which depends on the size of the pouch. Regurgitation may occur immediately after eating or several hours later. Halitosis is a common feature. Chronic cough, deglutitive cough, or recurrent pneumonia suggests associated aspiration. Weight loss may be seen, particularly if there is a large pouch.

Complications of Zenker diverticula are rare. Squamous cell carcinoma has been described with an incidence of up to 1.5%,[36] and might be related to chronic stasis. Significant bleeding from ulcerated mucosa in the diverticulum has been reported and can be treated endoscopically.[37] Bezoars and fistula formation have also been reported.[38]

Esophagram is needed to confirm the diagnosis of Zenker diverticulum (Figure 5-4). Dynamic fluoroscopy, however, is preferable to static imaging. Small diverticula might be seen only transiently during deglutition, and therefore can be missed by static films. Aspiration is also better witnessed by dynamic imaging. It is helpful to rotate the patient during the course of the study because the superimposed barium column in the esophageal lumen can make it difficult to identify small diverticula. Endoscopy has a limited role in diagnosing a Zenker diverticulum, as the opening is not always apparent endoscopically.

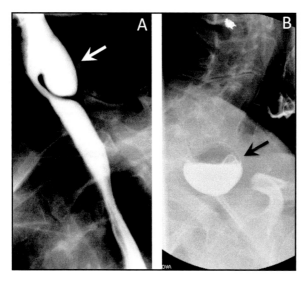

Figure 5-4. Two radiographic views of Zenker diverticula. In panel A, the arrow indicates a Zenker diverticulum during the barium swallow. In panel B, the arrow indicates retention of barium in the diverticulum.

Treatment

Zenker diverticula may be treated surgically or endoscopically (rigid or flexible endoscope). The favored approach depends on several factors, including body mass index, neck length, size of the pouch, and need for additional surgery.[39,40]

Surgical Approach

The surgical approach is through a left cervical incision. The diverticulum is freed, and a cricopharyngeal myotomy is performed. The diverticulum can be resected if particularly large, it can be fixed to the hypopharyngeal wall (diverticulopexy); or it can be invaginated into the esophageal lumen. These techniques lead to symptom resolution in 90% to 95% of patients, with a morbidity rate of 10.5%. The most common complications include recurrent laryngeal nerve injury, leak or perforation, fistula, and recurrent Zenker diverticulum.[41]

Rigid Endoscopic Approach

With the neck in an overextended position, a rigid diverticuloscope is passed transorally and the common septum separating the pouch from the esophageal lumen is identified. Division of the septum is then performed using one of various techniques, including electrocautery (known as Dohlman technique), CO_2 laser, stapling, or harmonic scalpel. The success rate of the rigid endoscopic approach, combining all septal division modalities, is about 90%, and the complication rate (including dental injury and perforation) is 7% to 8%.[41]

Flexible Endoscopic Approach

Unlike with the rigid endoscope, the neck does not need to be extended for the flexible endoscopic technique. A transparent hood can be used to improve visualization, and a nasogastric tube is passed though the esophageal lumen to protect the anterior esophageal wall during myotomy. There are a variety of options for dividing the septum, including needle knife and hook knife, argon plasma coagulation, and mono- and bipolar forceps. Cricopharyngeal myotomy via flexible endoscopy does not require general anesthesia, and can be performed over one or more sessions to reduce the risk of complications. Resolution of symptoms is seen in >90% of patients, the rate of recurrence or persistence is <20%, and the median overall complication rate is 6%.[42] Bleeding is the most common complication (5%), and the risk of perforation is about 4%.

GLOBUS PHARYNGEUS

Definition

Globus is a common and benign sensation that there is something retained in the throat. The sensation is usually located anteriorly between the sternal notch and thyroid cartilage. It is perceived in a variety of ways, including a lump, retained food, or mucus in the throat, but is sometimes described as throat tightness or a choking sensation. It has no association with structural or motor function abnormalities, and cannot be diagnosed in the presence of gastro-esophageal reflux disease (GERD). When first described, it was called globus hystericus because it was thought to be a psychological problem of women. We now know that not to be the case.

Pathophysiology

While the pathogenesis of globus is not known, a number of possibilities have been proposed. They include cricopharyngeal spasm, motor dysfunction of the pharynx or esophagus, gastro-esophageal reflux, esophageal hypersensitivity, or psychological problems. The most widely accepted, but by no means proven, etiology for globus is gastroesophageal reflux. The odds ratio for someone with globus having reflux symptoms (regurgitation and/or heartburn) is reported to be 11.6 (95% CI, 7.1 to 19.1).[43] The few adequately controlled studies exploring the relationship between intraesophageal pH testing and globus are conflicting. They range from showing no difference in acid exposure between globus sufferers and controls[44] to the incidence of globus increasing with the amount of acid exposure.[45] Properly controlled therapeutic trials with H2 antagonists or proton pump inhibitors (PPIs) have not demonstrated their efficacy in the treatment of globus.[46,47] A related hypothesis is that cervical heterotopic gastric mucosa (inlet patch) might trigger globus. In a small, randomized, sham-controlled trial, symptom improvement was better in those who had the inlet patch ablated than in the sham group.[48] However, the majority of globus sufferers do not have an inlet patch. There is some evidence that esophageal hypersensitivity underlies globus. Patients with globus are more sensitive to electrical stimulation or balloon dilation of the esophagus, and they almost universally sense the stimulus at or near the suprasternal notch rather than substernally.[49] The role of psychological factors in the genesis of globus is dubious since no psychiatric illnesses or psychological profiles are specific for globus. Still, there is some evidence that life stress might participate in the genesis of globus and exacerbate the symptom.[50] The notion that globus arises from UES hypertonicity or contraction caused by physiological or psychological stimuli is pretty much disproven. However, in a recent study using high-resolution manometry, the amplitude of respiratory oscillation in UES resting pressure appears to be greater in those with globus than in controls.[51] Whether this plays a role in the genesis of globus is unclear. There is essentially no good evidence supporting the hypothesis that globus arises from pharyngeal or esophageal motor dysfunction. The upshot of all these studies is that we really do not know what causes globus and that the pathogenesis is likely to be multifactorial.

Diagnosis

The diagnosis of globus is made primarily on clinical history. Criteria for the diagnosis of globus have been presented by the Rome III consensus group (Table 5-3).[52] In practice, it is essential to differentiate globus from dysphagia or odynophagia, because these entities portend more

TABLE 5-3
DIAGNOSTIC CRITERIA FOR GLOBUS ACCORDING TO ROME III[52]
In the preceding 6 months, at least 6 weeks of symptoms that need not be consecutive
• Persistent or intermittent, nonpainful sensation of a lump or foreign body in the throat
• Presence of the sensation between meals
• Absence of dysphagia or odynophagia
• Absence of evidence that GERD is causing the symptom
• Absence of histopathology-based esophageal motility disorder

worrisome pathological processes. All patients with globus should have a careful exam of the neck and nasolaryngoscopy to rule out the unlikely presence of a pharyngeal neoplasm. The use of other diagnostic testing with upper gastrointestinal (GI) endoscopy, barium studies, or intraesophageal pH testing is best reserved for patients with other symptoms like dysphagia, odynophagia, hoarseness, or weight loss.

Epidemiology

Globus is exceedingly frequent, being reported in up to 46% of seemingly normal people.[53] It is uncommon below the age of 20 years and peaks in middle age. It is just as prevalent in men as women in the community,[53] but women are more likely to seek medical attention for globus.

Treatment

Our poor understanding of its pathogenesis and our lack of efficacious treatments make the management of globus difficult. The patient should be counseled that globus is a benign condition that might persist for years. Despite a paucity of evidence to support it, a PPI treatment trial may be tried. The patient must understand that PPIs might not be effective and, if so, the drug should be stopped. Studies suggesting that globus might arise from hypersensitive esophageal sensory afferents imply that drugs that modulate sensory pathways might be of some benefit.

REFERENCES

1. Leopold NA, Daniels SK. Supranuclear control of swallowing. *Dysphagia*. 2010;25:250-257.
2. Ertekin C, Tarlaci S, Aydogdu I, et al. Electrophysiological evaluation of pharyngeal phase of swallowing in patients with Parkinson's disease. *Mov Disord*. 2002;17:942-949.
3. Strand EA, Miller RM, Yorkston KM, Hillel AD. Management of oro-pharyngeal dysphagia symptoms in amyotrophic lateral sclerosis. *Dysphagia*. 1996;11:129-139.
4. Juel VC, Massey JM. Myasthenia gravis. *Orphanet J Rare Dis*. 2007;2:1-13.
5. Jaradeh S. Dystrophies and myopathies (including oculopharyngeal). In: Shaker R, Belafsky PC, Postma GN, Easterling C, eds. *Principles of Deglutition*. New York, NY: Springer; 2013:421-430.
6. Buchbinder R, Forbes A, Hall S, Dennett X, Giles G. Incidence of malignant disease in biopsy-proven inflammatory myopathy. A population-based cohort study. *Ann Intern Med*. 2001;134:1087-1095.
7. Lazarus CL. Effects of chemoradiotherapy on voice and swallowing. *Curr Opin Otolaryngol Head Neck Surg*. 2009;17:172-178.
8. Flowers HL, Silver FL, Fang J, Rochon E, Martino R. The incidence, co-occurrence, and predictors of dysphagia, dysarthria, and aphasia after first-ever acute stroke. *J Commun Disord*. 2013;46:238-248.

9. Osawa A, Maeshima S, Matsuda H, Tanahashi N. Functional lesions in dysphagia due to acute stroke: discordance between abnormal findings of bedside swallowing assessment and aspiration on videofluorography. *Neuroradiology.* 2013;55:413-421.

10. Kalf JG, de Swart BJ, Bloem BR, Munneke M. Prevalence of oropharyngeal dysphagia in Parkinson's disease: a meta-analysis. *Parkinsonism Relat Disord.* 2012;18:311-315.

11. Chen A, Garrett CG. Otolaryngologic presentation of amyotrophic lateral sclerosis. *Otolaryngol Head Neck Surg.* 2005;132:500-504.

12. Conti-Fine BM, Milani M, Kaminski HJ. Myasthenia gravis: past, present, and future. *J Clin Invest.* 2006; 116:2843-2854.

13. Willig TN, Paulus J, Lacau Sint Guily J, Beon C, Navarro J. Swallowing problems in neuromuscular disorders. *Arch Phys Med Rehabil.* 1994;75:1175-1181.

14. Gallaugher AR, Wilson CL, Daniels SK. Cerebro-vascular accidents and dysphagia. In: Shaker R, Belafsky PC, Postma GN, Easterling C, eds. *Principles of Deglutition.* New York, NY: Springer; 2013:381-394.

15. Dalakas MC, Hohlfeld R. Polymyositis and dermatomyositis. *Lancet.* 2003;362:971-982.

16. Kahrilas PJ, Logemann JA, Krugler C, Flanagan E. Volitional augmentation of upper esophageal sphincter opening during swallowing. *Am J Physiol.* 1991;260:G450-G456.

17. Born LJ, Harned RH, Rikkers LF, Pfeiffer RF, Quigley EM. Cricopharyngeal dysfunction in Parkinson's disease: role in dysphagia and response to myotomy. *Mov Disord.* 1996;11:53-58.

18. Leonard R, Kendall K, McKenzie S. UES opening and cricopharyngeal bar in nondysphagic elderly and non-elderly adults. *Dysphagia.* 2004;19:182-191.

19. Massey BT. Cricopharyngeal achalasia. In: Shaker R, Belafsky PC, Postma GN, Easterling C, eds. *Principles of Deglutition.* New York, NY: Springer; 2013:515-528.

20. Cook IJ and Kahrilas PJ. AGA technical review on management of oropharyngeal dysphagia. *Gastroenterology.* 1999;116:455-478.

21. Dantas RO, Cook IJ, Dodds WJ, Kern MK, Lang IM, Brasseur JG. Biomechanics of cricopharyngeal bars. *Gastroenterology.* 1990;99:1269-1274.

22. Cruse JP, Edwards DA, Smith JF, Wyllie JH. The pathology of a cricopharyngeal dysphagia. *Histopathology.* 1979;3:223-232.

23. Conklin JL. Evaluation of esophageal motor function with high-resolution manometry. *J Neurogastroenterol Motil.* 2013;19:281-294.

24. Patel B, Mathur AK, Dehom S, Jackson CS. Savary dilation is a safe and effective long-term means of treatment of symptomatic cricopharyngeal bar: a single center experience. *J Clin Gastroenterol.* 2014;48:500-504.

25. Wang AY, Kadkade R, Kahrilas PJ, Hirano I. Effectiveness of dilation for symptomatic cricopharyngeal bar. *Gastrointest Endosc.* 2005;61:148-152.

26. Ozgursoy OB, Salassa JR. Manofluorographic and functional outcomes after endoscopic laser cricopharyngeal myotomy for cricopharyngeal bar. *Otolaryngol Head Neck Surg.* 2010;142:735-740.

27. Hatlebakk JG, Castell JA, Spiegel J, Paoletti V, Katz PO, Castell DO. Dilatation therapy for dysphagia in patients with upper esophageal sphincter dysfunction—manometric and symptomatic response. *Dis Esophagus.* 1998;11:254-259.

28. Terre R, Valles M, Panades A, Mearin F. Long-lasting effect of a single botulinum toxin injection in the treatment of oropharyngeal dysphagia secondary to upper esophageal sphincter dysfunction: a pilot study. *Scand J Gastroenterol.* 2008;43:1296-1303.

29. Shaw DW, Cook IJ, Jamieson GG, Gabb M, Simula ME, Dent J. Influence of surgery on deglutitive upper esophageal sphincter mechanics in Zenker's diverticulum. *Gut.* 1996;38:806-811.

30. Fenoglio-Preiser CM, Noffsinger AE, Stemmermann GN, Lantz PE, Listrom MB, Rilke FO. *Gastrointestinal Pathology: An Atlas and Text.* 2nd ed. Philadelphia, PA: Lippincott Williams and Wilkins; 1999.

31. Cook IJ, Gabb M, Panagopoulos V, et al. Pharyngeal (Zenker's) diverticulum is a disorder of upper esophageal sphincter opening. *Gastroenterology.* 1992;103:1229-1235.

32. Cook IJ, Blumbergs P, Cash K, Jamieson GG, Shearman DJ. Structural abnormalities of the cricopharyngeus muscle in patients with pharyngeal (Zenker's) diverticulum. *J Gastroenterol Hepatol.* 1992;7:556-562.

33. Fulp SR and Castell DO. Manometric aspects of Zenker's diverticulum. *Hepatogastroenterology.* 1992;39:123-126.

34. Watemberg S, Landau O, Avrahami R. Zenker's diverticulum: reappraisal. *Am J Gastroenterol.* 1996;91:1494-1498.

35. Ferreira LE, Simmons DT, Baron TH. Zenker's diverticula: pathophysiology, clinical presentation, and flexible endoscopic management. *Dis Esoph.* 2008;21:1-8.

36. Bradley PJ, Kochaar A, Quarashi MS. Pharyngeal pouch carcinoma: real or imaginary risks. *Ann Otol Rhinol Laryngol.* 1999;108:1027-1032.

37. Flicker MS, Weber HC. Endoscopic hemostasis in a case of bleeding from Zenker's diverticulum. *Gastrointest Endosc.* 2010; 71:869-871.

38. Sen P, Kumar G, Bhattacharyya AK. Pharyngeal pouch: associations and complications. *Eur Arch Otorhinolaryngol.* 2006;263:463-468.

39. Bloom JD, Bleier BS, Mizra N, Chalian AA, Thaler ER. Factors predicting endoscopic exposure in Zenker's diverticulum. *Ann Otol Rhinol Laryngol.* 2010;119:736-741.

40. Mantsopoulos K, Psychogios G, Künzel J, Zenk J, Iro H, Koch M. Evaluation of the different transcervical approaches for Zenker diverticulum. *Otolaryngol Head Neck Surg.* 2012;146:725-729.

41. Yuan Y, Zhao YF, Hu Y, Chen FQ. Surgical treatment of Zenker's diverticulum. *Dig Surg.* 2013;30:207-218.

42. Dzeletovic I, Ekbom D, Baron TH. Flexible endoscopic and surgical management of Zenker's diverticulum. *Expert Rev Gastroenterol Hepatol.* 2012;6:449-465.

43. Hori K, Kim Y, Sakurai J, et al. Non-erosive reflux disease rather than cervical inlet patch involves globus. *J Gastroenterol.* 2010;45:1138-1145.

44. Wilson JA, Heading RC, Maran AG, Pryde A, Piris J, Allan PL. Globus sensation is not due to gastro-oesophageal reflux. *Clin Otolaryngol Allied Sci.* 1987;12:271-275.

45. Locke GR 3rd, Talley NJ, Fett SL, Zinsmeister AR, Melton LJ 3rd. Prevalence and clinical spectrum of gastroesophageal reflux: a population-based study in Olmsted County, Minnesota. *Gastroenterology.* 1997;112:1448-1456.

46. Kibblewhite DJ, Morrison MD. A double-blind controlled study of the efficacy of cimetidine in the treatment of the cervical symptoms of gastroesophageal reflux. *J Otolaryngol.* 1990;19:103-109.

47. Dumper J, Mechor B, Chau J, Allegretto M. Lansoprazole in globus pharyngeus: double-blind, randomized, placebo-controlled trial. *J Otolaryngol Head Neck Surg.* 2008;37:657-663.

48. Bajbouj M, Becker V, Eckel F, et al. Argon plasma coagulation of cervical heterotopic gastric mucosa as an alternative treatment for globus sensations. *Gastroenterology.* 2009;137:440-444.

49. Chen CL, Szczesniak MM, Cook IJ. Evidence for oesophageal visceral hypersensitivity and aberrant symptom referral in patients with globus. *Neurogastroenterol Motil.* 2009;21:1142-e96.

50. Harris MB, Deary IJ, Wilson JA. Life events and difficulties in relation to the onset of globus pharyngis. *J Psychosom Res.* 1996;40:603-615.

51. Kwiatek MA, Mirza F, Kahrilas PJ, Pandolfino JE. Hyperdynamic upper esophageal sphincter pressure: a manometric observation in patients reporting globus sensation. *Am J Gastroenterol.* 2009;104:289-298.

52. Galmiche JP, Clouse RE, Bálint A, et al. Functional esophageal disorders. *Gastroenterology.* 2006;130:1459-1465.

53. Thompson WG, Heaton KW. Heartburn and globus in apparently healthy people. *Can Med Assoc J.* 1982; 126:46-48.

6

Esophageal Hypersensitivity

Jose M. Remes-Troche, MD and Ronnie Fass, MD

KEY POINTS

- Esophageal hypersensitivity is common, affecting a variety of esophageal disorders that appear to demonstrate a "sensory component," such as noncardiac chest pain (NCCP), functional heartburn, nonerosive reflux disease (NERD), and even refractory gastroesophageal reflux disease.

- Several techniques have been used to diagnose esophageal hypersensitivity, including acid perfusion, balloon distension, electrical stimulation, and recently, multimodal stimulation.

- There are no specific treatments for esophageal hypersensitivity. Consequently, treatment of patients with esophageal hypersensitivity as the underlying mechanism primarily include nonorgan-specific pain modulators such as tricyclic antidepressants (TCAs), selective serotonin reuptake inhibitors (SSRIs), serotonin-norepinephrine reuptake inhibitors (SNRIs), trazodone, theophylline, and others.

Currently, esophageal hypersensitivity is considered to be one of the main underlying mechanisms for a variety of esophageal disorders. In addition to functional esophageal disorders, such as functional chest pain (FCP), functional heartburn, and possibly globus sensation and functional dysphagia, esophageal hypersensitivity has been suggested to play an important role in nonerosive reflux disease (NERD), the hypersensitive esophagus, and refractory gastroesophageal reflux disease (GERD).[1] Esophageal hypersensitivity is not considered a distinct disorder, but rather a potential mechanism for the development of various esophageal disorders.

Definition

Visceral hypersensitivity is a phenomenon in which the conscious perception of a visceral stimulus is enhanced independent of the intensity of the stimulus. Esophageal hypersensitivity is

Rao SSC, Parkman HP, McCallum RW, eds.
Handbook of Gastrointestinal Motility and Functional Disorders (pp 77-88).

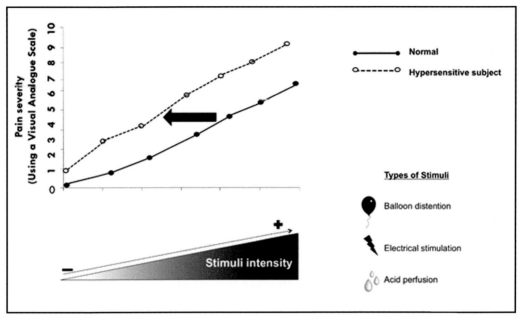

Figure 6-1. The "shift to the left" of esophageal sensation during multimodal stimuli is diagnostic of esophageal hypersensitivity.

defined as the perception of nonpainful esophageal stimuli as being painful and painful esophageal stimuli as being more painful (Figure 6-1). Peripheral and central mechanisms have been proposed to be responsible for visceral hypersensitivity in patients with noncardiac chest pain (NCCP).

Epidemiology

The epidemiology of esophageal hypersensitivity is not completely understood. In patients with FCP, who account for approximately 35% of those with NCCP, 75% to 80% demonstrate esophageal hypersensitivity. The degree of esophageal hypersensitivity in patients with other esophageal disorders is even less clear. It is estimated that about 75% of the patients with functional heartburn, as was defined by the Rome II criteria, demonstrate esophageal hypersensitivity to acid perfusion.[3] In addition, 86% of the NERD patients, as documented by normal endoscopy and abnormal pH test, demonstrate esophageal hypersensitivity to acid perfusion.

HYPERSENSITIVITY IN ESOPHAGEAL DISORDERS

Esophageal hypersensitivity has been described in several esophageal disorders, primarily those that fall under the category of functional esophageal disorders. They include FCP, functional heartburn, functional dysphagia, and those with globus sensation. Recent studies have also documented esophageal hypersensitivity in patients with NERD, refractory GERD, and the hypersensitive esophagus. Richter et al[4] were the first to describe the presence of esophageal hypersensitivity in patients with NCCP undergoing graded balloon distension. In their study, the authors performed esophageal balloon distension to evaluate sensory thresholds for pain in patients with NCCP using a latex balloon that was attached to a manometric catheter and filled with air. In this study, the authors found that a higher percentage of patients reported chest pain compared to healthy controls (60% vs. 20%). Further studies confirmed the important role of esophageal hypersensitivity

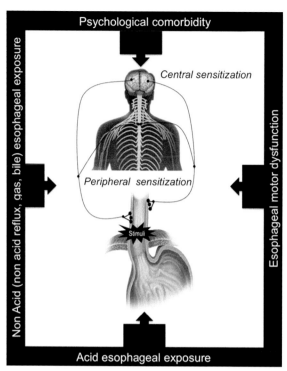

Figure 6-2. A schematic model of esophageal hypersensitivity. Several pathophysiological mechanisms have been described for esophageal hypersensitivity. The figure represents a "black box" where each side of the box represents a mechanism related to esophageal hypersensitivity. Although one side may play a predominant role, all of them are interconnected.

in symptom generation of patients with NCCP, and specifically FCP, using impedance planimetry, electrical stimulation, and acid perfusion.[5,6]

Repeated studies in patients with functional heartburn who use either esophageal balloon distention or electrical stimulation have consistently demonstrated a lower perception threshold for pain compared with that in patients with other presentations of GERD.[7] Furthermore, objective neurophysiological measures of esophageal-evoked potential latency revealed that functional heartburn patients achieve equivalent latency and amplitude responses with reduced afferent input, suggesting heightened esophageal sensitivity. Increased mechanoreceptor sensitivity to balloon distention seems to be a general phenomenon in functional heartburn, while only a subset of patients shows increased chemoreceptor sensitivity to acid.

In general, assessment of esophageal sensitivity in NERD patients has yielded evidence for reduced perception thresholds for painful stimuli (chemical, mechanical, electric, and thermal).[8-10] However, results are difficult to compare due to different sensory testing protocols and stimuli. Furthermore, many studies evaluated so-called "NERD patients" without excluding the functional heartburn group. In addition, it has been demonstrated that the proximal esophagus in NERD patients is more sensitive to acid perfusion as compared to the distal esophagus. This may provide one of the explanations for the strong relationship between proximal esophageal migration of acid reflux and symptom generation in GERD patients.

Pathophysiology

It has been hypothesized that peripheral sensitization of esophageal sensory afferents subsequently leads to heightened responses to physiologic or pathologic stimuli of the esophagus. In addition, central sensitization at the brain level or the dorsal horn of the spinal cord may modulate afferent neural function and thus enhance perception of intraesophageal stimuli (Figure 6-2).[2] What causes peripheral or central sensitization remains to be determined. Studies have shown that

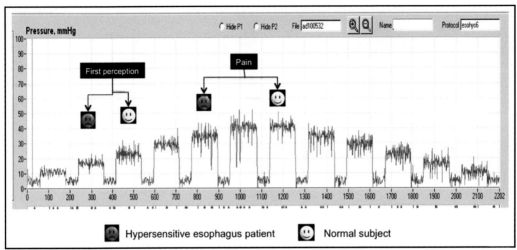

Figure 6-3. Reported sensory perception thresholds for first perception and pain during esophageal barostat distention in a patient with a hypersensitive esophagus (red sad face) and those typically seen in a normal subject (yellow smile face). The pressures that induce perception and pain are lower in patients as compared to controls. (The x-axis shows time in seconds and the y-axis shows pressure in mm Hg.)

acute tissue irritation results in subsequent peripheral and central sensitization, which is manifested as increased background activity of sensory neurons, lowering of nociceptive thresholds, changes in stimulus-response curves, and enlargements of receptive fields. Peripheral sensitization involves a reduction in the esophageal pain threshold and an increase in the transduction processes of primary afferent neurons. Esophageal tissue injury, inflammation, spasm, or repetitive mechanical stimuli can all sensitize peripheral afferent nerves. The presence of esophageal hypersensitivity can be subsequently demonstrated long after the original stimulus is no longer present and the esophageal mucosa has healed (Figure 6-3).

Peripheral Sensitization

The evidence supporting that esophageal hypersensitivity is due to peripheral sensitization is based on studies that demonstrate lower sensory thresholds after multimodal esophageal stimulation in patients with FCP and functional heartburn. In addition, increased expression of receptors that are located in the esophageal mucosa in response to intra-luminal stimuli has been shown to influence nociceptive signaling. Furthermore, the presence of dilated intracellular spaces (DIS) on esophageal mucosal biopsies of patients with gastroesophageal disease are also suggestive of peripheral mechanisms of enhanced acid sensitivity.[11]

Among all esophageal receptors, the TRPV1 seems a particularly attractive candidate for the receptor that mediates the sensation of heartburn during acid perfusion. The TRPV1 receptor is a cation channel that is expressed by sensory afferents and is activated by heat, acid, or ethanol, triggering a burning sensation. Furthermore, studies have shown that esophageal instillation of the TRPV1 receptor agonist capsaicin induces retrosternal and epigastric burning in a dose-dependent fashion. These findings suggest that increased TRPV1 expression has a potential (albeit peripheral) role in mediating heartburn in patients with GERD. Studies also have shown that adenosine can induce visceral hyperalgesia in healthy humans and is a possible neuromediator in the pathogenesis of FCP.

Central Sensitization

Recent developments in neuroimaging have led to the exploration of central mechanisms of chest pain in patients. By monitoring blood flow as a marker of cortical activity during esophageal balloon distention, investigators identified paralimbic and limbic structures such as the insular, anterior cingulate, and prefrontal cortices as visceral pain centers. Electrical stimulation of the proximal and distal esophagus, before and after acid exposure in 7 patients with FCP and 19 healthy volunteers, showed that the FCP group had lower esophageal pain thresholds, which decreased further and persisted for a longer duration when exposed to acid instillation. This suggests a central enhancement of sensory input. Also, cortical-evoked potential studies demonstrated that some patients with chest pain and visceral hypersensitivity have sensitized esophageal afferents, while others are hypervigilant to esophageal sensations, further suggesting a central perturbation of pain regulation.

Central Factors That Modulate Esophageal Hypersensitivity

The degree of central sensitization can be modulated by factors other than acid exposure. For example, psychological stress may play an important role in symptom generation of GERD patients. In a Gallup Poll, 64% of individuals with heartburn reported that stress increased their symptoms.

A substantial subset of patients with GERD demonstrates psychological disturbances such as depression, anxiety, and somatization, which may interact with environmental stress to produce increased perceptions of reflux symptoms, even in the absence of a concomitant increase in esophageal acid exposure. Major life stressors have been shown in a longitudinal study to predict symptom exacerbations in patients with heartburn. Interventions aimed at reducing stress in patients with GERD (eg, hypnosis, progressive muscle relaxation technique) have been shown to result in subjective improvement in reflux symptom ratings and significant reduction in total esophageal acid exposure.[12]

Acute stress has been shown to enhance perceptual responses to intraesophageal acid stimuli, even in the absence of a detectable increase in peripheral stress markers. Increased perceptual responses to intraluminal acid are associated with increased emotional responses to the stressor but are not related to the presence or absence of esophageal mucosal injury. Similarly, sleep deprivation has also been shown to enhance perception of intraesophageal acid. The mechanism by which sleep deprivation leads to enhanced perception of esophageal stimuli is unknown. It is possible that sleep deprivation has a profound effect on patients' mood or attention. Alternatively, esophageal mucosal inflammation predisposes GERD patients to accentuated nociceptive response after sleep deprivation. It is possible that stressful events, such as sleep deprivation, anxiety, and others, may lead to alteration of the descending inhibitory or excitatory pathways that modulate spinal transmission of nociceptive signals.

Diagnosis

Several diagnostic techniques have been developed to assess esophageal hypersensitivity. Most of them assess either chemosensitivity to acid or mechanosensitivity to balloon distension. Other techniques that have been used include electrical and thermal stimulation. Recently, multimodal probes were developed to provide in one session thermal, electric, chemical, and mechanical stimuli.

Acid Perfusion Test

The acid perfusion test was originally devised to distinguish between chest pain of cardiac and esophageal origin. However, since the initial description, many modifications have been made to the original Bernstein test. Although the basic principle of the test remained similar, many investigators have tried different acid perfusion rates, concentrations, and durations in the hope of increasing the sensitivity of the test. Furthermore, some have even suggested the addition of bile salts to the acid solution. Others required that, for a result to be positive, the acid-induced symptoms should quickly disappear with the reinfusion of saline or bicarbonate.

Many attempts were made to change the test from a qualitative to a quantitative tool. Time to onset of symptoms during acid perfusion was used to compare the extent of chemosensitivity to acid between GERD and Barrett's esophagus patients. In one study, the authors placed a manometry catheter 10 cm above the upper border of the lower esophageal sphincter (LES) to ensure sufficient exposure of the esophageal mucosa to acid. Saline was infused initially for 2 minutes, and then without the patient's knowledge, 0.1 HCl acid was infused for 10 min at a rate of 10 mL/min. Patients were instructed to report whenever their typical symptoms were reproduced. Esophageal chemosensitivity was assessed by both the duration until typical symptom perception was induced (expressed in seconds) and the total sensory intensity rating reported by the subject at the end of the acid perfusion by using a verbal descriptor scale. The scale consisted of a 20-cm vertical bar flanked by descriptors of increasing intensity (no sensation, faint, very weak, weak, very mild, mild moderate, barely strong, slightly intense, strong, intense, very intense, and extremely intense). Placement of words along each scale was determined from their relative log intensity rating in a normative study. The validity of these scales for assessing the perceived intensity of visceral sensations has been established.

An acid perfusion test intensity score (cm × s) was then calculated as follows:

$$I \times T / 100$$

where I is the total intensity rating at the end of the acid perfusion and T is the duration of reporting of typical symptom perception during the test. For convenience, the score was divided by 100.

Electrical Stimulation

Electrical stimulation of the esophagus has been used by very few research groups to study esophageal sensitivity and cortical responses to different intensities of intraesophageal stimuli. The technique has yet to be standardized, and published protocols are difficult to compare. The technique is currently used only as a research tool.

Electrical stimulation of the esophageal mucosa is performed using a stainless steel electrode attached to a standard manometric catheter assembly. Electrical stimuli are applied repeatedly in a series of 24 stimuli (duration 200 µs at 0.2 Hz). A reference electrode is placed on the abdominal wall. Electrical stimulation of the upper and lower esophagus can be achieved with 2 pairs of electrodes located at 5 and 20 cm proximal to the tip of the catheter. The ascending stimulus paradigm includes stimuli that are delivered at a frequency of 0.2 Hz at intensities between 0 and 100 mA. Severity and qualitative perceptual responses are usually assessed by a verbal descriptor. The sensory threshold is the intensity (measure in mA) at which the participant reports faint sensation, and the pain threshold is the intensity at which the participant reports an intense sensation. Different stimulus paradigms have been used in various studies.

Balloon Distention

Balloon distention has been used primarily for research purposes to determine perception thresholds for pain (Figure 6-4).[13] This modality has been used extensively in studies of various functional bowel disorders, most notably irritable bowel syndrome (IBS), functional dyspepsia, and NCCP.

The introduction of the electronic barostat, a computer-driven, volume-displacement device, has helped to ensure proper location of the balloon, regardless of the inflation paradigm that was used. The basic principle of the barostat is to maintain a constant pressure within the balloon/bag in the lumen despite muscular contractions and relaxations. To maintain a constant pressure, the barostat aspirates air with contractions and injects air with relaxations. Presently, many prefer the use of a polyethylene bag to that of a latex balloon. Bags are infinitely compliant and show no increase in intrabag pressure until about 90% of the maximum bag volume has been achieved. In contrast, latex balloons resist inflation and thus show a rapid increase in intraballoon pressure with a small volume of distention. When the pressure increases above the elastance threshold, the balloon becomes plastic and accommodates large volumes of air with very little change in

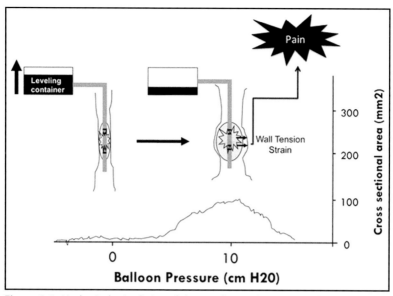

Figure 6-4. Mechanical stimulation of the esophagus that includes dynamic balloon distension using impedance planimetry equipment. The esophageal probe is a 6-mm diameter plastic tube that contains 4 ring electrodes (2 outer and 2 inner) and 5 side holes. A thin latex balloon, 5 cm long, is tied to the probe, enclosing the 4 ring electrodes. Balloon pressure is increased by using intermittent phasic distentions at increments of 6 mm Hg. This is done by raising the leveling container and infusing 0.018% NaCl (at 37°C) into the balloon. Each inflation is maintained for 2 minutes, after which the balloon is deflated by lowering the leveling container. One minute after each inflation, the subjects are asked to grade their sensations using a Likert-type scale. (0 = no sensation; 1 = sensation of fullness or distension; 2 = moderate discomfort; and 3 = pain.)

pressure. For tubular organs in the GI tract, such as the esophagus, experts recommend the use of a cylindrical (rather than a spherical) bag with a fixed length.

Various distention protocols have been used in different studies. Like any other technique that assesses esophageal sensation, balloon distention has yet to be standardized. Slow-ramp distention is an ascending method that involves slow (the rate varies from one study to another) increase in volume or pressure of the balloon, usually until the desired perceptual response has been reported by the subject. In contrast, phasic distentions are rapid inflations of the balloon that can be delivered in a random sequence of a double-random staircase. The latter includes 2 series of distention stimuli (staircases), and the computer alternates between the 2 staircases on a random basis. With the tracking method, the barostat is programmed to deliver a series of intermittent phasic stimuli separated by an interpulse rest period within an interactive stimulus tracking procedure. If the subject indicates a sensation below the tracked intensity, then the following stimulus will increase in pressure. If the subject reports the desired sensation, then the following pressure step is randomized to stay the same or decrease. The random element is placed to mask the relationship between ratings and subsequent stimulus change and, therefore, decrease potential scaling bias.

Commonly, qualitative and quantitative perceptual responses are evaluated during balloon distention studies. Qualitative perceptual responses include symptom reports in response to balloon distention, such as chest pain, heartburn, bloating, and fullness, among others.

Heartburn is a common sensation that occurs during balloon distention and may mimic the patient's typical heartburn symptom. Quantitative perceptual responses are commonly obtained during slow-ramp distention and include the minimal distention volume or pressure at which the individual first reports moderate sensation (innocuous sensation), discomfort, and pain (aversive sensation). Discomfort threshold is commonly defined as the first unpleasant esophageal sensation, and the pain threshold is defined as the first sensation of pain.

An increased rate of balloon distention results in reported perception at lower volumes or pressures. Longer durations of balloon distention are more likely to elicit sensation than are shorter durations. Elderly subjects demonstrate diminished visceral pain perception, and female patients seem to have lower perception thresholds for pain compared with male patients. The proximal esophagus has been suggested to be more sensitive to chemical and mechanical stimuli than is the distal esophagus. In addition, reduced sensitivity to intraluminal stimuli has been demonstrated in specific patient populations, such as those with Barrett's mucosa or esophageal stricture.

Multimodal Stimulation Device

Recently, probes that combine a battery of different stimuli have been introduced. These probes, multimodal devices, may include any combination of stimuli: chemical (acid), mechanical (balloon), electrical, and thermal (cold and hot). One such device includes a probe with a distal bag, electrodes for electrical stimuli that are mounted on the outer surface of the bag, and a pump system that recirculates water through 2 channels in the probe that end inside the bag (cool or hot water).[14] While this diagnostic technique has been validated, it is unclear whether sequential stimulations, although of different types, may affect subjects' pain perception. It is possible that one type of stimulus may sensitize the esophageal sensory afferents to the second type of stimulus. Furthermore, it is still unknown how these highly elaborated stimulation models represent clinical scenarios that have been studied.

Treatment

Esophageal hypersensitivity has been primarily treated with different pain modulators (Figure 6-5). The most commonly used pain modulators are antidepressants: tricyclic antidepressants (TCAs), selective serotonin reuptake inhibitors (SSRIs), serotonin-norepinephrine reuptake inhibitors (SSNRIs), and trazodone. These drugs can modulate central hyperalgesia and, to some degree, peripheral hyperalgesia.[15]

Tricyclic Antidepressants

Tricyclic antidepressants have been demonstrated to be efficacious in controlling esophageal pain in both healthy subjects and patients with esophageal disorders.[16] Thus far, this class of drugs has been successfully used in patients with FCP, those with globus sensation, and those with NCCP and an esophageal motor disorder. The effect on the latter group is presumed to be mediated by inhibition of calcium channels in addition to the visceral analgesic effect, resulting also in a muscle relaxant-like effect.

For pain modulation, TCAs are commonly given in low doses. The range of initial therapeutic dose reported from different trials was 10 to 50 mg/day, and the range of a maximal therapeutic dose was 25 to 150 mg/day. Based on our experience, it is recommended that the TCA dose be slowly titrated to a maximum of 30 to 50 mg/day. The incremental increase in dosing should be based on symptom improvement and development of side effects. In general, patients are initiated on 10 mg once a day, given at bedtime. Because of the anticholinergic and sedative side effects of TCAs, they are commonly administered at bedtime.

Side effects from TCA treatment develop in about 30% to 100% of patients. These side effects are related to the TCA's main receptor activity. Tertiary amines (such as amitriptyline and imipramine) are commonly associated with side effects, as compared with secondary amines (such as nortriptyline and desipramine), due to their greater receptor affinity. Side effects of TCAs include urinary retention, dry mouth, drowsiness, constipation, blurred vision, orthostatic hypotension, confusion and mental status change in the elderly, sexual dysfunction, and tachycardia. Tricyclic antidepressants should be prescribed with caution in patients with cardiovascular disease. The

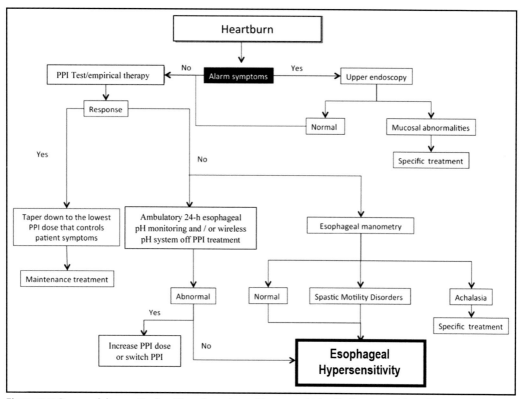

Figure 6-5. Proposed diagnostic algorithm of esophageal hypersensitivity. Notice the position of pain modulators.

antihistaminic property of the TCAs may result in sedation and weight gain. If side effects emerge, the dose could be decreased, or the patient can be switched to a different TCA because of their different receptor activity.[17] Of all TCAs, desipramine has the lowest anticholinergic and sedative adverse effects. Thus, this drug may be considered an alternative to amitriptyline or imipramine for patients who develop side effects.

Selective Serotonin Reuptake Inhibitors

SSRIs have demonstrated clinical efficacy in patients with a variety of esophageal disorders such as FCP, esophageal hypersensitivity, NERD, and heartburn unresponsive to proton pump inhibitor (PPI) treatment.

During a single-blinded, placebo-controlled trial, 30 subjects with NCCP were randomized to receive sertraline or placebo for 8 weeks (started at 50 mg and adjusted to a maximum of 200 mg). Patients with major depression and panic disorder were excluded. By using intention-to-treat analysis, the investigators found that sertraline induced a significant reduction in pain scores as compared with placebo. Side effects occurred in 27% of patients and included delayed ejaculation, decreased libido, and restlessness.[18]

Paroxetine has also been evaluated for NCCP. In a double-blind, placebo-controlled trial, subjects were randomized to paroxetine vs. placebo (27 and 23 patients, respectively) for 8 weeks. Paroxetine-treated patients showed a greater improvement on a physician-rated scale, but not on self-rated pain scores. In another study, 69 adults with NCCP were randomly assigned to treatment with cognitive behavioral therapy, paroxetine, or placebo. In this study, paroxetine was not found to be more effective than placebo.

A recent study demonstrated that citalopram (20 mg, given intravenously in a single dose) reduced chemical and mechanical esophageal hypersensitivity without altering esophageal motility.

Another study demonstrated the efficacy of fluoxetine in improving symptoms of patients with heartburn and normal endoscopy who failed once-daily PPI. The authors found that the medication was mostly effective for patients with a normal esophageal pH test rather than those with an abnormal test. This double-blind, placebo-controlled randomized trial demonstrated the value of an SSRI (fluoxetine) in improving symptoms of a very challenging group of patients (NERD unresponsive to a PPI daily). It is likely that these patients suffered from functional heartburn and thus were not truly GERD patients. Regardless, this study is an important addition to the literature of refractory GERD and functional esophageal disorders. It demonstrated the value of fluoxetine, an SSRI, as a pain modulator in patients with heartburn who failed PPI treatment and, specifically, those with functional heartburn. However, more studies are needed to substantiate the authors' findings.

The recommended initial and maximal doses of SSRIs are as follows: (1) fluoxetine, 10 to 20 mg/day and 20 to 80 mg/day, respectively; (2) fluoxetine, 25 to 50 mg/day and 50 to 300 mg/day, respectively; (3) paroxetine, 10 to 20 mg/day and 20 to 60 mg/day, respectively; and (4) sertraline, 25 to 50 mg/day and 50 to 200 mg/day, respectively. SSRIs have only 5-HT activity and, as a result, are better tolerated than TCAs. Their main side effects are nausea, gastric discomfort, vomiting, anorexia, and diarrhea. Decreased libido, delayed orgasm, hyperhidrosis, somnolence or insomnia, drowsiness, fatigue, and weight gain have also been reported.

Overall, the studies using SSRIs as pain modulators in esophageal disorders are scarce, relatively small, and use different evaluative tools. Thus, they are difficult to compare.

Trazodone

Trazodone has been evaluated for the treatment of NCCP. As with TCAs, the visceral analgesic effect of the drug has been evaluated in these patients. Trazodone (100 to 500 mg, 4 times a day, orally) for 6 weeks significantly improved the symptoms of patients with NCCP and esophageal dysmotility as compared with placebo. However, esophageal motility abnormalities remained unchanged. A small, open-label study reported symptom control and improved esophageal motility in patients with NCCP and distal esophageal spasm (DES) following treatment with both trazodone and clomipramine.

Serotonin-Norepinephrine Reuptake Inhibitors

Of all SNRIs, only venlafaxine has been studied in an esophageal disorder. In a randomized, double-blind, placebo-controlled, crossover trial, venlafaxine (75 mg/day) significantly improved symptoms in patients with FCP (48% therapeutic gain) as compared with placebo. In a systematic review, it was demonstrated that venlafaxine is the most efficacious antidepressant for reducing esophageal pain and improving global health assessment.

The side effects of SNRIs resemble those of SSRIs. In the case of venlafaxine, agitation, diarrhea, increased liver enzymes, hypertension, and hyponatremia may develop.

Adenosine Antagonists

Adenosine has been identified as a mediator of visceral pain, including esophageal pain. In healthy volunteers, adenosine induced angina-like pain shortly after infusion. It has been demonstrated that adenosine can induce esophageal hypersensitivity and decrease esophageal distensibility in humans.

Theophylline, a xanthine derivative, has been shown to inhibit adenosine-induced angina-like chest pain and adenosine-induced pain in other regions of the body. A study using an esophageal balloon distention protocol and impedance planimetry demonstrated that intravenous theophylline increased thresholds for sensation and pain in 755 of subjects with FCP. Similar results were documented in patients with functional chest pain who received oral theophylline for a period of 3 months. In another study, it was shown that oral doses of theophylline, 200 mg twice daily, were more effective than placebo for preventing chest pain in 19 subjects with FCP.[19] The use of theophylline to treat patients with NCCP should be weighed against potential toxicity and side effects of the drug.

Other Pain Modulators

Ondansetron, a 5-HT3 antagonist that is used as an antiemetic, has been shown to increase esophageal perception thresholds for pain in patients with NCCP.[20]

The selective 5-HT4 receptor agonist tegaserod has been demonstrated to reduce both chemo-receptor sensitivity to acid and mechanoreceptor sensitivity to balloon distention in patients with functional heartburn.

Octreotide, a synthetic analog of somatostatin, has been shown to increase rectal and sigmoid perception thresholds for pain in subjects with IBS and healthy subjects. It has been postulated that the effect of octreotide is mediated through the activation of somastotatin receptors at the spinal cord and/or the supraspinal level. Octreotide, administered at 100 mg subcutaneously, was found to significantly increase perception thresholds for pain as compared with placebo in healthy subjects undergoing intraesophageal balloon distention. Unfortunately, due to cost and the lack of an oral formulation, octreotide is rarely utilized for NCCP in clinical practice.

Treatment for globus sensation with gabapentin (300 mg 3 times daily) was assessed in patients who failed to respond to standard-dose PPI. A significant improvement was observed in 66% of the subjects.

Pregabalin is a second-generation $\alpha_2\delta$ ligand that is approved for the treatment of neuropathic pain and epilepsy. In a placebo-controlled, double-blind, randomized crossover trial, pregabalin was able to attenuate the development of acid-induced esophageal hypersensitivity in 15 healthy volunteers. The authors used the following dosing schedule: 75 mg twice daily for 3 days, 150 mg twice daily for 1 day, and 150 mg on the morning of the esophageal pain assessment.

Nonmedical Therapy

A number of psychological techniques have been used in the treatment of NCCP. Cognitive behavioral therapy (CBT) is based on the model of attribution approach. The goal of treatment is to correct the misattributions regarding physical symptoms (eg, chest pain) as being harmful. Patients must adopt the belief that psychological factors cause chest pain and attribute the chest pain to panic attacks, anxiety, and/or other psychological factors. Cognitive behavioral therapy has been reported to be effective in the treatment of NCCP.

Hypnotherapy has been recently evaluated in the treatment of NCCP patients. An 80% improvement in symptoms, with a significant reduction in pain intensity, has been demonstrated among patients who were receiving 12 sessions of hypnotherapy, compared to only 23% symptom improvement in the control group. Hypnotherapy also resulted in a significantly greater improvement in overall well-being in addition to a reduction in medication usage. The study concluded that hypnotherapy appears to have a role in treating NCCP and that further studies are needed.

REFERENCES

1. Dickman R, Maradey-Romero C, Fass R. The role of pain modulators in esophageal disorders: no pain no gain. *Neurogastroenterol Motil.* 2014;26(5):603-610.
2. Fass R, Naliboff B, Higa L, et al. Differential effect of long-term esophageal acid exposure on mechano-sensitivity and chemosensitivity in humans. *Gastroenterology.* 1998;115(6):1363-1373.
3. Shapiro M, Green C, Bautista JM, et al. Functional heartburn patients demonstrate traits of functional bowel disorder but lack a uniform increase of chemoreceptor sensitivity to acid. *Am J Gastroenterol.* 2006;101(5):1084-1091.
4. Richter JE, Barish CF, Castell DO. Abnormal sensory perception in patients with esophageal chest pain. *Gastroenterology.* 1986;91(4):845-852.

5. Rao SS, Hayek B, Summers RW. Functional chest pain of esophageal origin: hyperalgesia or motor dysfunction. *Am J Gastroenterol.* 2001;96(9):2584-2589.

6. Sarkar S, Aziz Q, Woolf CJ, Hobson AR, Thompson DG. Contribution of central sensitisation to the development of non-cardiac chest pain. *Lancet.* 2000;356(9236):1154-1159.

7. Fass R, Tougas G. Functional heartburn: the stimulus, the pain, and the brain. *Gut.* 2002;51(6):885-892.

8. Fass R, Naliboff BD, Fass SS, et al. The effect of auditory stress on perception of intraesophageal acid in patients with gastroesophageal reflux disease. *Gastroenterology.* 2008;134(3):696-705.

9. Hobson AR, Furlong PL, Aziz Q. Oesophageal afferent pathway sensitivity in non-erosive reflux disease. *Neurogastroenterol Motil.* 2008;20(8):877-883.

10. Rodriguez-Stanley S, Robinson M, Earnest DL, Greenwood-Van Meerveld B, Miner PB, Jr. Esophageal hypersensitivity may be a major cause of heartburn. *Am J Gastroenterol.* 1999;94(3):628-631.

11. Remes-Troche JM, Chahal P, Mudipalli R, Rao SSC. Adenosine modulates oesophageal sensorimotor function in humans. *Gut.* 2009;58(8):1049-1055.

12. McDonald-Haile J, Bradley LA, Bailey MA, Schan CA, Richter JE. Relaxation training reduces symptom reports and acid exposure in patients with gastroesophageal reflux disease. *Gastroenterology.* 1994;107(1):61-69.

13. Peghini PL, Katz PO, Castell DO. Imipramine decreases oesophageal pain perception in human male volunteers. *Gut.* 1998;42(6):807-813.

14. Drewes AM, Schipper KP, Dimcevski G, et al. Multimodal assessment of pain in the esophagus: a new experimental model. *Am J Physiol Gastrointest Liver Physiol.* 2002;283(1):G95-103.

15. Broekaert D, Fischler B, Sifrim D, Janssens J, Tack J. Influence of citalopram, a selective serotonin reuptake inhibitor, on oesophageal hypersensitivity: a double-blind, placebo-controlled study. *Aliment Pharmacol Ther.* 2006;23(3):365-370.

16. Prakash C, Clouse RE. Long-term outcome from tricyclic antidepressant treatment of functional chest pain. *Dig Dis Sci.* 1999;44(12):2373-2379.

17. Ostovaneh MR, Saeidi B, Hajifathalian K, et al. Comparing omeprazole with fluoxetine for treatment of patients with heartburn and normal endoscopy who failed once daily proton pump inhibitors: double-blind placebo-controlled trial. *Neurogastroenterol Motil.* 2014;26(5):670-678.

18. Varia I, Logue E, O'Connor C, et al. Randomized trial of sertraline in patients with unexplained chest pain of noncardiac origin. *Am Heart J.* 2000;140(3):367-372.

19. Rao SS, Mudipalli RS, Remes-Troche JM, Utech CL, Zimmerman B. Theophylline improves esophageal chest pain: a randomized, placebo-controlled study. *Am J Gastroenterol.* 2007;102(5):930-938.

20. Tack J, Sarnelli G. Serotonergic modulation of visceral sensation: upper gastrointestinal tract. *Gut.* 2002;51(Suppl 1):i77-80.

Section II

Gastric Disorders

Symptoms of Gastric Dysmotility
Nausea, Vomiting, Abdominal Pain, Postprandial Fullness, and Early Satiety

William L. Hasler, MD

KEY POINTS

- Nausea, vomiting, abdominal pain, postprandial fullness, and early satiety are symptoms commonly reported by patients with a diverse range of conditions and etiologies.

- The pathogenesis of symptoms in gastric functional and motor disorders include contributions from gastric sensorimotor factors, CNS dysfunction, psychological dysfunction, inflammatory mediators, and genetic factors.

- Evaluation of patients with unexplained upper GI symptoms includes a careful history and physical examination with directed laboratory, structural, and GI functional testing to define the cause of symptoms and potentially direct clinical decisions.

- Several scoring instruments have been devised to quantify symptoms and characterize symptom clusters in gastroparesis and functional dyspepsia. The FDA has released industry guidance recommendations for appropriate questionnaire development that will be considered in the generation of newer surveys for inclusion in the design of clinical trials of novel therapies.

INTRODUCTION

Definition of Symptoms

Many symptoms are reported by patients with suspected upper gut motility or functional disorders. *Nausea* is an urge to vomit and is perceived in the throat or epigastrium. *Vomiting*

Rao SSC, Parkman HP, McCallum RW, eds.
Handbook of Gastrointestinal Motility and Functional Disorders (pp 91-105).

(emesis) is the forceful oral ejection of gut contents and may occur with or without nausea. *Retching* also is forceful but without oral content expulsion. *Abdominal pain* is the feeling experienced by something that hurts the body region below the chest. *Postprandial fullness* is the perception of being satisfied after eating. Early satiety is the sense of feeling full before completing a normal-sized meal. *Dyspepsia* is used to characterize the sensation of difficult digestion, and includes pain, fullness, early satiety, and sometimes nausea and vomiting.[1]

Differential Diagnosis of Clinical Disorders With These Symptoms

Nausea and Vomiting

Nausea and vomiting are caused by many conditions affecting the abdomen, central nervous system (CNS), and other body functions (Table 7-1). Medications, including cancer chemotherapies, usually elicit nausea and vomiting soon after initiating therapy. Infections are prominent triggers for acute emesis. Viruses (norovirus, rotavirus, adenoviruses) and bacteria (*Staphylococcus aureus*, *Bacillus cereus*) cause acute enteritis. Luminal mechanical processes (gastric or small bowel obstruction, superior mesenteric artery syndrome, gastric volvulus, antral webs, Crohn's disease, abdominal irradiation) and intraperitoneal disorders (biliary colic, cholecystitis, pancreatitis, appendicitis, hepatitis) are prevalent causes of nausea and vomiting. Nausea and vomiting are noted during 50% to 70% of pregnancies. Hyperemesis gravidarum, presenting as relentless vomiting with fluid and electrolyte abnormalities, complicates < 5% of pregnancies. Other metabolic causes include uremia, diabetic ketoacidosis, hyper- and hypoparathyroidism, hyperthyroidism, and Addison disease. Postoperative nausea and vomiting complicate 17% to 37% of operations. Nausea and vomiting are promoted by CNS processes (malignancy, infarction, hemorrhage, infection), anxiety and depression, motion sickness, labyrinthine disorders, and dysautonomias. Rare causes include fatty liver of pregnancy, cardiac disease (myocardial infarction, heart failure), acute graft versus host disease, excess ethanol intake, acute intermittent porphyria, and disorders of fatty acid oxidation.

Gut motor disorders commonly cause nausea or emesis. Gastroparesis presents with symptoms of gastric retention with documented delayed gastric emptying in the absence of obstruction. Gastroparesis most often is idiopathic but also occurs with diabetes, after gastric surgeries (fundoplication, bariatric surgery, gastric or esophageal resection), connective tissue disease, amyloidosis, neurologic conditions (Parkinson disease, muscular dystrophy), ischemia, and cancer (paraneoplastic gastroparesis). Chronic intestinal pseudoobstruction presents with similar symptoms but often with more severe nutritional consequences and bowel habit disturbances. Etiologies of pseudoobstruction include connective tissue disorders, infiltrative disease, neurologic conditions, paraneoplastic manifestations, and idiopathic disease.

Functional gastroduodenal disorders causing nausea and vomiting have been defined by expert panels. The Rome III criteria for cyclic vomiting syndrome are (1) stereotypical episodes of vomiting regarding onset (acute) and duration (< 1 week); (2) >3 episodes in the past year; and (3) absent nausea and vomiting between episodes.[2] Supportive criteria include a personal or family history of migraine headaches. Cannabinoid hyperemesis syndrome is a subset of cyclic vomiting that presents after use of large amounts of marijuana (3 to 5 times daily) over 2 to 19 years.[3] The Rome III definition of chronic idiopathic nausea includes (1) bothersome nausea occurring several times weekly; (2) not often associated with vomiting; and (3) with absent endoscopic abnormalities or metabolic disease to explain nausea.[2] The Rome III definition of functional vomiting includes (1) average >1 weekly vomiting episodes and (2) absent eating disorder, rumination, psychiatric disease, self-induced vomiting, chronic cannabinoid use, CNS abnormalities, and metabolic diseases to explain recurrent vomiting.[2] Criteria for the 3 disorders are fulfilled for the last 3 months, with symptom onset >6 months before diagnosis.

TABLE 7-1	
DIFFERENTIAL DIAGNOSIS OF NAUSEA AND VOMITING	

ETIOLOGY	*Endocrine/Metabolic Disease*
	Nausea and vomiting of pregnancy/ hyperemesis gravidarum
Medications	Thyroid and parathyroid disease
Cancer chemotherapy	Uremia
Nonsteroidal anti-inflammatory agents/aspirin	Ketoacidosis
Opiates	Addison disease
Antibiotics	
Anti-Parkinsonian/restless legs syndrome drugs	*Postoperative Nausea and Vomiting*
Anticonvulsants	*CNS and Peripheral Neural Conditions*
Cardiac antiarrhythmics/antihypertensives	Malignancy
Diuretics	Infarction
Antidiabetics	Hemorrhage
Antidepressants	Infection
Oral contraceptives	Motion sickness
Smoking cessation drugs	Labyrinthine disease
Infections	*Motility Disorders*
Viral gastroenteritis	Gastroparesis
Bacterial gastroenteritis	Chronic intestinal pseudoobstruction
Opportunistic infections (immunosuppression)	
Nongastrointestinal	*Functional Gastroduodenal Disorders*
	Cyclic vomiting syndrome
Organic GI/Intraperitoneal Conditions	Chronic idiopathic nausea
Gastric/small bowel obstruction	Functional vomiting
Superior mesenteric artery syndrome	Rumination syndrome
Volvulus	
Antral web	*Miscellaneous*
Peptic ulcer disease	Fatty liver of pregnancy
Crohn's disease	Myocardial infarction/heart failure
Pancreatitis	Ethanol intoxication
Cholecystitis	Graft versus host disease
Appendicitis	Acute intermittent porphyria
Hepatitis	Disorders of fatty acid oxidation
Abdominal irradiation	

Though it does not cause emesis, another condition, rumination syndrome, is included in the differential diagnosis because many patients are referred for refractory "vomiting." Rumination syndrome is characterized by the Rome Foundation as the repeated, effortless regurgitation of recently ingested food followed by its rechewing and reswallowing or oral expulsion.[2] Patients with

TABLE 7-2 **DIFFERENTIAL DIAGNOSIS OF** **UNEXPLAINED CHRONIC UPPER ABDOMINAL PAIN**	

ETIOLOGY	
Acid/Peptic Disorders GERD Erosive esophagitis Peptic ulcer disease	*Mesenteric Ischemia*
	Medications Antibiotics Hormonal treatments Iron supplements Potassium supplements
Gastroesophageal Malignancy	
Pancreaticobiliary Disease Chronic pancreatitis Pancreatic cancer Sphincter of Oddi dysfunction	*Motility Disorders* Gastroparesis Chronic intestinal pseudoobstruction
Inflammatory/Infiltrative Disease Gastroduodenal Crohn's disease Amyloidosis Sarcoidosis	*Functional Dyspepsia* Postprandial distress syndrome Epigastric pain syndrome

other functional bowel disorders may note nausea or vomiting in addition to lower gastrointestinal (GI) symptoms.

Abdominal Pain

Upper abdominal pain may result from several organic and functional disorders (Table 7-2). Ulcer disease is a consequence of *Helicobacter pylori* infection or analgesic medications. Gastroesophageal reflux disease (GERD) may cause epigastric pain instead of heartburn in some cases. Gastroesophageal malignancy is a rare cause of upper abdominal pain. Findings of upper endoscopy in patients with uninvestigated dyspepsia include erosive esophagitis in 13%, peptic ulcer in 8%, and cancer in only 0.3% of patients.[4] Pancreaticobiliary causes include chronic pancreatitis, pancreatic neoplasm, and sphincter of Oddi dysfunction. Gastroduodenal Crohn's disease, amyloidosis, sarcoidosis, and mesenteric ischemia present with unexplained upper abdominal pain. Other medication causes of abdominal pain include antibiotics, hormonal therapies, and iron and potassium supplements.

The most common etiology of upper abdominal pain is functional dyspepsia, which is defined by the Rome Foundation as (1) >1 of bothersome postprandial fullness, early satiation, or epigastric pain or burning and (2) no structural disease to explain symptoms.[2] A functional dyspepsia subset, the epigastric pain syndrome, focuses on patients with pain as the major symptom. Pain in epigastric pain syndrome is (1) localized to the epigastrium and is of at least moderate severity >1 time weekly; (2) is intermittent; (3) is not generalized or localized to other regions; (4) is not relieved by defecation or flatulence; and (5) does not fulfill criteria for biliary pain.[2] Characteristics supportive of this diagnosis include (1) pain that may have a burning quality, but without a retrosternal component; and (2) pain that is commonly induced or relieved by meals, but may occur while fasting. Criteria for functional dyspepsia or epigastric pain syndrome must be fulfilled for the last 3 months, with symptom onset >6 months before diagnosis.

Postprandial Fullness and Early Satiety

The differential diagnosis of postprandial fullness and early satiety overlaps with conditions causing nausea and vomiting. Induction of satiety is an intended mechanism of the benefits of some type 2 diabetes drug therapies (eg, exenatide), as well as medical and surgical morbid obesity treatments. A second functional dyspepsia subset, the postprandial distress syndrome, is defined as (1) bothersome postprandial fullness after ordinary-sized meals several times weekly and (2) early satiation that prevents finishing a regular meal several times weekly.[2] These criteria are fulfilled for the last 3 months, with symptom onset >6 months before diagnosis. Upper abdominal bloating or postprandial nausea or excessive belching supports this diagnosis. Factorial analyses of symptom groupings have stratified dyspepsia into 3 factors, with the first factor including fullness, bloating, and early satiety; the second factor including nausea and vomiting; and the third factor including discomfort, pain, belching, and reflux.[5]

Demographic and Clinical Symptom Features in Motility and Functional Disorders

Dysmotility syndromes like gastroparesis present with variable degrees of many symptoms. Nausea is reported by 79% to 93% of gastroparetics, while vomiting is noted by 68% to 84%. Among 393 patients, nausea was the predominant symptom of 34% of gastroparesis patients, while vomiting was predominant in 9% and retching in 0.3%.[6] In another single-center cohort, vomiting frequencies averaged 7.3 per day in people with diabetes vs 3.5 in idiopathic patients.[7] The prevalence of abdominal pain in gastroparesis ranges from 42% to 90%. Two-thirds of both diabetic and idiopathic patients report moderate to severe pain, on average, with associated increases in opiate use.[6] Pain is the predominant symptom noted by 21% of gastroparetics. Gastroparesis pain is postprandial in 24% to 80% of cases, but also is nocturnal in 74% and constant in 38%.[8] Gastroparesis pain often is described as burning, vague, crampy, sharp, or pressure-like, and occurs daily in 43% of patients. Early satiety is described by 60% to 86% of gastroparetics. Fullness, early satiety, and/or anorexia are considered predominant by 12% of gastroparesis patients, with most of these reporting some fullness descriptor as the main symptom.

Symptoms of gastroparesis may be indistinguishable from those of functional gastroduodenal disorders. In one report, 91% of patients with idiopathic gastroparesis satisfied criteria for postprandial distress syndrome, while 34% fulfilled criteria for chronic idiopathic nausea, and 39% had symptoms of functional vomiting.[9] Thus, distinguishing diagnoses of gastroparesis from functional gastroduodenal disorders may be artificial. Like gastroparesis, most functional dyspepsia patients report intermittent symptoms that are exacerbated by meals.[1] Postprandial fullness and bloating are the most common symptoms experienced by functional dyspeptics, while pain, early satiety, and nausea are noted less often.

SYMPTOM PATHOPHYSIOLOGY IN MOTILITY AND FUNCTIONAL DISORDERS

Gut sensorimotor impairments, inflammation, neuropsychiatric dysfunction, and other activities are proposed pathogenic factors of upper GI symptoms (Table 7-3). Yet, underlying mechanisms of symptom induction in most patients with such symptoms remain unproved.

TABLE 7-3
PATHOGENIC FACTORS UNDERLYING UPPER GASTROINTESTINAL SYMPTOMS

FACTOR	
Gastric Emptying Sbnormalities	*Nonsensorimotor Abnormalities*
Delayed gastric emptying	*Helicobacter pylori* gastritis
Rapid gastric emptying	Increased gastroesophageal acid reflux
Abnormal proximal gastric emptying	Duodenal eosinophil and macrophage infiltration
	Obesity
Other Gastrointestinal Sensorimotor Abnormalities	Menstrual cycle hormonal variations
Blunted fundic accommodation	Altered CNS processing
Heightened gastric sensitivity to distention and nutrients	Anxiety
	Depression
Heightened duodenal sensitivity to lipids and acid	Prior sexual or physical abuse
	Genetic factors

Gastric Emptying Impairments

Delays in gastric emptying are mandated for diagnosis of gastroparesis and are observed in about 40% with functional dyspepsia. Among patients with suspected gastroparesis, severities of overall and individual symptoms (including nausea, vomiting, upper abdominal pain, postprandial fullness, and early satiety), health care utilization, and quality of life were similar with prolonged vs. normal 2- and 4-hour gastric retention.[10] Yet in a subset with idiopathic gastroparesis, slightly lesser degrees of nausea, vomiting, retching, discomfort, and overall symptom severity were noted in those with mild (10% to 20% 4-hour retention) vs. severe (>35% 4-hour retention) impairments. On regression analyses, those with pronounced emptying delays had more severe vomiting and used more antiemetic drugs, suggesting gastric transit defects may contribute to some clinical manifestations of idiopathic gastroparesis. However, percentages of idiopathic gastroparetics satisfying criteria for the distinct Rome III gastroduodenal disorders were similar, with mild, moderate, and severe emptying delays confirming that their diagnoses do not depend on degrees of gastric retention. Likewise, in functional dyspepsia studies, emptying only weakly associates with fullness and does not relate to pain or nausea. Furthermore, emptying delays do not correlate with symptom severity when postprandial distress syndrome or epigastric pain syndrome are considered separately. However, other reports observe closer associations of fullness and pain with delayed emptying when symptoms are quantified during scintigraphy testing. Nevertheless, symptoms reported by those with normal vs. delayed emptying overlap so much that no symptom profile can predict the rate of gastric retention. Complicating these observations is the recent characterization of rapid gastric emptying in subsets of patients with functional dyspepsia, diabetes, or cyclic vomiting syndrome. In these individuals, symptoms are indistinguishable from those with delayed emptying. One modeling study concluded only 10% of the variance in postprandial dyspepsia relates to gastric emptying.[11]

Similarly, it has been difficult to relate symptom reductions during treatment of gastroparesis or functional dyspepsia to normalization of delayed emptying. Metoclopramide and domperidone produce long-term symptom benefits even when initial prokinetic effects wane, likely because of their additional antiemetic actions. In functional dyspepsia, symptom improvements on cisapride, an older prokinetic, do not correlate with emptying acceleration. Gastric electrical stimulation reduces vomiting but does not reliably affect gastric emptying in gastroparesis and shows similar efficacy in those with delayed versus normal emptying. A meta-analysis reported inferior responses to the motilin agonist erythromycin versus metoclopramide; a systematic review calculated benefits in only 43% of gastroparetics given erythromycin.[12] Further, in small controlled trials, symptom benefits of pyloric botulinum toxin injection were not superior to placebo. These reports suggest that pure prokinetic treatments without central antiemetic effects (erythromycin, pyloric botulinum toxin) may be less effective than agents with combined prokinetic and antiemetic action (metoclopramide, domperidone).

Other Gastrointestinal Sensorimotor Disturbances

Researchers have examined other gut sensorimotor parameters as potential causes of symptoms in these disorders. Blunting of fundic accommodation after eating is seen in 40% of functional dyspeptics (especially postprandial distress syndrome); enhanced sensitivity to gastric distention is found in 34%.[1] In functional dyspepsia, delayed emptying relates to nausea, vomiting, and fullness, while impaired accommodation correlates with pain, early satiety, and weight loss and hypersensitivity to distention with weight loss and belching.[13] In another report, the prevalence of prolonged gastric retention was greatest (38%) with fullness as a predominant symptom; hypersensitivity was noted most (44%) with predominant pain, while impaired accommodation was found in 79% with predominant early satiety.[14] Blunted gastric accommodation and heightened perception during gastric nutrient perfusion also have been seen with functional vomiting and gastroparesis. Other factors proposed to promote symptoms in functional dyspepsia include heightened perception of duodenal lipid and acid perfusion.

Nonsensorimotor Causes of Symptoms

Factors unrelated to sensorimotor function have been studied as pathogenic factors in gastroparesis and functional dyspepsia symptom development. Benefits observed with *H pylori* eradication in small patient subsets suggest this infection is a minor risk factor for functional dyspepsia. Increased acid reflux on esophageal pH testing in >33% of epigastric pain syndrome patients reflects an overlap with GERD. Functional dyspepsia may present after acute gastroenteritis. Duodenal mucosal eosinophilic and macrophage infiltration with increased cytokine production relates to functional dyspepsia symptoms, especially with postinfectious disease and with increased early satiety and fullness, suggesting potential roles for inflammation.[15] Obesity predicts gastroparesis severity, perhaps from activated inflammatory pathways. Gastroparesis symptoms are increased during the luteal phase of the menstrual cycle, reflecting possible hormonal participation. A positron emission tomography investigation reported impaired anterior cingulate cortex activation during gastric distention in functional dyspepsia, suggestive of altered brain processing of visceral information.[16] Scores for anxiety and depression correlate with symptom intensities in gastroparesis. As in irritable bowel syndrome (IBS), women with idiopathic gastroparesis may report prior physical or sexual abuse. Though these findings do not prove psychological dysfunction causes upper GI symptoms, they do show interactions between the CNS and gut manifestations of this disorder. Epidemiologic and genetic polymorphism studies indicate a subset of functional dyspeptics has a heritable tendency to develop symptoms.

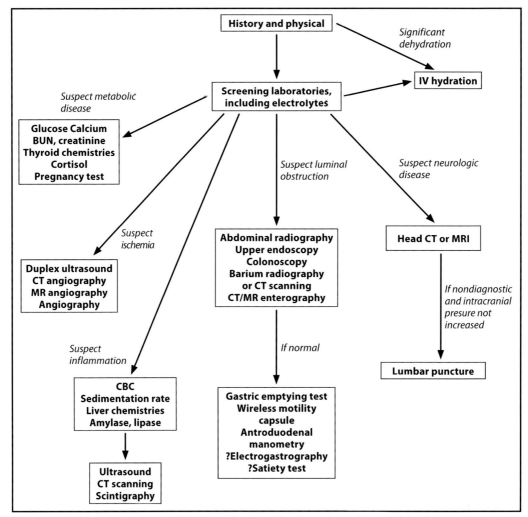

Figure 7-1. This is a proposed general algorithm for evaluating the patient with unexplained upper GI symptoms. Most importantly, the decision to proceed with structural and functional testing to assess the cause of the clinical presentation should be directed by a careful history and physical examination.

EVALUATION OF SYMPTOMS

Diagnosing the cause of unexplained upper GI symptoms requires a careful history and physical exam in concert with directed laboratory, structural, and functional testing (Figure 7-1).

Initial History, Physical Examination, and Laboratory Testing

The history helps define the etiology of unexplained symptoms. Drugs, toxins, and infections often cause acute symptoms, while established illnesses evoke chronic complaints. Gastroparesis and gastric obstruction cause emesis within 1 hour of eating; vomiting occurs later with small bowel obstruction. Vomiting within minutes of eating prompts consideration of behavioral causes, like rumination. Vomiting of old food residue suggests either pyloric obstruction or gastroparesis, while feculent emesis occurs with more distal blockage; emesis of undigested food is consistent with a proximal cause (Zenker diverticulum, achalasia). Hematemesis raises concern for an ulcer, malignancy, or Mallory-Weiss tear. Intracranial disease is considered if there are

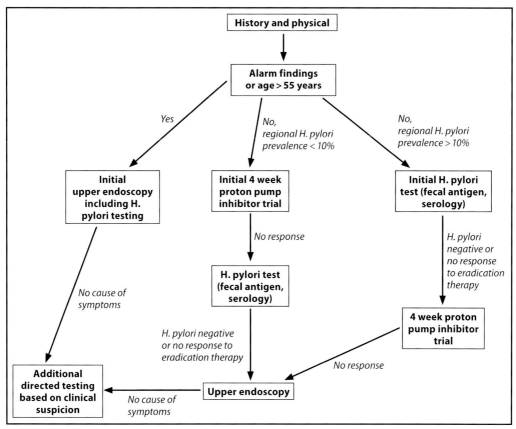

Figure 7-2. This is a proposed algorithm for evaluating the patient with unexplained dyspepsia.

associated headaches or visual field defects, while vertigo is reported with labyrinthine causes. Pain associated with cough, sore throat, hoarseness, or chest pain mimicking angina suggests GERD. Abdominal pain with functional dyspepsia may be meal induced, while that relieved by defecation or associated with changes in bowel habit is consistent with IBS. Alarm features with unexplained abdominal pain that warrant further investigation include unexplained weight loss, recurrent vomiting, occult or gross bleeding, jaundice, palpable mass or adenopathy, and a family history of GI neoplasm.

The physical examination complements the history, but often is normal with motor and functional disorders. Orthostatic hypotension and reduced skin turgor from intravascular fluid depletion result from recurrent emesis. Poor dentition, pharyngeal erythema, or wheezing may be noted with atypical GERD. Pulmonary abnormalities raise concern for aspiration in patients with vomiting, especially with impaired mentation. Absent bowel sounds are consistent with acute ileus or severe intestinal pseudoobstruction; high-pitched rushes suggest bowel obstruction. A succussion splash upon abrupt lateral movement may be heard on auscultation of patients with gastroparesis or gastric obstruction. Tenderness or involuntary guarding raises suspicion of inflammation, but many functional dyspeptics exhibit nonspecific upper abdominal tenderness. Malignant causes of pain are suggested by detecting occult fecal blood, masses, hepatomegaly, or lymphadenopathy. Finding papilledema, visual field loss, or focal neural abnormalities with unexplained emesis warrants evaluation for neurologic disease.

Laboratory findings provide diagnostic information and can inform initial management. Hypokalemia or metabolic alkalosis may indicate the need for oral or intravenous replenishment. Iron deficiency anemia warrants testing to exclude mucosal injury. Leukocytosis suggests

Figure 7-3. This is an endoscopic photograph of retained intragastric food residue in a patient with diabetic gastroparesis taken 16 hours after last consuming a solid meal.

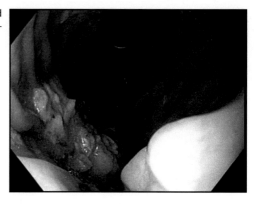

inflammation, while leukopenia occurs with viral infection. Abnormal pancreatic or liver chemistries raise concern for pancreaticobiliary disease. Hypoalbuminemia results from chronic disease or protein-losing enteropathy; low prealbumin suggests malnutrition. Pregnancy testing, thyroid chemistries, serum calcium, and fasting cortisol levels are obtained for suspected endocrine or metabolic causes. Serologies screen for celiac sprue or connective tissue disease. Serum protein electrophoresis, urine paraproteins, and angiotensin-converting enzyme levels are measured if infiltrative disorders (amyloidosis, sarcoidosis) are considered. Paraneoplastic autoantibodies are positive with cancer-associated motility disorders or autoimmune ganglionitis. Testing to exclude porphyria, urea cycle defects, or fatty acid disorders sometimes are obtained for unexplained cyclical emesis, especially with symptom onset before 2 years old, associated neurologic findings, hypoglycemia, anion gap metabolic acidosis, or hyperammonemia.[17] Perform lumbar puncture tests for suspected meningitis or neoplasia after excluding masses on CNS imaging.

Managing patients < 55 years old with unevaluated dyspepsia who do not report alarm features depends on the local *H pylori* prevalence (Figure 7-2). In areas with < 10% prevalence, an initial 4-week trial of an acid-suppressing drug (eg, proton pump inhibitor [PPI]) is advocated. For nonresponders, a test-and-treat approach is initiated with determination of *H pylori* status by fecal antigen or blood serology. *H pylori*–positive patients are given therapy to eradicate the infection. For regions with *H pylori* prevalence > 10%, the PPI trial is bypassed and *H pylori* testing is performed, with subsequent prescription of an acid suppressant given to those who do not respond to *H pylori* treatment or those who are negative for the infection.

Structural Testing

Testing to define structural abnormalities is indicated if the initial evaluation is nondiagnostic and empiric therapies are ineffective. Supine and upright abdominal radiographs show small intestinal air-fluid levels and reduced colonic air with bowel obstruction vs. diffusely dilated small and large bowel loops with ileus or chronic pseudoobstruction. Pneumoperitoneum suggests visceral perforation. Endoscopy detects ulcers, malignancy, and retained food residue in gastroparesis; it also affords the ability to biopsy abnormal-appearing tissue (Figure 7-3). Upper endoscopy is recommended to exclude malignancy or ulcers in patients with uninvestigated dyspepsia older than age 55 years or who have alarm factors, and for dyspepsia patients who fail acid suppressants or *H pylori* eradication. Small bowel barium radiography or computed tomography (CT) scans can diagnose partial bowel obstruction. CT and magnetic resonance imaging (MRI) enterography provide superior definition of internal bowel wall structure and can characterize inflammation in Crohn's disease and other disorders with luminal narrowing. Colonoscopy or contrast enema radiography detects partial colonic obstruction. Ultrasound or CT defines intraperitoneal inflammation and mass lesions. Scintigraphy can assess for biliary causes of symptoms. CT findings of gastroduodenal dilation with a diminished distance between the superior mesenteric artery and

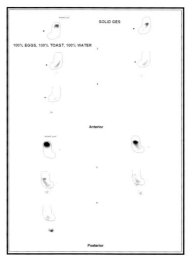

Figure 7-4. These images are sample anterior (upper panels) and posterior (lower panels) scintiscans from a gastric emptying study in a patient with unexplained nausea and vomiting after consuming a ^{99m}Tc-labelled egg substitute meal. Her 2-hour retention was 93%, and her 4-hour retention was 40%; these values are consistent with a diagnosis of gastroparesis.

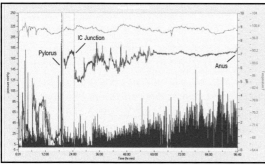

Figure 7-5. This is a sample wireless motility capsule recording from a diabetic patient with unexplained nausea and vomiting. The recording from the pH sensor (red line) shows evidence of delayed gastric emptying (20 hours; normal < 5 hours) as well as slow colon transit (71 hours; normal < 59 hours), reflecting detection of generalized dysmotility. The pressure sensor (blue line) presents motor activity in the three gut regions.

aorta suggest superior mesenteric artery syndrome. Duplex ultrasound, mesenteric angiography, CT, or MRI is useful for suspected ischemia. Head CT or MRI can delineate intracranial disease.

Tests of Gastroduodenal Function

Functional etiologies of symptoms are considered after structural disease is excluded. Clinicians can empirically treat patients with agents that stimulate gut motility. Alternatively, tests of gastroduodenal function may be performed to characterize motor dysfunction.

Gastric emptying tests are ordered to exclude gastroparesis (and rapid transit in some cases). Scintigraphy involves consuming a ^{99m}Tc-sulfur colloid label bound to digestible solid food (Figure 7-4). A standardized protocol using an egg substitute meal has been promoted by major societies; with this technique, > 60% gastric retention at 2 hours and/or > 10% at 4 hours are diagnostic of gastroparesis in the appropriate setting. Measuring emptying of a radiolabeled liquid complements information provided by solid-phase scanning, increasing detection of abnormal emptying by up to 26%. Gastric scintigraphy also characterizes rapid emptying. Other techniques also can measure gastric emptying. A wireless motility capsule (WMC) can be swallowed and transmit luminal pH and pressure data to a receiver worn by the patient. Wireless motility capsule gastric emptying is measured from the time of ingestion to the time a pH reading of near neutrality is recorded, reflecting passage into the duodenum. Wireless motility capsule testing also can quantify small intestine and colon transit and pressure patterns (Figure 7-5). Gastric emptying breath testing involves measuring $^{13}CO_2$ in breath samples after consuming a nonradioactive 13_C-labelled substrate (octanoate, *Spirulina platensis*). Ultrasound, MRI, and single photon emission computed tomography (SPECT) can quantify gastric emptying, but have limitations that

Figure 7-6. This is a sample antroduodenal manometry recording of fasting motor activity from a healthy individual showing a phase III component of the migrating motor complex originating in the antrum and propagating normally through the duodenum.

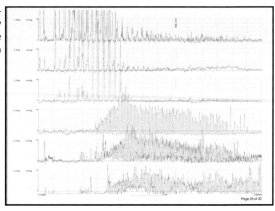

restrict their clinical applicability. Gastric accommodation and/or regional intragastric distribution after eating can be characterized using MRI, SPECT, or specialized scintigraphy methods.

Other gut function tests are performed in centers with expertise in dysmotility disorders. Antroduodenal manometry quantifies fasting and fed motor activity and responses to prokinetic drugs using fluoroscopically or endoscopically placed catheters with solid-state or water-perfused pressure sensors (Figure 7-6). Manometry is performed in patients (1) with unexplained symptoms (especially when other tests are unrevealing), (2) who did not respond to therapy, or (3) who are being considered for surgeries or enteral versus parenteral nutrition. Findings in gastroparesis include blunting of fasting and fed antral contractions and, in some cases, increased pyloric activity. Manometry can discriminate myopathic (low contractile amplitudes with normal morphology) vs. neuropathic (chaotic, uncoordinated burst contractions) small bowel dysmotility profiles. R waves on antroduodenal manometry in some rumination patients appear as simultaneous early postprandial contractions in all pressure sites. Rumination also can be identified by esophageal impedance with high-resolution manometry. Electrogastrography (EGG) employs cutaneous electrodes applied over the stomach to measure gastric slow-wave activity. Normal EGGs exhibit uniform 3-cycle-per-minute waveforms that increase in amplitude after water or meal ingestion. Rhythm disruptions like tachygastria (frequency >4 cycles per minute) or bradygastria (<2 cycles per minute) or a lack of fed signal amplitude increase are observed in some nauseated patients. Satiety testing involves consuming water or liquid nutrients until maximal fullness is reported. Volumes ingested are reduced in functional dyspeptics with early satiety, reflecting either impaired accommodation or enhanced gastric sensation. Roles for EGG and satiety testing in clinical decision making need to be defined.

Symptom Scoring Systems

Several symptom scoring systems have been employed as outcome measures in trials of gastroparesis and dyspepsia therapies (Table 7-4). Older studies quantified vomiting frequencies and intensities, total symptom scores, and visual analog scales. The Patient Assessment of Upper Gastrointestinal Disorders Symptoms (PAGI-SYM) survey was introduced to measure gastroparesis, dyspepsia, and GERD symptoms. This instrument enumerates 20 symptoms in 6 subscales (heartburn/regurgitation, fullness/early satiety, nausea/vomiting, bloating, upper abdominal pain, lower abdominal pain) from 0 (no symptoms) to 5 (most severe) recalled over 2 weeks.[18] The Gastroparesis Cardinal Symptom Index (GCSI) includes 9 questions from the PAGI-SYM to quantify gastroparesis severity. Gastroparesis Cardinal Symptom Index subscale scores for nausea/vomiting, fullness/early satiety, and bloating/distention are calculated to stratify patients by predominant symptom cluster. An updated version, the Gastroparesis Cardinal Symptom Index-Daily Diary, is composed of 11 questions, including an additional domain

TABLE 7-4
SYMPTOM SCORING SYSTEMS FOR GASTROPARESIS AND DYSPEPSIA

SURVEY	COMPOSITION	UTILITY
Patient Assessment of Upper Gastrointestinal Disorders Symptoms (PAGI-SYM)	20 symptoms in 6 subscales rated from 0 (no symptoms) to 5 (most severe) with 2-week recall	Valid and reliable survey to characterize symptoms in gastroesophageal reflux disease, dyspepsia, and gastroparesis
Gastroparesis Cardinal Symptom Index (GCSI)	9 symptoms in 3 subscales rated from 0 to 5 (subset of PAGI-SYM) with 2-week recall	Valid and reliable survey to characterize symptoms in gastroparesis
Gastroparesis Cardinal Symptom Index-Daily Diary (GCSI-DD)	11 symptoms in 4 subscales rated from 0 to 5 recalled daily	Update of GCSI includes pain severity, early satiety, nausea, postprandial fullness, and bloating that are responsive to gastroparesis treatment; a symptom composite is valid and responsive to treatment
Daily Diary of Gastroparesis Symptoms (GSDD)	Worst severity of nausea, early satiety, bloating, and upper abdominal pain from 0 (none) to 5 (very severe) recalled daily	Composite symptom score employed as a primary outcome measure in a clinical trial of a ghrelin agonist in gastroparesis
Gastrointestinal Symptom Rating Scale (GSRS)	15 items in 5 clusters rated from 1 (nontroublesome) to 7 (very troublesome)	Reliable measure of symptoms in irritable bowel syndrome and peptic ulcer disease
Leeds Dyspepsia Questionnaire (LDQ)	8 items, each with 2 stems, on the severity and frequency of dyspeptic symptoms over 6 months with a total range of scores from 0 to 40	Valid and reliable survey of the presence and severity of dyspepsia that is responsive to treatments
Rome III Modules	Self-reported questionnaire of 8 modules, including (i) functional dyspepsia module and (ii) nausea, vomiting, and belching disorders module	Facilitates diagnosis of functional gastroduodenal disorders in adult patients with unexplained upper GI symptoms

(pain/discomfort) queried daily, and shows good test-retest reliability, responsiveness to treatment, and relation to clinician-rated severity.[19] Related surveys like the Daily Diary of Gastroparesis Symptoms (GSDD) rating worst severities of nausea, early satiety, bloating, and pain have been employed in recent trials.[20]

Survey instruments also have been devised for dyspepsia. The Gastrointestinal Symptom Rating Scale consists of 15 items in 5 clusters scored from 1 (nontroublesome) to 7 (very troublesome) and has been used in dyspepsia and gastroparesis trials.[21] The Leeds Dyspepsia Questionnaire rates severities and frequencies of dyspeptic symptoms in relation to how bothersome they are.[22] Rome III modules classify patients into different functional disorders.

In 2009, the United States Food and Drug Administration (FDA) revised its recommendations to industry relating to developing patient-reported outcome (PRO) measures for clinical trials to support labeling claims.[23] Patient-reported outcomes should report on patient status without external interpretation by clinicians or others. Thus, PRO development should include open-ended input from the target patient population with no outside influence. The FDA commented that PRO instruments composed of single-item global items evaluating functional disorders are inadequate to support labeling claims and do not help understand effects of therapy on individual symptoms and signs. Other features considered by the FDA in reviewing PROs include reliability (temporal stability of scores, inter-interviewer consistency of scoring), validity (the instrument measures the concept of interest, relationships between items conform to a priori hypotheses), ability to detect change, data collection methodologies, patient comprehension, burden to patients and administrators, and recall period length. Nevertheless, the FDA emphasized that no single PRO development approach is necessarily correct. Most survey instruments in gastroparesis and functional dyspepsia trials do not strictly adhere to the FDA guidelines, as they did not originate from open-ended query of appropriate patient populations. Validation of newer survey instruments remains a focus of active investigation in this field.

CONCLUSION

Nausea, vomiting, pain, fullness, and early satiety are prevalent symptoms of patients with a range of organic, motility, and functional gastroduodenal disorders. Directed laboratory, structural, and functional testing can define an underlying diagnosis and suggest potential therapies. Additional studies will more definitively characterize and differentiate physiologic mechanisms for each symptom. Newer symptom assessment instruments will be validated for inclusion in clinical trial designs for patients with gastric motor or functional disease.

REFERENCES

1. Oustamanolakis P, Tack J. Dyspepsia: organic versus functional. *J Clin Gastroenterol.* 2012;46:175-190.
2. Tack J, Talley NJ, Camilleri M, et al. Functional gastroduodenal disorders. *Gastroenterology.* 2006;130:1466-1479.
3. Simonetto DA, Oxentenko AS, Herman ML, Szostek JH. Cannabinoid hyperemesis: a case series of 98 patients. *Mayo Clin Proc.* 2012;87:114-119.
4. Ford AC, Marwaha A, Lim A, Moayyedi P. What is the prevalence of clinically significant endoscopic findings in subjects with dyspepsia? Systematic review and meta-analysis. *Clin Gastroenterol Hepatol.* 2010;8:830-837.
5. Piessevaux H, De Winter B, Louis E, et al. Dyspeptic symptoms in the general population: a factor and cluster analysis of symptom groupings. *Neurogastroenterol Motil.* 2009;21:378-388.
6. Hasler WL, Wilson LA, Parkman HP, et al. Factors related to abdominal pain in gastroparesis: contrast to patients with predominant nausea and vomiting. *Neurogastroenterol Motil.* 2013;25:427-e301.
7. Cherian D, Parkman HP. Nausea and vomiting in diabetic and idiopathic gastroparesis. *Neurogastroenterol Motil.* 2012;24:217-e103.
8. Bielefeldt K, Raza N, Zickmund SL. Many faces of gastroparesis. *World J Gastroenterol.* 2009;15:6052-6060.
9. Parkman HP, Yates K, Hasler WL, et al. Clinical features of idiopathic gastroparesis vary with sex, body mass, symptom onset, delay in gastric emptying, and gastroparesis severity. *Gastroenterology.* 2011;140:101-115.
10. Pasricha PJ, Colvin R, Yates K, et al. Characteristics of patients with chronic unexplained nausea and vomiting and normal gastric emptying. *Clin Gastroenterol Hepatol.* 2011;9:567-576.
11. Delgado-Aros S, Camilleri M, Cremonini F, et al. Contributions of gastric volumes and gastric emptying to meal size and postmeal symptoms in functional dyspepsia. *Gastroenterology.* 2004;127:1685-1694.

12. Maganti K, Onyemere K, Jones MP. Oral erythromycin and symptomatic relief of gastroparesis: a systematic review. *Am J Gastroenterol.* 2003;98:259-263.

13. Karamanolis G, Caenepeel P, Arts J, Tack J. Determinants of symptom pattern in idiopathic severely delayed gastric emptying: gastric emptying rate or proximal stomach dysfunction? *Gut.* 2007;56:29-36.

14. Karamanolis G, Caenepeel P, Arts J, Tack J. Association of the predominant symptom with clinical characteristics and pathophysiological mechanisms in functional dyspepsia. *Gastroenterology.* 2006;130:296-303.

15. Walker M, Aggarwal K, Shim L, et al. Duodenal eosinophilia and early satiety in functional dyspepsia: confirmation of a positive association in an Australian cohort. *J Gastroenterol Hepatol.* 2014;29:474-479.

16. Van Oudenhove L, Vandenberghe J, Dupont P, et al. Abnormal regional brain activity during rest and (anticipated) gastric distension in functional dyspepsia and the role of anxiety: a H215O-PET study. *Am J Gastroenterol.* 2010;105:913-924.

17. Li BU, Lefevre F, Chelimsky GG, et al. North American Society for Pediatric Gastroenterology, Hepatology, and Nutrition consensus statement on the diagnosis and management of cyclic vomiting syndrome. *J Pediatr Gastroenterol Nutr.* 2008;47:379-393.

18. Rentz AM, Kahrilas P, Stanghellini V, et al. Development and psychometric evaluation of the patient assessment of upper gastrointestinal symptom severity index (PAGI-SYM) in patients with upper gastrointestinal disorders. *Qual Life Res.* 2004;13:1737-1749.

19. Revicki DA, Camilleri M, Kuo B, et al. Evaluating symptom outcomes in gastroparesis clinical trials: validity and responsiveness of the Gastroparesis Cardinal Symptom Index-Daily Diary (GCSI-DD). *Neurogastroenterol Motil.* 2012;24:456-e216.

20. McCallum RW, Lembo A, Esfandyari T, et al. Phase 2b, randomized, double-blind 12-week studies of TZP-102, a ghrelin receptor agonist for diabetic gastroparesis. *Neurogastroenterol Motil.* 2013;25:e705-e717.

21. Parkman HP, Van Natta M, Abell TL, et al. Effect of nortriptyline on symptoms of idiopathic gastroparesis: the NORIG randomized clinical trial. *JAMA.* 2013;310:2640-2649.

22. Moayyedi P, Duffett S, Braunholtz D, et al. The Leeds Dyspeptia Questionnaire: a valid tool for measuring the presence and severity of dyspepsia. *Aliment Pharmacol Ther.* 1998;12:1257-1262.

23. US Department of Health and Human Services Food and Drug Administration. Guidance for industry: Patient-reported outcome measures: Use in medical product development to support labeling claims. www.fda.gov/downloads/Drugs/Guidances/UCM193282.pdf. Published December 2009.

Gastroparesis

Sameer Dhalla, MD, MHS and Pankaj Jay Pasricha, MD

KEY POINTS

- Gastroparesis should be suspected in a patient with nausea, vomiting, bloating, early satiety, and abdominal pain where no obvious structural or mucosal cause can be found on upper endoscopy or upper gastrointestinal series.

- The pathophysiology of gastroparesis remains an active area of investigation and involves some combination of vagal neuropathy and an inflammatory infiltration of the enteric nerves and smooth muscle in the stomach leading to mechanical dysfunctions in solid food accommodation and forward propagation of food.

- Gastric scintigraphy is the most well-established diagnostic test to identify gastroparesis.

- Diabetes and recent abdominal surgery are the most common risk factors; however, more than one-third of patients have no identifiable risk factor.

- Treatment involves a multimodal strategy of diet, prokinetic medications, antiemetic medications, pain control, and electrical stimulation.

DEFINITION

Gastroparesis is an important motility disorder of the stomach characterized by delayed gastric emptying in the absence of mechanical outlet obstruction. The symptoms of gastroparesis include nausea, vomiting, bloating, early satiety, and abdominal pain, along with an impaired quality of life.[1] In research studies and in clinical practice, symptom severity is tracked using the Gastroparesis Cardinal Symptom Index (GCSI) (Table 8-1).[2] Diabetes is a major underlying cause for gastroparesis and requires specific therapy for glycemic control when present. Many other patients lack a clear explanation for their symptoms and are labeled idiopathic.

Rao SSC, Parkman HP, McCallum RW, eds.
Handbook of Gastrointestinal Motility and Functional Disorders (pp 107-114).
© 2015 Taylor & Francis Group.

QUESTION	GCSI SYMPTOMS*
1.	Nausea (feeling sick to your stomach as if you were going to vomit or throw up)
2.	Retching (heaving as if to vomit, but nothing comes up)
3.	Vomiting
4.	Stomach fullness
5.	Not able to finish a normal-sized meal
6.	Feeling excessively full after meals
7.	Loss of appetite
8.	Bloating (feeling like you need to loosen your clothes)
9.	Stomach or belly visibly larger

*Each symptom is scored on a 5-point Likert scale: 0=absent, 1=very mild, 2=mild, 3=moderate, 4=severe, 5=very severe. Adjustments are made for those on feeding tubes who are not eating.

TABLE 8-1. GASTROPARESIS CARDINAL SYMPTOM INDEX (GCSI)

PATHOPHYSIOLOGY

The emptying of solid foods and liquids from the stomach is a highly integrated physiologic process. Liquids tend to rapidly empty first, during which time solid food is stored in the proximal stomach (fundus) in an initial lag phase. The fundus relaxes during feeding to accommodate the food bolus.[3] After the lag phase, transfer to the distal stomach (antrum) allows for grinding of solid food into chyme in a process called trituration. Chyme is then pumped across a variably resistant pylorus into the duodenum at a rate influenced by nutritional content of the chyme and neurohumoral feedback onto the fundus and antrum. Gastric programs in both fed and fasting are controlled by the myenteric plexus with its system of intrinsic primary afferents, interneurons, and motor neurons. In turn, the myenteric plexus is regulated by vagal efferents, with their nuclei in the dorsal motor vagal (DMV) complex in the brainstem. Myenteric motor neurons are of two broad types: 1) excitatory, with the main neurotransmitter being acetylcholine and 2) inhibitory, with the main neurotransmitter being nitric oxide. Gastric contractile rhythm is set by an electrical slow wave (normally around 3 Hz) generated by specialized pacemaker cells known as the interstitial cells of Cajal (ICC).[4] ICC are also important in transducing neural signaling to the ultimate effector, the smooth muscle. Diseases such as diabetes, scleroderma, parkinsonism, and paraneoplastic disorders may affect any or all of these elements. Derangements of these ICC, the enteric and autonomic nervous systems (peripherally or centrally), or smooth muscles lead to various pathophysiological abnormalities, including altered frequency of the gastric electrical slow wave on electrogastrography (ie, tachygastria, bradygastria, or chaotic rhythm), increased pyloric contractility, antral hypomotility, and decreased fundic accommodation.[5]

We are just beginning to understand the pathological basis of these abnormalities. Studies of full-thickness gastric biopsies in refractory diabetic gastroparesis and idiopathic gastroparesis patients identified ICC dropout, decreased density of nerve fibers, smooth muscle fibrosis, changes in neurotransmitters, and a myenteric immune infiltrate in the muscle later.[6] Of these, changes in the ICC appear to correlate best with delays in gastric emptying. However, the pathogenesis of symptoms such as nausea and vomiting remain properly understood.

DIAGNOSIS

When gastroparesis is suspected clinically by patient risk factors and symptoms, the first step is to exclude mechanical obstruction via an upper endoscopy or radiography. Thereafter, gastric scintigraphy is the most widely accepted modality to objectively characterize delayed gastric emptying. The consensus test consists of scintigraphy at 0, 1, 2, and 4 hours using of a standardized meal containing radiolabeled Eggbeaters with jam, toast, and water.[7] In preparation for this test, drugs that accelerate (metoclopramide, domperidone, erythromycin) or delay (narcotic analgesics, anticholinergics) gastric emptying should be discontinued for 48 to 72 hours prior to the examination. If hyperglycemia is present due to diabetes or critical illness, the test should be delayed until relative euglycemia (blood glucose <275) can be achieved.[8] With this test, gastroparesis is defined as less than 40% emptying at 2 hours or less than 90% at 4 hours. Shorter-duration, solid-phase testing and liquid emptying alone have been shown to be less sensitive.[9] Although the use of liquid gastric emptying as an adjunctive measure to solid gastric emptying yields additional patients (up to 35% in one study),[10] it is not clear what the pathophysiological or clinical implications of this are.

An alternative modality that has not found widespread use or utility includes the wireless motility capsule (WMC, marketed as SmartPill [Given Imaging Ltd]). The WMC simultaneously measures pH, temperature, and pressure. Emptying of the capsule from the stomach is denoted by a precipitous rise in pH as the capsule transitions from an acidic gastric environment to the bicarbonate-rich small bowel lumen. Using a cutoff of 5 hours for gastric emptying time, WMC yielded sensitivity of 65% and specificity of 87% for diagnosis of gastroparesis as compared to 4-hour gastric scintigraphy.[11]

EPIDEMIOLOGY

The incidence and prevalence of gastroparesis vary by gender. The age-adjusted prevalence is estimated to be 9.8/100,000 persons in men and 37.8/100,000 persons in women.[12] Diabetics are at an increased risk for gastroparesis, which is far more for type I (30×) than type 2 (8×). Over a 10-year period, population-based studies suggest that 5.2% of type I diabetics, 1% of type II diabetics, and 0.2% of nondiabetics develop gastroparesis.[13] These figures may be underestimated, as many patients with delayed gastric emptying remain undiagnosed; one prognostic model suggests that the true prevalence in the community could be as high as 1.8%.[14]

The mean age at onset is 33.7 years. The etiologies seen in one study of 146 gastroparetics found 36% to be idiopathic, 29% diabetic, 13% postsurgical (particularly where vagus nerve injury is suspected), 7.5% Parkinson disease, 4.8% collagen vascular disease, 4.1% intestinal pseudoobstruction, and 6% miscellaneous causes (Figure 8-1).[15] More recent findings from the National Institutes of Health (NIH)–sponsored Gastroparesis Consortium of 401 patients as of March 15, 2010, demonstrated 61% to be idiopathic, 33% diabetic, and only 7% due to other causes.[16] The differences could be explained by referral bias, but both case series demonstrate a high proportion of idiopathic patients where no obvious reversible etiology can be identified.

Figure 8-1. Etiology of gastroparesis.

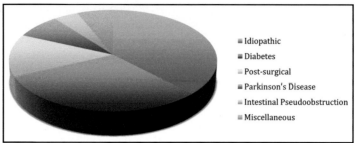

- Idiopathic
- Diabetes
- Post-surgical
- Parkinson's Disease
- Intestinal Pseudoobstruction
- Miscellaneous

TREATMENT

Nutrition

Gastroparesis can lead to poor oral intake, leading to weight loss and calorie/micronutrient deficiency in up to 64% of surveyed gastroparetic patients.[17] Nutritional support strategies depend on the severity of symptoms. For mild to moderate symptoms, transition to small, more frequent meals that are low in fat and fiber—and perhaps even liquefied—which may counteract some of the dysfunctional gastric motor activities described earlier. A "stepped" approach to gastroparesis is widely recommended but not robustly validated.[18]

In more severe cases of malnutrition, enteral support may be provided by a jejunal feeding tube, either directly or as an extension of a gastrostomy tube. A trial of nasojejunal feeding should precede endoscopic or surgical feeding tube placement because of the possible co-occurrence of small bowel dysmotility, even precluding jejunal feeding. In these most severe cases, parenteral nutrition may be the only option for the patient; however, this is to be avoided as long as possible because of the increased risk of morbidity and mortality from infections and thromboses.[19,20] Although often suggested as a benefit, the role of "venting" via the gastrostomy tube has not been rigorously evaluated.

Prokinetic Therapy

Prokinetic drugs are traditionally the first-line therapy for gastroparesis based on their ability to accelerate gastric emptying. However, there is generally little correlation between the degree of delay in gastric emptying and severity of symptoms; further, many drugs that produce improvement in gastric emptying do not necessarily improve symptoms (eg, the mitemcinal trial). The beneficial effects of some prokinetics (metoclopramide and domperidone) may be in large part due to their centrally mediated antiemetic effect.[4,21]

Metoclopramide, a prokinetic and antinausea agent approved by the United States Food and Drug Administration (FDA) for treatment of diabetic gastroparesis, is a potent central and peripheral dopamine receptor antagonist. The FDA recommends only short-term treatment (4 to 12 weeks), as metoclopramide crosses the blood/brain barrier, producing central nervous system (CNS) side effects such as anxiety, agitation, somnolence, insomnia, and extrapyramidal symptoms including, in rare cases, intractable tardive dyskinesia.[22,23] Older people and women should be especially cautious in its use.

Domperidone, another dopamine (D2) antagonist, enhances stomach contraction by antagonizing the peripheral receptors in the stomach. Its utility is similar to that of metoclopramide, but without the CNS side effects, and is widely available in most countries. In a systematic review in diabetic gastroparesis, 64% of patients noted symptom reductions, 67% reported decreased hospitalizations, and 60% exhibited accelerated emptying. Although the drug is not approved in the United States, the FDA makes it available for use via an investigational new drug application.[24] However, recent concerns about its cardiovascular adverse effects (it prolongs the QT interval) have led the European Medicines Agency (EMA) to issue much more stringent guidelines, limiting its use to small doses for less than 1 week.[25]

Erythromycin, a macrolide antibiotic, also mimics the action of motilin, an endogenous gastro-intestinal hormone that augments interdigestive gastric and intestinal peristaltic contractions. While it improves gastric emptying when given acutely over a few days and its use for gastroparesis has been hallowed over time, limited controlled trials have failed to show an effect in either acute treatment or after 2 weeks of treatment.[26,27] Low concentrations of erythromycin stimulate neural motilin receptors and peristaltic activity, while higher doses can stimulate motilin receptors directly on the muscle.[28,29] Thus, although the usual dose is 2 to 3 mg/kg (125 to 250 mg in most adults) given every 8 hours, at the higher doses, intestinal motility may be inhibited and gastric accommodation may be impaired.[30] Adverse effects of erythromycin include stomach pain, electrocardiographic QTc prolongation, and interactions with drugs metabolized by the CYP3A4 pathway. Azithromycin, another macrolide, has also been used for gastroparesis, but in the absence of controlled trials and given its similarity of action to erythromycin, its beneficial effects are not clear. However, it may have a better safety profile.[31]

Other Medical Therapies

Since most patients with moderate or severe gastroparesis cannot be managed by simple pro-kinetics alone, a variety of empirical medications mainly directed at the predominant symptom of nausea and vomiting are used. Among these, 5-HT3 antagonists such as ondansetron are commonly used in doses of 4 to 8 mg every 8 hours as needed for adults. In patients with vomiting, the orally disintegrating tablets may provide an advantage; sustained-release dermal delivery formulations (granisetron) may also be useful in this instance. Additional medications for symptomatic relief of nausea include prochlorperazine, promethazine, dimenhydrate, and others. These drugs exert their antinauseant effects via a combination of different receptors, including dopamine (D2), histamine (H1), and muscarinic (M1), with the predominant effect (and adverse effects) varying by drug class.[32] Some of these are also available as rectal or dermal formulations. In addition to the expected pharmacological adverse effects (eg, sedation and dryness of mouth), some of these drugs (such as promethazine) can be habit forming and they are best used for "rescue" rather than round-the-clock. A second-line drug that can be useful in patients with refractory nausea is dronabinol, the cannabinoid agonist that is also a potent appetite stimulant, used in doses of 5 to 20 mg a day. Some of the side effects are to be expected and include marijuana-like highs and binge eating, which could lead to more vomiting.

Neuromodulator therapies are also emerging as useful for the treatment of gastroparesis for a variety of symptoms, particularly pain. They include tricyclic antidepressants (eg, nortriptyline). Although anecdotal evidence suggested a beneficial effect, the largest controlled trial to date for nortriptyline in idiopathic gastroparesis showed no improvement over placebo in overall symptoms or the portion of the GCSI related to abdominal discomfort or symptoms overall.[33] However, this does not preclude a role for pain, as these drugs have established efficacy in neuropathic pain. Another particularly useful antidepressant to consider is mirtazapine, which has potent 5-HT3 antagonist activity as well as analgesic and appetite stimulation properties.[34,35] However, it has not been formally tested in gastroparesis patients.

Opioid narcotics should be avoided in these patients, as they will further delay gastric emptying, worsen nausea, and potentially cause paradoxical hyperalgesia as part of the narcotic bowel syndrome.

Nonpharmacological Therapy

Injection of botulinum toxin, a potent neuromuscular inhibitor, into the wall of the gastric pylorus during an upper endoscopy was first proposed because of a manometric phenomenon in a subset of diabetic gastroparetic patients where the pyloric tone and contractions were markedly increased. While small, open-label trials demonstrated a symptomatic benefit, placebo-controlled studies demonstrated no improvement in symptoms, despite improvement in gastric emptying.[36,37] Other attempts to target the pylorus include surgical pyloromyotomy, which in short-term observations suggests considerable improvement in emptying as well as symptoms, particularly of vomiting.[38]

Endoscopic placement of a self-expanding metal stent across the pylorus has also been proposed, but as with all other attempts to improve gastric emptying, it remains to be seen what the long-term benefit on symptoms really is.

Gastric electrical stimulators (GES) have been used for more than a decade for refractory nausea and vomiting in patients with gastroparesis. The underlying rationale has evolved from trying to "pace" gastric motility to modulating vagal afferents. However, evidence for their benefit remains equivocal, and the device has remained restricted under the Humanitarian Device Exemption clause of the FDA. Two controlled, partially blinded, crossover studies have yielded less-than-rigorous proof of benefit in the randomized phase of the studies, although subsequent open-label observations have been used to justify the benefits. It also appears that the device may be beneficial to diabetic but not idiopathic gastroparesis. Concerns with gastric neurostimulator implantation include risk of pocket site infections related to a foreign body, the high upfront cost, and the differential benefit based on phenotype. Dependence on narcotics prior to implantation is also a poor prognostic sign.[21] Improvements in technology are awaited before we can see the real potential of this promising approach.

Acupuncture and electroacupuncture have been proposed as a therapy for nausea; it is the most well-studied form of complementary and alternative medicine for gastroparesis. A single-blinded, sham-controlled, randomized trial of 19 diabetic gastroparesis patients demonstrated improvement not just in the GCSI score (which was persistent after the end of acupuncture therapy), but also an improvement in solid-phase gastric emptying on scintigraphy when comparing treatment to the sham-control group. Data are still limited in this area, but newer modes of therapy are under development in the area of cutaneous electrical stimulation.[39]

EVALUATION AND TREATMENT ALGORITHM

Step 1: Gastroparesis is suspected in a patient with nausea, vomiting, and abdominal discomfort
Perform esphagogastroduodenoscopy to exclude mechanical obstruction.
Identify and manage reversible causes of delayed gastric emptying (eg, hyperglycemia, narcotics)

Step 2: Confirm diagnosis
Perform 4-hour gastric scintigraphy

Step 3: Lifestyle modification
Nutritional counseling and surveillance
Rescue nutritional therapy (eg, transgastric jejunal feeding tube)

Step 4: Medications
Metoclopramide (with caution); trial of erythromycin and antinauseants
Neuromodulator medications for persistent nausea and abdominal pain despite prokinetic therapy

Step 5: Endoscopic and surgical therapy for medically refractory patients (limited evidence of benefit)
Gastric electrical stimulator
Pyloroplasty

REFERENCES

1. Parkman HP, Hasler WL, Fisher RS. American Gastroenterological Association medical position statement: diagnosis and treatment of gastroparesis. *Gastroenterology.* 2004;127(5):1589-1591.
2. Revicki DA, Rentz AM, Dubois D, et al. Development and validation of a patient-assessed gastroparesis symptom severity measure: the Gastroparesis Cardinal Symptom Index. *Aliment Pharmacol Ther.* 2003;18(1): 141-150.
3. Collins PJ, Horowitz M, Cook DJ, Harding PE, Shearman DJ. Gastric emptying in normal subjects: a reproducible technique using a single scintillation camera and computer system. *Gut.* 1983;24(12):1117-1125.
4. Khoo J, Rayner CK, Jones KL, Horowitz M. Pathophysiology and management of gastroparesis. *Expert Rev Gastroenterol Hepatol.* 2009;3(2):167-181.
5. Thazhath SS, Jones KL, Horowitz M, Rayner CK. Diabetic gastroparesis: recent insights into pathophysiology and implications for management. *Expert Rev Gastroenterol Hepatol.* 2013;7(2):127-139.
6. Grover M, Bernard CE, Pasricha PJ, et al. Clinical-histological associations in gastroparesis: results from the Gastroparesis Clinical Research Consortium. *Neurogastroenterol Motil.* 2012;24(6):531-539, e249.
7. Abell TL, Camilleri M, Donohoe K, et al. Consensus recommendations for gastric emptying scintigraphy: a joint report of the American Neurogastroenterology and Motility Society and the Society of Nuclear Medicine. *Am J Gastroenterol.* 2008;103(3):753-763.
8. Camilleri M, Parkman HP, Shafi MA, Abell TL, Gerson L. Clinical guideline: management of gastroparesis. *Am J Gastroenterol.* 2013;108(1):18-37; quiz 38.
9. Pathikonda M, Sachdeva P, Malhotra N, Fisher RS, Maurer AH, Parkman HP. Gastric emptying scintigraphy: is four hours necessary? *J Clin Gastroenterol.* 2012;46(3):209-215.
10. Ziessman HA, Chander A, Clarke JO, Ramos A, Wahl RL. The added diagnostic value of liquid gastric emptying compared with solid emptying alone. *J Nucl Med.* 2009;50(5):726-731.
11. Kuo B, McCallum RW, Koch KL, et al. Comparison of gastric emptying of a nondigestible capsule to a radiolabelled meal in healthy and gastroparetic subjects. *Aliment Pharmacol Ther.* 15 2008;27(2):186-196.
12. Jung HK, Choung RS, Locke GR, 3rd, et al. The incidence, prevalence, and outcomes of patients with gastroparesis in Olmsted County, Minnesota, from 1996 to 2006. *Gastroenterology.* 2009;136(4):1225-1233.
13. Choung RS, Locke GR, 3rd, Schleck CD, Zinsmeister AR, Melton LJ, 3rd, Talley NJ. Risk of gastroparesis in subjects with type 1 and 2 diabetes in the general population. *Am J Gastroenterol.* 2012;107(1):82-88.
14. Rey E, Choung RS, Schleck CD, Zinsmeister AR, Talley NJ, Locke GR, 3rd. Prevalence of hidden gastroparesis in the community: the gastroparesis "iceberg." *J Neurogastroenterol Motil.* 2012;18(1):34-42.
15. Soykan I, Sivri B, Sarosiek I, Kiernan B, McCallum RW. Demography, clinical characteristics, psychological and abuse profiles, treatment, and long-term follow-up of patients with gastroparesis. *Dig Dis Sci.* 1998;43(11): 2398-2404.
16. Parkman HP, Yates K, Hasler WL, et al. Clinical features of idiopathic gastroparesis vary with sex, body mass, symptom onset, delay in gastric emptying, and gastroparesis severity. *Gastroenterology.* 2011;140(1):101-115.
17. Parkman HP, Yates KP, Hasler WL, et al. Dietary intake and nutritional deficiencies in patients with diabetic or idiopathic gastroparesis. *Gastroenterology.* 2011;141(2):486-498, 498 e481-487.
18. Hejazi RA, McCallum RW. Treatment of refractory gastroparesis: gastric and jejunal tubes, Botox, gastric electrical stimulation, and surgery. *Gastrointest Endosc Clin N Am.* 2009;19(1):73-82, vi.
19. Abell TL, Malinowski S, Minocha A. Nutrition aspects of gastroparesis and therapies for drug-refractory patients. *Nutr Clin Pract.* 2006;21(1):23-33.
20. Cutts TF, Luo J, Starkebaum W, Rashed H, Abell TL. Is gastric electrical stimulation superior to standard pharmacologic therapy in improving GI symptoms, healthcare resources, and long-term health care benefits? *Neurogastroenterol Motil.* 2005;17(1):35-43.
21. Oh JH, Pasricha PJ. Recent advances in the pathophysiology and treatment of gastroparesis. *J Neurogastroenterol Motil.* 2013;19(1):18-24.
22. Parkman HP, Hasler WL, Fisher RS. American Gastroenterological Association technical review on the diagnosis and treatment of gastroparesis. *Gastroenterology.* 2004;127(5):1592-1622.
23. Tonini M, Cipollina L, Poluzzi E, Crema F, Corazza GR, De Ponti F. Review article: clinical implications of enteric and central D2 receptor blockade by antidopaminergic gastrointestinal prokinetics. *Aliment Pharmacol Ther.* 2004;19(4):379-390.

24. Dumitrascu DL, Weinbeck M. Domperidone versus metoclopramide in the treatment of diabetic gastroparesis. *Am J Gastroenterol.* 2000;95(1):316-317.

25. CMDh confirms recommendations on restricting use of domperidone-containing medicines [Press Release]. European Medicines Agency, April 25, 2014. http://www.ema.europa.eu/ema/index.jsp?curl=pages/news_and_events/news/2014/04/news_detail_002083.jsp.

26. Arts J, Caenepeel P, Verbeke K, Tack J. Influence of erythromycin on gastric emptying and meal related symptoms in functional dyspepsia with delayed gastric emptying. *Gut.* 2005;54(4):455-460.

27. Samsom M, Jebbink RJ, Akkermans LM, Bravenboer B, vanBerge-Henegouwen GP, Smout AJ. Effects of oral erythromycin on fasting and postprandial antroduodenal motility in patients with type I diabetes, measured with an ambulatory manometric technique. *Diabetes Care.* 1997;20(2):129-134.

28. Coulie B, Tack J, Peeters T, Janssens J. Involvement of two different pathways in the motor effects of erythromycin on the gastric antrum in humans. *Gut.* 1998;43(3):395-400.

29. Van Assche G, Depoortere I, Thijs T, Janssens JJ, Peeters TL. Concentration-dependent stimulation of cholinergic motor nerves or smooth muscle by [Nle13]motilin in the isolated rabbit gastric antrum. *Eur J Pharmacol.* 1997;337(2-3):267-274.

30. Bruley des Varannes S, Parys V, Ropert A, Chayvialle JA, Roze C, Galmiche JP. Erythromycin enhances fasting and postprandial proximal gastric tone in humans. *Gastroenterology.* 1995;109(1):32-39.

31. Potter TG, Snider KR. Azithromycin for the treatment of gastroparesis. *Ann Pharmacother.* 2013;47(3):411-415.

32. Abell TL, Bernstein RK, Cutts T, et al. Treatment of gastroparesis: a multidisciplinary clinical review. *Neurogastroenterol Motil.* 2006;18(4):263-283.

33. Parkman HP, Van Natta ML, Abell TL, et al. Effect of nortriptyline on symptoms of idiopathic gastroparesis: the NORIG randomized clinical trial. *JAMA.* 2013;310(24):2640-2649.

34. Kast RE, Foley KF. Cancer chemotherapy and cachexia: mirtazapine and olanzapine are 5-HT3 antagonists with good antinausea effects. *Eur J Cancer Care.* 2007;16(4):351-354.

35. Yeephu S, Suthisisang C, Suttiruksa S, Prateepavanich P, Limampai P, Russell IJ. Efficacy and safety of mirtazapine in fibromyalgia syndrome patients: a randomized placebo-controlled pilot study. *Ann Pharmacother.* 2013;47(7-8):921-932.

36. Arts J, Holvoet L, Caenepeel P, et al. Clinical trial: a randomized-controlled crossover study of intrapyloric injection of botulinum toxin in gastroparesis. *Aliment Pharmacol Ther.* 2007;26(9):1251-1258.

37. Friedenberg FK, Palit A, Parkman HP, Hanlon A, Nelson DB. Botulinum toxin A for the treatment of delayed gastric emptying. *Am J Gastroenterol.* 2008;103(2):416-423.

38. Hibbard ML, Dunst CM, Swanstrom LL. Laparoscopic and endoscopic pyloroplasty for gastroparesis results in sustained symptom improvement. *J Gastrointest Surg.* 2011;15(9):1513-1519.

39. McNearney TA, Sallam HS, Hunnicutt SE, Doshi D, Chen JD. Prolonged treatment with transcutaneous electrical nerve stimulation (TENS) modulates neuro-gastric motility and plasma levels of vasoactive intestinal peptide (VIP), motilin and interleukin-6 (IL-6) in systemic sclerosis. *Clin Exp Rheumatol.* 2013;31(2 Suppl 76): 140-150.

9

Functional Dyspepsia

Jan Tack, MD, PhD

KEY POINTS

- Early satiation, postprandial fullness, epigastric pain, and epigastric burning are the cardinal functional dyspepsia (FD) symptoms.

- Functional dyspepsia can be subdivided into post-prandial distress syndrome (PDS) and epigastric pain syndrome (EPS).

- The underlying pathophysiology in FD is probably multifactorial, involving disorders of motility and sensitivity of the stomach and duodenum, as well as altered brain processing of afferent stimuli.

- The most important peripheral mechanisms for functional dyspepsia include impaired gastric accommodation to a meal, hypersensitivity to gastric distention, delayed gastric emptying, *Helicobacter pylori* infection, altered duodenal sensitivity to lipids or acid, and abnormal intestinal motility.

- In those diagnosed with *H pylori* infection, eradication is recommended, although the symptom impact is often limited and delayed.

- Proton pump inhibitors (PPIs) are the preferred initial treatment for EPS, while prokinetics are advocated for PDS.

- Tricyclic antidepressants can be used for refractory symptoms, especially in EPS.

DEFINITION

Dyspepsia refers to a heterogeneous group of symptoms, which are centrally located in the upper abdomen. Over time, the symptoms that are considered to be part of dyspepsia have varied, ranging from postprandial fullness, early satiation, epigastric pain, upper abdominal bloating, and nausea to even heartburn, regurgitation, anorexia, belching, or vomiting.[1] When additional

Rao SSC, Parkman HP, McCallum RW, eds.
Handbook of Gastrointestinal Motility and Functional Disorders (pp 115-122).
© 2015 Taylor & Francis Group.

Figure 9-1. Definition of dyspepsia and sequence of uninvestigated, organic, and functional dyspepsia.

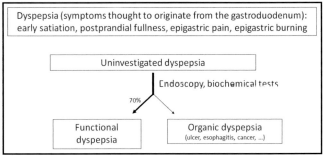

investigations are performed in patients with dyspeptic symptoms, they may identify an underlying organic disease that explains the symptoms. These subjects are diagnosed with an organic cause of dyspepsia. However, in the majority of subjects with dyspeptic symptoms, routine investigations will reveal no organic abnormality, and these patients are diagnosed with FD. Patients with dyspeptic symptoms in whom diagnostic investigations have not yet been performed are referred to as having uninvestigated dyspepsia (Figure 9-1).[1]

The definitions of dyspepsia, as well as functional dyspepsia, have varied with time during the last 2 decades, based on the type and number of symptoms that are considered indicative of dyspepsia. In the most recent consensus definitions, symptoms suggestive of gastroesophageal reflux disease (GERD) are considered separate from dyspepsia, and the cardinal symptoms considered typical of dyspepsia have undergone progressive restrictions.[2-4]

The most recent consensus was published in the Rome III definitions, which defined dyspepsia as a group of symptoms that are considered to arise from the gastroduodenum.[4] Only 4 symptoms are invariably considered to have a gastroduodenal origin: postprandial fullness, early satiation, epigastric pain, and epigastric burning, although several other symptoms may coexist.[4] Consequently, functional dyspepsia is defined as the presence of early satiation, postprandial fullness, epigastric pain, or epigastric burning in the absence of underlying organic or metabolic disease that is likely to explain the symptoms, with an additionally required history of at least 3 months of active symptoms and an onset of at least 6 months earlier.[4]

Furthermore, the Rome III consensus considered FD to be a condition with highly variable symptom presentation, underlying pathophysiology, and therapeutic approach. Hence, it was proposed to subdivide FD into PDS (meal-related dyspeptic symptoms characterized by postprandial fullness and early satiation) and EPS (meal-unrelated dyspeptic symptoms characterized by epigastric pain and epigastric burning).[4]

DIAGNOSIS

Although the differential diagnosis of dyspepsia is extremely wide, including virtually all upper gastrointestinal tract diseases, the diagnostic approach to the patient with dyspeptic symptoms is relatively simple in the vast majority of cases. In patients presenting with one or more of the cardinal dyspeptic symptoms, detailed clinical history taking aims at determining the full symptom profile and at verifying the absence of alarm symptoms (weight loss, nocturnal pain, nonsteroidal anti-inflammatory [NSAID] use, family history of gastric or esophageal cancer or celiac disease). For each symptom, the location, mode of onset, intensity, character, and precipitating or relieving factors should be reviewed. Typically, FD symptoms are triggered or worsened by ingestion of a meal, although this may not always be perceived as such by the patient.[5] Careful history taking should also aim at recognizing coexisting or dominant GERD symptoms, and this can be helped

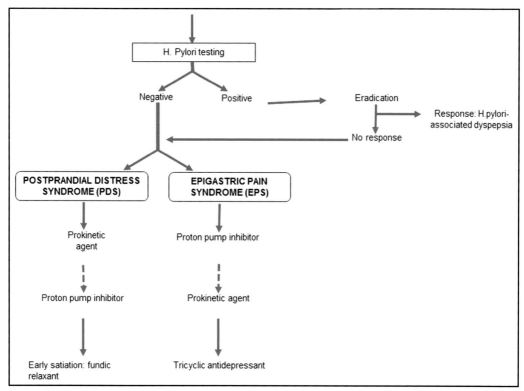

Figure 9-2. Proposed management algorithm for functional dyspepsia based on *H pylori* detection and distinction of EPS and PDS according to the Rome III definitions.

by using heartburn descriptor questions.[6] In the case of typical GERD symptoms, the patient should be managed as GERD, as dyspeptic symptoms may also respond.

Physical examination of the dyspeptic patient will be normal in the majority of cases. The clinician may choose to manage the symptoms as "uninvestigated dyspepsia" by starting empiric treatment without additional investigations (Figure 9-2). This is an option when there are no alarm symptoms and when organic disease seems less likely. In all other cases, upper gastrointestinal endoscopy with biopsies is the key technical examination, but will turn out normal in the vast majority of cases. Often, additional biochemical testing will be considered, although there is no evidence that this is cost effective.[1]

Abdominal ultrasound is often considered a complementary examination in patients with dyspeptic symptoms, but in the absence of symptoms suggestive of biliary tract disease, it is not cost effective. In refractory patients, or when weight loss or other severe symptoms accompany dyspeptic symptoms, additional evaluations such as abdominal computed tomography (CT) scan or angiography, small bowel radiography, psychiatric assessment, and advanced reflux and motility testing can be considered.[1]

EPIDEMIOLOGY

Epidemiological studies, using the variable definitions of dyspepsia that have been applicable over time, reported extremely high prevalence, with over 20% of subjects in the general population experiencing dyspeptic symptoms in the broad sense. However, only a minority of these will come to medical attention.[7]

More recent epidemiological studies, using the more restrictive Rome III criteria, have shown population prevalence of uninvestigated dyspepsia ranging between 15% and 20%, and FD (those with negative endoscopy) ranging between 11% and 16% of the total adult population.[8] In addition, these epidemiological studies have provided strong support for the existence of PDS and EPS as separate subentities in the general population, as both were present with only limited overlap. However, in patients who consult and are diagnosed with FD, major overlap between PDS and EPS exists, which hampers its applicability in clinical practice.[8]

Pathophysiological Mechanisms

A large variety of pathophysiological mechanisms have been implicated in symptom generation in FD. The most important peripheral mechanisms include impaired gastric accommodation to a meal, hypersensitivity to gastric distention, delayed gastric emptying, *H pylori* infection, altered duodenal sensitivity to lipids or acid, and abnormal intestinal motility.[9] In addition, several central nervous mechanisms have been implicated, including lack of activation of antinociceptive pathways, anxiety, depression, and somatization.[10]

Impaired Gastric Accommodation

Accommodation of the stomach to a meal, triggered by ingestion of a meal and enabling storage of food in the proximal stomach without a rise in intragastric pressure, is controlled by a vagovagal reflex pathway. Recent studies used intragastric manometry to demonstrate that meal ingestion triggers a drop in intragastric pressure followed by a gradual recovery of pressure during ongoing nutrient ingestion, which parallels the occurrence of meal-induced satiation.[11] Using a variety of techniques (gastric barostat, scintigraphy, ultrasound, single photon emission CT) or noninvasive surrogate markers (nutrient volume tolerance testing) indicates that approximately 40% of FD patients have impaired accommodation.[9] In case of impaired accommodation, meal ingestion is associated with a higher intragastric pressure, which activates tension-sensitive mechanoreceptors, leading to early satiation and potentially weight loss.[9,12] The causes of impaired accommodation are unknown, but an increased prevalence is reported in FD patients with a postinfectious symptom onset, presumably through impaired nitrergic nerve function.[12]

Hypersensitivity to Gastric Distension

Functional dyspepsia patients as a group are hypersensitive to distention of the proximal stomach.[9,12] Symptom generation is thought to involve activation of tension-sensitive mechanoreceptors and may, just as impaired accommodation, respond to gastric relaxant therapy.[9,12] Recent studies have implicated impaired accommodation as a contributor to postprandial hypersensitivity to gastric distention.[13]

Delayed Gastric Emptying

Approximately one-third of FD patients have delayed solid gastric emptying, but its contribution to symptom generation, as well as the distinction from gastroparesis, have remained controversial.[9,12] Gastroparesis is defined as the presence of delayed gastric emptying in the absence of a mechanical obstruction and has been associated with symptoms of nausea and vomiting, early satiety, postprandial fullness, bloating, and upper abdominal pain.[14] However, the correlation of emptying rate with symptoms is poor in both conditions.[12,15] A study from the Mayo Clinic has reported rapid gastric emptying in a large subset of FD patients, but others were unable to confirm this as a prevalent finding.[12,16]

Altered Duodenal Sensitivity and Integrity

Several small-scale studies reported that FD patients are hypersensitive to duodenal lipid or acid perfusion.[12] Studies using duodenal pH monitoring, again in small patient groups, showed increased duodenal acid exposure in FD compared to healthy controls, and this was attributable to impaired duodenal acid clearance.[12] A recent study reported decreased duodenal mucosal integrity in FD, potentially related to prolonged acid stasis, with changes in tight junction protein expression and low-grade inflammatory changes.[17] Another potential contributor to loss of intestinal mucosal integrity, as seen in FD, is acute psychological stress.[18]

Altered Central Nervous System Processing

FD patients, as well as dyspeptic symptoms in the general population, are characterized by elevated prevalence of anxiety disorders, depressive disorders, somatoform disorders, and a recent or remote history of abuse.[10] In tertiary care FD patients, symptom severity is more strongly correlated to psychosocial factors (especially depression, abuse history, and somatization) than to abnormalities of gastric sensorimotor function.[19] However, this is not sufficient to establish a causal role for psychosocial factors in the generation of dyspeptic symptoms. Mechanistic studies showed a close relationship between psychosocial factors and visceral hypersensitivity in particular, and this is associated with differential processing of gastric stimuli in the central nervous system.[10,19,20]

TREATMENT

A firm diagnosis of FD is only possible after a negative endoscopy in patients with dyspeptic symptoms. However, empirical therapy with acid-suppressive therapy or *H pylori* infection of those who show evidence of infection is often applied prior to endoscopy in those without alarm symptoms and a lower probability of organic disease based on age and absence of NSAID use.[1]

After a negative upper endoscopy, reassurance and communication of a confident and positive diagnosis are probably of primary importance in FD. Dietary recommendations (more frequent, smaller-sized meals that are low in fat content) are also frequently recommended, but this has not been studied systematically. Other common lifestyle adjustments, such as avoidance of coffee, alcohol, and NSAIDs and smoking cessation, also have not been studied. Pharmacotherapy will be considered in the vast majority of patients, and a large number of options are available, all of them with limited efficacy.

H pylori *Eradication*

In those FD patients who are infected with *H pylori*, a small but statistically significant benefit is observed after eradication. A Cochrane meta-analysis showed a yield of eradication in terms of symptom relief over placebo of approximately 10%, and this occurs only after 6 to 11 months.[21] As the subgroup of infected FD patients is progressively declining in Western populations, the gain of eradication also becomes smaller. On the other hand, *H pylori* eradication can induce sustained remission, may protect against peptic ulcer and gastric cancer, and is relatively inexpensive.[1,21]

Acid-Suppressive Therapy

A meta-analysis of controlled trials with proton pump inhibitors (PPIs) in FD showed a benefit of 13% over placebo, and this gain was found in those with concomitant heartburn and those with epigastric pain, but not in those with motility-like symptoms.[22] Hence, this therapy is attractive in the EPS group but not in the PDS group according to the Rome III classification.[4]

Prokinetic Drugs

Prokinetics, drugs that enhance gastric contractility, are widely used in the treatment of FD. A meta-analysis reported significant benefit for prokinetics over placebo, with a relative risk reduction of 33% and a number to treat of 6, but concerns were raised about publication bias.[23] Prokinetics are a heterogeneous class of agents, with dopamine 2 receptor (D2) antagonists and 5-HT4 receptor agonists being the most classical agents. Both metoclopramide and domperidone are D2 antagonists, but metoclopramide has been associated with neurological adverse effects and domperidone with QT interval prolongation.[24] Itopride, a novel D2 antagonist that also has cholinesterase inhibitory effects, failed to show consistent efficacy in phase 3 studies.[24]

Cisapride, a widely used 5-HT4 receptor agonist, was withdrawn due to QT prolongation and fatal arrhythmias.[24] More recent studies with other 5-HT4 agonists like tegaserod or mosapride failed to show convincing benefit. Motilin and ghrelin receptors are other targets for the development of prokinetics, but to date, convincing efficacy has not been shown.[24]

Acotiamide (Z-338) is a novel compound with fundus-relaxing and gastroprokinetic properties based on a mechanism of action that differs from other gastroprokinetic agents. Acotiamide is an antagonist of the inhibitory muscarinic type 1 and type 2 (M1/M2) autoreceptors on cholinergic nerve endings and is a cholinesterase inhibitor.[24] The drug is available for the treatment of FD in Japan based on a 4-week controlled study.[25] Acotiamide is currently under evaluation for the treatment of PDS in a phase 3 program in Europe.

Activation of 5-HT1A receptors relaxes the proximal stomach through inhibition of cholinergic tone.[22,25] Buspirone, a 5-HT1A receptor agonist used in the treatment of panic attacks, showed benefit over placebo in a small placebo-controlled pilot study in FD, and this was attributed to enhancement of meal-induced accommodation.[25,26] A clinical trial investigated a similar compound, tandospirone, which showed a significant benefit over placebo that was not attributable to anxiolytic or antidepressant effects.[27]

Psychotropic Agents

Psychotropics, especially antidepressants, are frequently used second-line drugs in functional disorders, including FD. A systematic review suggested efficacy for these drugs, but the quality of the available trials was suboptimal.[26] A recent large, controlled trial with the serotonin/noradrenaline reuptake inhibitor venlafaxine in 160 FD patients failed to show any benefit over placebo.[27] The anxiolytics buspirone and tandospirone were shown to be beneficial in FD, but their effects may have been attributable to their fundus-relaxing properties.[28,29]

Psychological Therapies

Psychological therapies such as hypnotherapy and cognitive behavioral therapy are advocated as rescue therapy for refractory FD symptoms, but truly convincing evidence of their efficacy has not really been delivered.[30]

Management Algorithm

In FD patients with mild symptoms, reassurance and lifestyle advice may be sufficient. In those with persisting or more severe symptoms, testing for *H pylori* and eradication when positive is the next recommended step (see Figure 9-2). Because symptom relief is often delayed, additional symptomatic therapy may be required. With the Rome III subdivision of FD, recommendations for specific initial pharmacotherapy were made.[4] In EPS patients, 1 to 2 months of PPI therapy is the preferred initial approach, while in PDS patients, a prokinetic is favored as initial therapy. The access to prokinetics varies strongly among countries but, if available, acotiamide is probably the agent of choice. In case of insufficient response, a switch in therapeutic class or combination therapy can be considered.

In patients with refractory epigastric pain, a trial of a low-dose tricyclic antidepressant such as amitriptyline can be considered, although strong evidence is lacking. In those with important early satiation and perhaps weight loss, fundic relaxants like buspirone or tandospirone can be used. In refractory patients who accept psychological therapies, cognitive behavioral therapy or hypnotherapy can be offered.

REFERENCES

1. Oustamanolakis P, Tack J. Dyspepsia: organic versus functional. *J Clin Gastroenterol.* 2012;46(3):175-190.
2. Drossman DA, Thompson GW, Talley NJ, et al. Identification of subgroups of functional gastrointestinal disorders. *Gastroenterol Int.* 1990;3:159-172.
3. Talley NJ, Stanghellini V, Heading RC, Koch KL, Malagelada JR, Tytgat GN. Functional gastroduodenal disorders. *Gut.* 1999;45 Suppl 2:II 37-42.
4. Tack J, Talley NJ, Camilleri M, et al. Functional gastroduodenal disorders. *Gastroenterology.* 2006;130:1466-1479.
5. Bisschops R, Karamanolis G, Arts J, et al. Relationship between symptoms and ingestion of a meal in functional dyspepsia. *Gut.* 2008;57:2387-2393.
6. Tack, J, Caenepeel, P, Arts, J, Lee K-J, Sifrim D, Janssens J. Prevalence of acid reflux in functional dyspepsia and its association with symptom profile. *Gut.* 2005;54:1370-1376.
7. Mahadeva S, Goh KL. Epidemiology of functional dyspepsia: a global perspective. *World J Gastroenterol.* 2006;12(17):2661-2666.
8. Tack J, Talley NJ. Functional dyspepsia: symptoms, definitions and validity of the Rome III criteria. *Nat Rev Gastroenterol Hepatol.* 2013;10(3):134-141.
9. Tack J, Bisschops R, Sarnelli G. Pathophysiology and treatment of functional dyspepsia. *Gastroenterology.* 2004;127:1239-1255.
10. Van Oudenhove L, Aziz Q. The role of psychosocial factors and psychiatric disorders in functional dyspepsia. *Nat Rev Gastroenterol Hepatol.* 2013;10(3):158-167.
11. Janssen P, Verschueren S, Giao Ly H, Vos R, Van Oudenhove L, Tack J. Intragastric pressure during food intake: a physiological and minimally invasive method to assess gastric accommodation. *Neurogastroenterol Motil.* 2011;23(4):316-322, e153-154.
12. Vanheel H, Farré R. Changes in gastrointestinal tract function and structure in functional dyspepsia. *Nat Rev Gastroenterol Hepatol.* 2013;10(3):142-149.
13. Farré R, Vanheel H, Vanuytsel T, et al. Functional dyspepsia, hypersensitivity to postprandial distention correlates with meal-related symptom severity. *Gastroenterology.* 2013;145(3):566-573.
14. Masaoka T, Tack J. Gastroparesis: current concepts and management. *Gut Liver.* 2009;3(3):166-173.
15. Janssen P, Harris MS, Jones M, et al. The relation between symptom improvement and gastric emptying in the treatment of diabetic and idiopathic gastroparesis. *Am J Gastroenterol.* 2013;108(9):1382-1391.
16. Delgado-Aros S, Camilleri M, Cremonini F, Ferber I, Stephens D, Burton DD. Contributions of gastric volumes and gastric emptying to meal size and postmeal symptoms in functional dyspepsia. *Gastroenterology.* 2004;127(6):1685-1694.
17. Vanheel H, Vicario M, Vanuytsel T, et al. Impaired duodenal mucosal integrity and low-grade inflammation in functional dyspepsia. *Gut.* 2014;63:262-271.
18. Vanuytsel T, van Wanrooy S, Vanheel H, et al. Psychological stress and corticotropin-releasing hormone increase intestinal permeability in humans by a mast cell-dependent mechanism. *Gut.* 2013 Oct 23. doi: 10.1136/gutjnl-2013-305690. [Epub ahead of print].
19. Van Oudenhove L, Vandenberghe J, Geeraerts B, et al. Determinants of symptoms in functional dyspepsia: gastric sensorimotor function, psychosocial factors or somatisation? *Gut.* 2008;57(12):1666-1673.
20. Fischler B, Tack J, De Gucht V, et al. Heterogeneity of symptom pattern, psychosocial factors and pathophysiological mechanisms in severe functional dyspepsia. *Gastroenterology.* 2003;124:903-910.
21. Moayyedi P, Soo S, Deeks JJ, et al. Eradication of Helicobacter pylori for non-ulcer dyspepsia. *Cochrane Database Syst Rev.* 201116;(2):CD002096. doi: 10.1002/14651858.CD002096.pub5.
22. Moayyedi P, Delaney BC, Vakil N, et al. The efficacy of proton pump inhibitors in nonulcer dyspepsia: a systematic review and economic analysis. *Gastroenterology.* 2004;127:1329-1337.
23. Moayyedi P, Shelly S, Deeks J, et al. Pharmacological interventions for non-ulcer dyspepsia. Cochrane Database Syst Rev. 2011;2:CD001960.

24. Camilleri M, Tack JF. Current medical treatments of dyspepsia and irritable bowel syndrome. *Gastroenterol Clin North Am.* 2010;39(3):481-493.

25. Matsueda K, Hongo M, Tack J, Saito Y, Kato H. A placebo-controlled trial of acotiamide for meal-related symptoms of functional dyspepsia. *Gut.* 2012;61(6):821-828.

26. Hojo M, Miwa H, Yokoyama T, et al. Treatment of functional dyspepsia with antianxiety or antidepressive agents: systematic review. *J Gastroenterol.* 2005;40:1036-1042.

27. van Kerkhoven LA, Laheij RJ, Aparicio N, et al. Effect of the antidepressant venlafaxine in functional dyspepsia: a randomized, double-blind, placebo-controlled trial. *Clin Gastroenterol Hepatol.* 2008;6:746-752.

28. Tack J, Janssen P, Masaoka T, Farré R, Van Oudenhove L. Efficacy of buspirone, a fundus-relaxing drug, in patients with functional dyspepsia. *Clin Gastroenterol Hepatol.* 2012;10(11):1239-1245.

29. Miwa H, Nagahara A, Tominaga K, et al. Efficacy of the 5-HT1A agonist tandospirone citrate in improving symptoms of patients with functional dyspepsia: a randomized controlled trial. *Am J Gastroenterol.* 2009; 104(11):2779-2787.

30. Soo S, Moayyedi P, Deeks J, Delaney B, Lewis M, Forman D. Psychological interventions for non-ulcer dyspepsia. Cochrane Database Syst Rev. 2011;18:CD002301.

10

Dumping Syndrome

Patrick Berg, BS and
Richard W. McCallum, MD, FACP, FRACP (AUST), FACG, AGAF

KEY POINTS

- Dumping syndrome (DS) involves the rapid gastric transit of chyme from the stomach into the small bowel, and DS symptoms can be classified as early (30 minutes after ingestion) and/or late (1 to 3 hours after ingestion).

- DS should be considered in the setting of undiagnosed abdominal pain and/or diarrhea.

- The symptoms of DS can be clinically indistinguishable from gastroparesis, and a radionuclide gastric emptying test is important to distinguish between the two.

- Treatment approach starts with dietary changes, and may extend to acarbose and anticholinergics, with octreotide (a somatostatin) being the final medical option.

The underlying mechanism of DS is rapid gastric emptying. DS is a syndrome that causes a specific set of gastric and vasomotor symptoms. There are many etiologies that cause DS. Before the *Helicobacter pylori* era, gastric surgeries, with or without vagotomy, were the main cause. Currently, diabetes mellitus (DM) and an idiopathic subgroup are predominant etiologies of rapid gastric emptying, of which, many patients have symptoms of DS. The symptoms of DS include both gastric and vasomotor symptoms as a result of the rapid release of chyme into the intestines. These sequelae can be separated into early symptoms (30 minutes after ingestion) and late symptoms (1 to 3 hours after ingestion). Gastrointestinal symptoms may include epigastric cramps, bloating, distention, gas, borborygmi, pain, nausea, vomiting, and diarrhea. Vasomotor symptoms may consist of fatigue, lightheadedness, palpitations, diaphoresis, hypotension, headache, pallor, and possibly syncope. For both early and late DS, symptoms can be debilitating. Abdominal symptoms are due to small bowel distention and hypercontractility. Vasomotor symptoms of early DS involve the excessive secretion of GI hormones, as well as a fluid shift from systemic to GI

Rao SSC, Parkman HP, McCallum RW, eds.
Handbook of Gastrointestinal Motility and Functional Disorders (pp 123-134).

circulation. Systemic symptoms of late DS are more related to a reactive hypoglycemia. Treatment for DS consists initially of dietary changes and behavioral modification. Guar gum, pectin, fiber, and acarbose may also help. Anticholinergics (eg, dicyclomine or hyoscamine) can inhibit gastric emptying, as well as reduce abdominal pain by decreasing small bowel contractility. Following that, for severe cases, octreotide (somatostatin) is an effective treatment by inhibiting gastric emptying, small bowel secretions, and modifying splanchnic blood flow. The clinical impact of DS is anticipated to increase, due to an increasing number of gastric bypass surgeries performed for obesity, the rising incidence of DM, and as the "idiopathic" subgroup of DS receives more recognition.

Introduction

Since first being described in 1913, DS has been associated with surgical procedures on the stomach and small bowel. In the mid-1900s, before *H pylori* was discovered to be the common etiology of chronic peptic ulcer disease, DS was an adverse effect of surgeries routinely performed for the treatment and management of peptic ulcer disease. These surgeries included vagotomy and pyloroplasty, as well as Billroth I and Billroth II gastric resections. DS, therefore received abundant attention in the literature at this time.

With the discovery of *H pylori* as the causative agent of peptic ulcer disease in the 1980s and the advent of medical treatments for this condition, the frequency of gastric surgery declined. This led to a decreased prevalence of DS by the end of the 20th century. However, it has remained a common complication of gastric surgeries performed for other reasons, and the incidence of surgical DS is once again climbing due to gastric bypass surgery. In addition, DM continues to be a nonsurgical cause of DS, and an increasing number of idiopathic cases are being described.[1,2]

Symptoms

In DS, chyme rapidly passes through the stomach; partially undigested food is literally "dumped" into the small intestines (see Figure 10-1 for an illustration of gastric emptying mechanics). The subsequent neural and hormonal responses triggered by this event explain many of the symptoms.

Symptoms of DS are classified as either early or late, although many patients present with both forms. Early DS, which is present in a majority of DS patients, begins in the first 30 minutes following a meal. Vasomotor sequelae may lead to flushing, fatigue, lightheadedness, confusion, diaphoresis, palpitations, tachycardia, and headache. Abdominal symptoms include early satiety, fullness, epigastric or diffuse pain, cramping, bloating, borborygmi, nausea, and diarrhea. Vomiting is infrequent and, when present, probably triggered by abdominal pain.

Late DS is characterized by symptoms that occur 1 to 3 hours postprandially. These symptoms include perspiration, decreased concentration, altered levels of consciousness, hunger, pallor, and even syncope. Late DS is mainly explained by a reactive hypoglycemia. As food rapidly enters the duodenum, the intestines secrete an increased amount of glucagon-like peptide 1 (GLP-1) and gastric inhibitory polypeptide (GIP), which causes an excessive release of insulin from the pancreas. This results in hypoglycemia 1 to 3 hours after the meal. Bloating may also occur in the

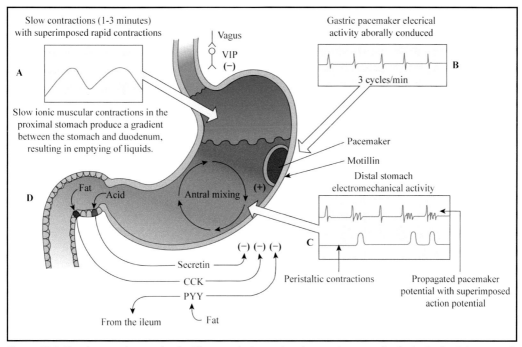

Figure 10-1. Gastric emptying mechanics. The area designated as the gastric pacemaker in the body of the stomach initiates slow wave impulses that travel toward the antrum. Food intake and hormones like motilin reinforce these impulses, increasing the likelihood that they achieve threshold voltages. Depolarization in this case causes smooth muscle contraction. A number of hormones released from the duodenum act to inhibit gastric contractions (secretin, cholecystokinin, peptide YY, and vasoactive intestinal polypeptide).

late phase as incompletely digested nutrients encounter colonic flora, which subsequently generates increased gas in the form of hydrogen and/or methane. Late DS may also include syncope.

Pathophysiology

Surgery

There are many etiologies of DS (Table 10-1). Surgical procedures that have been associated with DS include pyloroplasty, pyloromyotomy, antrectomy, and vagotomy. In the past, these surgeries were performed more frequently for complicated peptic ulcer disease. Each of these procedures has the potential to accelerate the transit of chyme through the stomach. A vagotomy inhibits the receptive relaxation of the gastric fundus following a meal and impairs pyloric contraction. Pyloroplasties and pyloromyotomies directly disrupt the inhibitory effect of the pylorus on gastric emptying. Antrectomies remove the inhibitory effects of both the pylorus and antrum, while significantly reducing gastric volume.

Other surgeries that lead to DS and are frequently performed in the current era include Nissen fundoplication, bariatric surgeries, and esophagectomy. Nissen fundoplication reduces the volume

TABLE 10-1 CAUSES OF DUMPING SYNDROME	
SURGICAL CAUSES	**NONSURGICAL CAUSES**
Roux-en-Y bypass	Diabetes mellitus
Nissen fundoplication	Cyclic vomiting syndrome
Vagotomy	Idiopathic
Esophagectomy	
Pyloroplasty	
Pylorectomy	
Antrectomy	
Gastrojejunostomy	

of the fundus that can accommodate ingestion, and thus promotes the rapid movement of contents to the antrum. In addition, accidental vagotomy, which may occur during the procedure, attributed to retraction, cautery, or entrapment in the wrap, can contribute to rapid gastric transit as previously described. Esophagectomy also involves transection of the vagus nerve. As for bariatric procedures, the Roux-en-Y bypass is the most common type in the United States. The goal of this procedure is to fashion a small gastric remnant; this gastric remnant is too small to accommodate a normal caloric load, thus limiting oral intake. However, the small pouch rapidly empties through the gastrojejunal anastomosis into the small bowel, inducing DS. Gastric bypass patients comprise an interesting population that experience DS, and as bypass surgeries become more frequent, working with this patient population will become increasingly important. Patients may initially view DS symptoms as favorable, since they contribute to weight loss. Thus, dietary counseling is very important to avoid malnutrition. It is estimated that with adequate dietary control, 85% of patients successfully adapt to their anatomy and volume limitations, leading to the resolution of symptoms by 18 months.[3]

Nonsurgical Etiologies

The importance of nonsurgical etiologies of DS is highlighted in a recent study from our research group that reviewed 223 gastric scintigraphy studies conducted at our tertiary gastrointestinal (GI) motility center in 2013. It was found that only 10% of patients with rapid gastric emptying had a surgical cause. On the other hand, 46.5% were diabetic, 31% had no identifiable cause (idiopathic), and 12.5% had cyclic vomiting syndrome (CVS).[1] One caveat, however, is that our university medical center does not have an established bariatric program.

Although long-standing DM is associated with gastroparesis, DM of shorter duration is thought to cause rapid gastric emptying.[5] This has been hypothesized to be due to early vagal damage, while over time with continued vagal and neuronal loss, gastroparesis may evolve. However, in our clinical practice we have not confirmed this concept, and we are finding rapid gastric emptying in all stages of DM.

CVS is also associated with rapid gastric emptying during the remission stage (when no vomiting is occurring). In one study, rapid gastric emptying was identified during this phase in 77% of patients.[6] Recent research from our team suggests that an elevated serum ghrelin level, found in CVS patients, mediates this effect.[7] Another theory focuses on impaired vagal function based

	TABLE 10-2
	HORMONES THAT MEDIATE DUMPING SYNDROME

HORMONE	PATHOPHYSIOLOGY
VIP	Dilates intestinal blood vessels, water and electrolyte secretion, increases bowel contractions
Serotonin	Dilates intestinal blood supply
Peptide YY	Unknown; elevated in DS, and direct infusion elicits symptoms
Bradykinin	Vasodilates intestinal and systemic blood vessels, increases blood vessel permeability
Norepinephrine	Mediates sympathetic symptoms
GLP-1	Synergistic effect stimulating the sympathetic nervous system; also stimulates insulin secretion and inhibits glucagon
GIP	Stimulates insulin secretion
Insulin	Causes reactive hypoglycemia in late DS

on decreased pancreatic polypeptide response to a "sham meal" test.[1] However, few of these CVS patients are symptomatic with DS.

The idiopathic subgroup of DS is not fully understood. One unifying concept may be that a gastroenteritis illness, suspected to be viral in origin, is the trigger. When questioned, almost half of idiopathic patients could identify such an illness heralding the onset of chronic dumping symptoms.[8] A possible sequelae of a viral GI illness could be damage to the duodenal mucosa and hence impairment of the duodenal receptors related to osmotic content, fat, and protein. Without the "braking" mechanism that these receptors induce, gastric emptying would be accelerated. However, in many idiopathic patients, no such history was elicited. Another theory is that the idiopathic group displays impaired vagal nerve function with loss of gastric accommodation to a meal and rapid movement to the antrum and small bowel.

Gastrointestinal Response to Rapid Gastric Transit

In early DS, rapid gastric transit causes a domino effect that explains the symptoms. During normal digestion, body fluids are shifted to the GI circulation and lumens, facilitating trituration and absorption. This is achieved by parasympathetic activation and GI hormone secretion in response to the presence of chyme in the intestines. In early DS, the large amount and hyperosmolar concentration of chyme that is rapidly expelled into the duodenum provides an unusually strong stimulus for both of these pathways. The resulting shift in fluid from general to GI circulation is so pronounced that systemic symptoms occur. Lightheadedness, pallor, headaches, confusion, and syncope are possible, with hypotension contributing in many cases. Some reflex sympathetic activation may also contribute to symptomatology, causing tachycardia and, if significant, palpitations. Abdominal symptoms such as pain, bloating, and cramping are attributable to abdominal distension, small bowel hyperactivity and hypercontractility, and increased gas production by colonic bacteria upon encountering partially digested chyme. Malabsorption also contributes to bloating, gas, and diarrhea.

Many hormones secreted from the GI tract have been shown to be elevated in patients with dumping symptoms when compared with normal subjects (Table 10-2). Examples that are important in early DS include vasoactive intestinal peptide (VIP) and serotonin.[9,10] Both of these hormones elevate in response to the presence of chyme in the intestines. VIP increases bowel contractions, dilates intestinal blood vessels, and secretes water and electrolytes into the intestinal lumen. These effects probably contribute to the fluid shift observed in DS, as well as to the rapid transit of the hyperosmolar chyme. Serotonin also dilates intestinal blood supply, and so may synergize with VIP. Interestingly, the most effective medical treatment for DS, octreotide (a somatostatin), antagonizes VIP and serotonin.

Late DS is mediated by a reactive hypoglycemia. Hormones such as GLP-1 and GIP, which stimulate the exaggerated release of insulin from the pancreas, are increased in late DS patients.[11] One to 3 hours after a meal, insulin levels are elevated out of proportion to counter regulatory mechanisms and glucose absorption from the GI tract—hypoglycemia prevails. Glucose levels can be less than 50 mg/dL at 2 to 3 hours in these patients based on glucose tolerance testing. Accompanying symptoms include confusion, headaches, weakness, palpitations, diaphoresis, and syncope.

EPIDEMIOLOGY

For surgical causes of DS, the incidence varies widely depending on the specific surgery performed. In general, 25% to 50% of all patients undergoing gastric surgery experience some of the symptoms of DS after surgery, with an increased risk for developing DS in females vs males. However, the symptoms tend to decrease over time as patients adapt with diet and behavior modification, and perhaps as "intestinal symbiosis" is achieved. Only 5% to 10% of patients describe their symptoms as significant, and 1% to 5% of patients report severe symptoms. The incidence of DS markedly decreased throughout the 1980s and 1990s due to the advent of medical therapies for peptic ulcer disease and the *H pylori* revolution, thus lessening the need for surgical treatment. However, DS continues to be a significant postoperative complication due to the continuing contribution from Nissen fundoplication and the increasing number of gastric bypass surgeries in the United States.[12]

In addition to surgical causes, DM and idiopathic DS contribute significantly to the current patient milieu that experiences DS. As the prevalence of DM2 continues to rise, it is likely that the number of Americans with DS will increase as well. The idiopathic subgroup is accounting for a larger proportion of the DS population as recognition of this new entity increases.

DIAGNOSIS

The Sigstad scoring system is helpful to diagnose DS (Table 10-3). A score over 7 is indicative of DS, while a score less than 4 makes DS unlikely. The Sigstad scoring system can also be used to monitor therapeutic success.

Diagnosis is based heavily on the clinical setting of postprandial symptomatology. In some cases, DS may be clinically indistinguishable from gastroparesis. In a recent study from our group, the incidence of rapid gastric transit and gastroparesis in patients referred to our tertiary motility center in 2013 was comparable.[4] Some clinical differentiation rests in the higher rate of nausea and vomiting in gastroparesis, and less severe abdominal pain than is present in DS. Diarrhea is also more frequent in DS. Due to the increasing prevalence of DM2, it is likely that the number of Americans with GI motility disorders will increase as well, and the necessity of distinguishing between these 2 entities will become an issue of increasing importance. Radionuclide scintigraphy is the crucial method to definitively distinguish between DS and gastroparesis.

Another diagnostic challenge is distinguishing between irritable bowel syndrome (IBS) and DS. Both processes include symptoms of abdominal pain, and the profound gastrocolic reflex occurring with DS mimics IBS. However, the systemic symptoms of DS should help to distinguish

TABLE 10-3

SIGSTAD SCORING SYSTEM

SYMPTOM	POINTS
Shock	5
Syncope, unconsciousness	4
Desire to lie down	4
Dyspnea	3
Weakness	3
Sleepiness, apathy	3
Palpitations	3
Restlessness	2
Dizziness	2
Headaches	1
Warm, clammy skin, pallor	1
Nausea	1
Fullness in abdomen	1
Borborygmi	1
Eructation	−1
Vomiting	−4
Score > 7 favors DS; score < 4 unlikely to be DS.	

between the two. Also, for diarrhea of unknown origin, DS would not be considered if bowel movements occur at night while fasting. Patients with IBS should be questioned regarding the Rome III diagnostic criteria of IBS. This criteria defines IBS as at least 3 months of episodic abdominal discomfort associated with a change in the consistency and frequency of stools. Relief of abdominal pain after defecation is also classic. Importantly, a diagnosis of IBS does not preclude concomitant DS.

Gastric emptying tests (GET) in the form of radionuclide scintigraphy are the gold standard for gastroenterologists to diagnose gastroparesis and DS. The standardized method involves the consumption of a scrambled egg substitute (equivalent to 2 large eggs) labeled with ^{99m}Tc sulphur-colloid, 2 slices of whole-wheat bread, and 120 mL of water. Anterior and posterior images of the stomach are taken immediately after eating, and then at 30 minutes and hourly for 4 hours (Figure 10-2). Gastric retention of gamma counts are calculated for each of the images, and the geometric mean is calculated. This method provides a concrete quantification of the magnitude of rapid emptying. Traditionally, rapid gastric emptying has been defined as < 35% isotope retention at 1 hour. Realistically, however, in the absence of other viable explanations for postprandial distress, < 50% retention at 1 hour may be a tenable explanation for the meal-driven symptoms. A gastric retention of < 20% at 2 hours may also be used for late DS. A practical way to approach analyzing a GET report is to never settle for a report of "no gastroparesis" or "normal gastric emptying." Personally reviewing the data is key to rule out rapid gastric emptying.

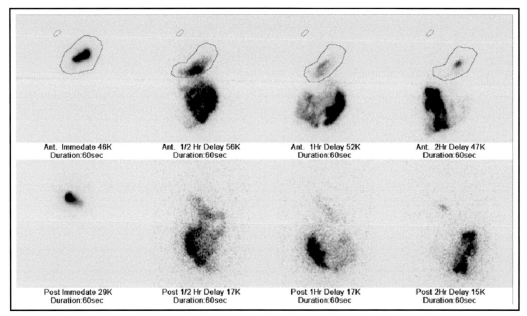

Ant. Immediate 46K Duration:60sec	Ant. 1/2 Hr Delay 56K Duration:60sec	Ant. 1Hr Delay 52K Duration:60sec	Ant. 2Hr Delay 47K Duration:60sec
Post Immedate 29K Duration:60sec	Post 1/2 Hr Delay 17K Duration:60sec	Post 1Hr Delay 17K Duration:60sec	Post 2Hr Delay 15K Duration:60sec

Figure 10-2. Gastric emptying test demonstrating rapid gastric emptying. Images were taken immediately after egg meal ingestion, at 30 minutes, 1 hour, and 2 hours. Anterior (above) and posterior (below) images are displayed. Note the decrease in gastric signal intensity beginning at 30 minutes, with increasing isotope signal coming from the small bowel over the course of the study.

The oral glucose challenge is also used to diagnose DS. It consists of a 10-hour (overnight) fast, followed by the ingestion of 50 g of glucose. Pulse and blood pressure are measured before, during, and after the exam in 30-minute intervals. The test is positive for DS if heart rate increases by 10 or more beats per minute. Hematocrit may also be measured; an increase of 3% in the first 30 minutes after ingestion indicates early DS. Hypoglycemia (glucose <60 mg/dL) 2 hours after ingestion is indicative of late DS. The oral glucose challenge test is 100% sensitive and 92% specific for DS.[13,14]

Other tests, such as endoscopy, barium studies with small bowel follow through, and abdominal ultrasound, are also performed both to understand the anatomy and to rule out other potential contributors to postprandial abdominal pain. For a diagnostic algorithm of DS, see Figure 10-3.

TREATMENT

Many effective techniques can be exploited to treat DS (see Table 10-4 for a summary of the treatment approach, and Figure 10-4 for a treatment algorithm). Lifestyle modification is the first line treatment for DS. Recommended changes include instituting a low-carbohydrate diet, favoring complex rather than simple carbohydrates, thereby decreasing chyme osmolarity. Protein and fat intake should be increased to compensate for and meet the caloric requirements of the body. Eating smaller and more frequent meals helps to decrease the volume of chyme, limiting abdominal symptoms. Consuming liquids 1 to 2 hours after meals reduces the gastric transit of meals. Another simple therapy is dietary fiber or Metamucil, which helps treat hypoglycemia. Dairy products have been found to exacerbate DS and should be avoided. Lying down for 30 minutes postprandially may be beneficial for those with vasomotor symptoms and is crucial in cases involving syncope. Many patients are able to alter diet to personal tastes and needs successfully, but when they cannot, other therapies exist.

Symptomatic treatment is an option. Treatment for diarrhea (eg, diphenoxylate), nausea (eg, promethazine), or antigas measures are helpful. Glucose tablets or hard candy at the onset of late

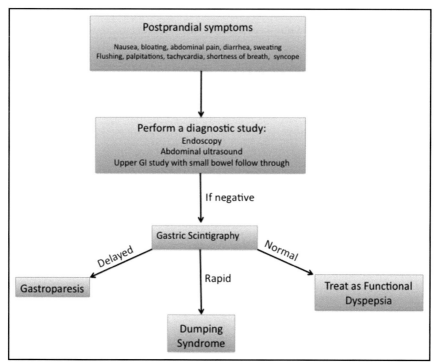

Figure 10-3. Diagnostic approach to dumping syndrome.

TABLE 10-4
TREATMENT APPROACH FOR DUMPING SYNDROME
DIETARY CHANGES
Diet low in carbohydrates, rich in fat and protein
Eat more, smaller meals
Separate solids and liquids
Fiber
LIFESTYLE CHANGES
Lie down for 30 minutes postprandially
MEDICATIONS
Metamucil
Guar gum
Pectin
Acarbose
Anticholinergics
Somatostatin analogues

Figure 10-4. Treatment approach to DS.

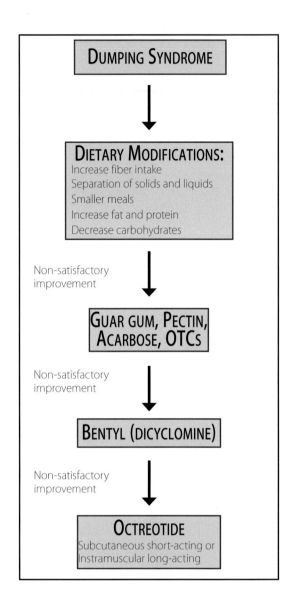

dumping symptoms may also abort symptoms. However, these treatments do not address the underlying mechanism.

Increasing the viscosity of the food to decrease the rate of gastric emptying can be achieved with Guar gum and pectin. Each is administered as 5 g doses 3 times a day (with meals). Pectin is a polysaccharide found in plant cell walls, and Guar gum is a water-soluble fiber. Guar gum, in particular, has also been used to treat DM because it regulates glucose levels and increases glucose tolerance. These effects may also be beneficial in late DS patients. Both are effective, but patients report poor taste, among other side effects. Consequently, patient compliance and satisfaction are often low.

Another treatment, acarbose, treats postprandial hypoglycemia effectively. Acarbose is an (alpha)-glycosidase inhibitor that interferes with the digestion of polysaccharides to monosaccharides at the brush border of the intestines.[15] This treatment helps resolve discomfort from the problematic absorption of carbohydrates that characterizes late DS. While it is successful in its role in preventing late DS, patients have reported some irritating GI side effects (bloating, diarrhea).

Anticholinergics (such as dicyclomine or hyoscamine) are the next major option. The main goal with these agents is to inhibit smooth muscle function, thus slowing gastric emptying and reducing contractility of the small bowel. Side effects are the sequelae of anticholingerics, including dry mouth, bladder retention, and glaucoma exacerbation. Bentyl (dicyclomine) is administered in 20- to 40-mg doses 30 minutes before the 3 main meals, and dosing can be titrated up if tolerated to gain more symptom control.

Octreotide is an option that can markedly improve quality of life, and therefore should be used for patients whose symptoms do not remit with the initial approaches that we have outlined. It is most effective at the onset of treatment, with most patients reporting dramatic improvement of symptoms at that time. However, some patients report diminishing benefit over several months. Octreotide is a somatostatin analog. It is a major inhibitor of gastric motility and slows both solid and liquid emptying.[16] It also inhibits insulin and blunts enteral hormone release (in particular, antagonizing VIP and serotonin). It contributes to vasomotor stability by decreasing postprandial splanchnic vasodilation.[17] Octreotide is administered in 50-mcg (25 to 100 mcg) doses subcutaneously 5 minutes before each meal. After initiating octreotide, dosing is adjusted to optimize the clinical response. Other agents (such as dicyclomine or hyoscamine) may still be used in the background to increase the efficacy, and may help decrease doses. Octreotide is also available in an intramuscular long-acting release (LAR) formula. The LAR formulation does not require frequent injections like subcutaneous octreotide does, and is therefore more convenient for patients. Thus, if subcutaneous octreotide is shown to be effective over the course of 1 to 2 months, a trial of LAR octreotide is justified. This option consists of a monthly injection of 20 or 40 mg of octreotide. However, during the latter weeks of the month, if efficacy becomes reduced, "back-up" subcutaneous injections may be necessary to restore symptom control for the whole month. From the studies that have been conducted, it appears that LAR octreotide is more effective in reducing DS symptoms. It may also cause greater weight gain.[18] Other possible side effects of octreotide include mild steatorrhea and gallstone formation. An abdominal ultrasound to asses for cholelithiasis is a good practice before starting octreotide.

Pasreotide (Novartis Pharmaceuticals) is the newest somatostatin analogue. Evidence suggests Pasreotide has greater potency with similar subcutaneous and intramuscular dosing strategies.

Surgical Treatment

The role of corrective surgery for DS is limited, although the idea could be entertained in the refractory setting depending on the initial surgery that resulted in DS. An example of a corrective surgery for DS is jejunal interposition surgery. This type of surgery has been proposed based on the concept of creating an iso- or antiperistaltic limb between the stomach and the jejunum,[19] delaying the transit of chyme from the stomach to the duodenum. However, these antiperistaltic or retrograde peristaltic limbs can also result in excessive retention. Realistically, surgery has not been meaningfully utilized in the clinical care of DS, although this theoretical approach is always discussed.

Conclusion

The causes of DS are varied, including gastric surgery, DM, and an idiopathic subgroup. Diagnosis is initially clinical, but a gastric scintigraphy study is mandatory for an accurate diagnosis, and an oral glucose challenge can also aid in diagnosis. Treatment should start conservatively with dietary modification and with options such as guar gum, acarbose, and anticholinergics.

Octreotide therapy is the final medical step and has all the credentials to address the pathophysiology of DS. In the future, the incidence of DS will likely increase due to bariatric surgery, to DM, and as idiopathic DS receives greater recognition. Familiarity with the syndrome is important to increase diagnostic and treatment efficacy.

REFERENCES

1. Hejazi HA, Patil H, McCallum RW. Dumping syndrome: Establishing criteria for diagnosis and identifying new etiologies. *Dig Dis Sci.* 2010;55:117-123.
2. Tack J, et al. Pathophysiology, diagnosis and management of postoperative dumping syndrome. *Nat Rev Gastroenter Hep.* 2009;6:583-590
3. Laurenius A, Olbers T, Naslund I, Karlsson J. Dumping syndrome following gastric bypass: Validation of the dumping symptom rating scale. *Obes Surg.* 2013;23(6):740-55. doi: 10.1007/s11695-012-0856-0.
4. Diaz JR, Bagherpour A, Reber J, et al. The increasing recognition of rapid gastric emptying by scintigraphy in patients referred to a tertiary center for suspected upper gastrointestinal motility disorder. Abstract submission to RSNA. 2014
5. Schwartz JG, et al. Rapid gastric emptying of a solid pancake meal in type II diabetic patients. *Diabetes Care.* 1996;19:468-71
6. Namin F, et al. Clinical, psychiatric and manometric profile of cyclic vomiting syndrome in adults and response to tricyclic therapy. *Neurogastroenterol Motil.* 2007;19:196-202.
7. Hejazi R, Lavenbarg T, McCallum R. Elevated serum ghrelin levels in adult patients with cyclic vomiting syndrome. *Am J Gastroenterol.* 2011;106(10):1858-9
8. Berg, P, Hall, M, Sarosiek, I, McCallum, R. Understanding the etiologies, clinical spectrum, and diagnostic challenge of dumping syndrome. *Gastroenterology.* 2013;144(5):S-734
9. Sagor GR, Bryant MG, Ghatei MA, Kirk R, Bloom SR. Release of vasoactive intestinal peptide in the dumping syndrome. *BMJ (Clin Res Ed).* 1981;282(6263):507-510.
10. Foxx-Orenstein A, Camilleria M, Stephens D, Burton D. Effect of a somatostaton analogue on gastric motor and sensory functions in healthy humans. *Gut.* 2003;52(11):1555–1561.
11. Yamamoto H, Mori T, Tsuchihashi H, et al. A possible role of GLP-1 in the pathophysiology of early dumping syndrome. *Dig Dis Sci.* 2005;50(12):2263-7.
12. Abell TL, Minocha A. Gastrointestinal complications of bariatric surgery: diagnosis and therapy. *Am J Med Sci.* 2006;331(4):214–218.
13. van der Kleij F, Vecht J, Lamers C, Masclee A. Diagnostic value of dumping provocation in patients after gastric surgery. *Scand J Gastroenterol.* 1996;31:1162–1166.
14. Ukleja A. Sumping Syndrome. *Practical Gastroenterology (UVA).* 2006;35:32-46.
15. Hasawega T, Yoneda M, Nakamura K, et al. Long-term effect of a-glucosidase inhibitor on late dumping syndrome. *J Gastroenterol and Hepatol.* 1998;13:1201–1206. doi: 10.1046/j.1440-1746.1998.01783.x
16. Hasler WL, Soudah HC, Owyang C. Mechanisms by which octreotide ameliorates symptoms in the dumping syndrome. *J Pharmacol Exp Ther.* 1996;277:1359–1365.
17. Li-Ling J, Irving M. Therapeutic value of octreotide for patients with severe dumping syndrome-a review of randomised controlled trials. *Postgrad Med J.* 2001;77(909):441-442. doi:10.1136/pmj.77.909.441.
18. Penning C, Vecht J, Masclee A. Efficacy of depot long-acting release octreotide therapy in severe dumping syndrome. *Aliment Pharmacol Ther.* 2005;22(10):963-9.
19. Vogel S, Hocking M, Woodward E. Clinical and radionuclide evaluation of Roux-Y diversion for postgastrectomy dumping. *Am J Surg.* 1988;155:57–62.

11

Cyclic Vomiting Syndrome

Thangam Venkatesan, MD and Erica A. Samuel, MD

KEY POINTS

- Cyclic vomiting syndrome (CVS) is a chronic functional disorder of unknown etiology and is characterized by stereotypic episodes of nausea and vomiting.

- CVS occurs in both children and adults and affects mostly whites in North America.

- Diagnosis is made with Rome III criteria in adults and North American Society for Pediatric Gastroenterology, Hepatology and Nutrition (NASPGHAN) criteria in children.

- CVS is associated with high rates of health care utilization and poor quality of life.

- Use of tricyclic antidepressants (TCAs) as prophylactic agents in adults and cyproheptadine in children < 5 years of age is effective in controlling symptoms.

DEFINITION

Cyclic vomiting syndrome (CVS) is a chronic functional disorder characterized by episodes of severe nausea and vomiting that alternate with symptom-free intervals.[1] Symptoms are often triggered by social stress; episodes can occur after the loss of a loved one, job-related stress, during exams, and even on vacations.[2] The etiology of CVS is not known, but several theories have been proposed, including genetic factors in children and marijuana use in adults. Patients also have many associated conditions, including a history of migraine and autonomic dysfunction and high rates of anxiety and depression.

While CVS is generally not life threatening, it is associated with significant morbidity. Many patients are often misdiagnosed as having viral gastroenteritis, gastroparesis, or even psychogenic vomiting given the lack of awareness in the medical community.[3] Approximately 20% of patients are subjected to surgical procedures such as cholecystectomies and appendectomies that fail to improve their symptoms. Affected adults also have multiple emergency department visits and hospitalizations for relief of symptoms, which pose a significant economic burden on limited health

Rao SSC, Parkman HP, McCallum RW, eds.
Handbook of Gastrointestinal Motility and Functional Disorders (pp 135-144).

care resources.[3] Prompt diagnosis, education about the disease, and treatment are essential and can reduce severity and frequency of episodes. This review on CVS will elucidate the epidemiology, historical perspective, clinical features, diagnosis, and available therapy in CVS and also provide a suggested algorithm for workup of recurrent vomiting.

HISTORY AND EPIDEMIOLOGY

Dr. Samuel Gee first described this syndrome in children in 1882 when he noted a pattern of "fitful vomiting in children."[4] He said, "These cases all seem to be of the same kind, their characteristic being fits of vomiting that recur after intervals of uncertain length. The intervals themselves are free from signs of disease. The vomiting continues for a few hours or days. When it has been severe the patients are left much exhausted."[4] Of interest, Charles Darwin, the noted scientist best known for his work on the theory of evolution, also seemed to have suffered from CVS, which spontaneously resolved in his 70s.[5] He also resorted to "water therapy" at the suggestion of his physician to no avail. The clinical description of CVS remains unchanged to the present day and is now characterized by the Rome III criteria.

CVS was initially thought to occur only in children, but it is now clear that CVS occurs in all age groups. It is also more common than originally thought; the estimated prevalence of CVS in children is 0.3% to 2.2%.[6] The incidence of CVS in Ireland (1.3 million children) was 3.15 cases per 100,000 children per year, which was much higher than expected. In a cross-sectional study of school-age children in Scotland, the prevalence was 1.9%.[7]

A similar study in Turkey of 1263 children aged 6 to 17 years showed a similar prevalence of 1.9%. To put this in perspective, the incidence of CVS is comparable to pediatric inflammatory bowel disease in Wisconsin.[8] The prevalence in adults is not known, and the absence of a unique diagnostic code for CVS hampers such a determination. In North America, CVS primarily affects Caucasians with a mean age of onset of 35 years in adults and 5 years in children.[9] There does not appear to be a clear gender predilection; some studies have identified a predominance of pediatric CVS in females and adult-onset CVS in males, although reports have been conflicting.[6]

CLINICAL FEATURES

The hallmark of CVS is a recurrent, stereotypical pattern of symptoms. Patients feel normal in between episodes, and symptoms frequently occur "out of the blue." Many patients report that episodes occur early in the morning, and some have noted a seasonal variation. Cyclic vomiting syndrome can be divided into 4 phases (Figure 11-1): the prodromal phase, the emetic phase, the recovery phase, and the asymptomatic phase, which was described by Fleisher et al.[10]

Phases of Cyclic Vomiting Syndrome

Episodes usually start with the prodromal phase, similar to those seen in migraine patients who will often have a premonition of an impending attack. Symptoms during this phase can include nausea, sweating, epigastric pain, fatigue, weakness, hot and cold flushes, shivering, intense thirst, loss of appetite, burping, lightheadedness, and paresthesias, and patients will describe an impending sense of doom. Patients also have symptoms of panic during this time and may have difficulty conversing. This phase can last from a few minutes to many hours and even days, and experts often prescribe the use of medications such as triptans, sedatives, and antiemetic agents to abort symptoms although there are no well-designed studies in CVS to support this approach. Patients can be tachycardic and hypertensive during an episode due to the adrenergic drive.

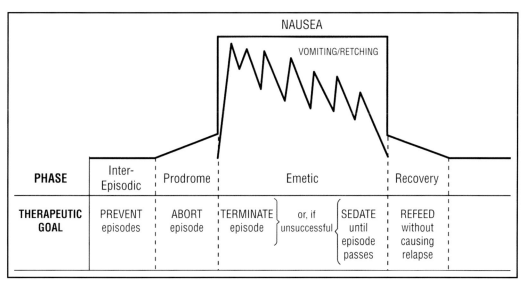

Figure 11-1. Phases of CVS. (Reprinted with permission from Fleisher DR, Gornowicz B, Adams K, et al. Cyclic vomiting syndrome in 41 adults: the illness, the patients, and problems of management. *BMC Medicine*. 2005; 3:20.)

The emetic phase is characterized by unrelenting nausea, retching, and vomiting in addition to the other gastrointestinal (GI) and autonomic symptoms. The frequency of vomiting can vary considerably from once every 2 hours to 20 times an hour or more. The majority of adults with CVS may experience significant abdominal pain, and this should not exclude a diagnosis of CVS. Other symptoms include hot sweats, chills, headache, photosensitivity, sensitivity to sounds, and diarrhea. Patients sometimes report an intense feeling of thirst and will often drink large amounts of water and subsequently vomit, called the "drinking and guzzling behavior." This appears to soothe their symptoms and should not be interpreted as being self-induced or as malingering. Patients often have altered consciousness during episodes that is frequently referred to as a "conscious coma," in which the patient is lethargic, listless, withdrawn, disoriented, and/or difficult to arouse. The patient can also seem very agitated and in a state of panic during an episode. A large proportion of patients report that extremely hot showers or baths alleviate their symptoms, at least temporarily, and this pattern of "compulsive hot water bathing" has been associated with marijuana use. In adults, the emetic phase typically lasts days; in children, it usually lasts hours to a couple of days.[11] Complications include dehydration, electrolyte abnormalities, Mallory-Weiss tears with subsequent GI bleeding, and very rarely esophageal perforation (Boerhaave syndrome) from the intense retching and vomiting.[12] This is followed by the recovery phase when patients return to baseline and are able to tolerate oral intake.

Triggers

Stressors are frequently responsible for triggering CVS episodes in both pediatric and adult populations.[13] Triggers can include infections, diet, lack of sleep, and psychological stressors, both positive and negative. Motion sickness and onset of menses have also been found to be trigger mechanisms.[12]

Subcategories of Cyclic Vomiting Syndrome

Subcategories of CVS have been identified, including CVS plus, catamenial CVS, and Sato's variant of CVS.[14] CVS plus is defined by the presence of at least 2 or more neuromuscular disease manifestations, including cognitive disorders, skeletal myopathy, cranial nerve dysfunction, and seizure disorders. Children with CVS plus are more likely to present at an earlier age and have dysautonomia-related disorders such as migraine, chronic fatigue, and neurovascular dystrophy.[15] Catamenial CVS coincides with a menstrual cycle, and the Sato's variant of CVS was described in children who presented with emesis, hypertension, and depression. With attacks, they were found to have transient hyperglycemia and glycosuria; elevated plasma adrenocorticotropic hormone (ACTH), cortisol, and urinary 17-OHCS excretion; and low plasma osmolality with hyponatremia.[14]

Comorbid Conditions

Adults with CVS have multiple comorbid conditions such as irritable bowel syndrome in 28%, anxiety in 47%, depression in 44%, migraine in 48%, syncope in 36%, photophobia in 29%, and other conditions including attention deficit disorder (ADHD), chronic fatigue syndrome, and seizures.[16] In a prospective study of 20 patients with CVS, 90% had impairment of the sympathetic nervous system with sudomotor dysfunction, postural tachycardia, or both.[17] These findings were validated by another study by McCallum et al. The study also confirmed that the majority of patients (57%) had rapid gastric emptying, which has been associated with autonomic dysfunction.[18] This significant burden of coexistent illness should be borne in mind when treating these patients.

Natural History of Symptoms

In a series of 88 children with CVS, 27% developed migraine headaches with cessation of vomiting, 7% evolved into abdominal migraine, and the majority (65%) became asymptomatic and outgrew their symptoms completely with time. Pediatric patients who develop symptoms later in childhood may have a shorter duration of CVS symptoms.[19]

The natural history of CVS in adults is not known, but approximately 40% of patients lose the typical periodicity and can develop interepisodic nausea and dyspepsia over time, which is referred to as "coalescent CVS" by experts in the field.[10] A careful history and assessment of the patient's symptoms can aid in making an accurate diagnosis, as all patients will have the classic "on-off" pattern at symptom onset.

PATHOPHYSIOLOGY

The pathophysiology of CVS is unknown, and both environmental and genetic factors seem to play a role. Pedigree analysis by Boles et al in 80 subjects (mostly children) with CVS revealed a clustering of various functional conditions such as migraine, depression, irritable bowel, and hypothyroidism in over 50% of matrilineal relatives vs. patrilineal relatives. Subsequent studies in children sequencing the mitochondrial genome in Haplogroup H individuals by the same author revealed a significant association between CVS and two mitochondrial DNA single-nucleotide polymorphisms (mt DNA SNPs) 16519 T and 3010A. The presence of both these SNPs was associated with 17-fold increased odds of having CVS. A similar study was then performed in children and adults with CVS, but adults with CVS did not have the mitochondrial SNPs of interest. The authors concluded that CVS might be biologically different based on onset of symptoms. However, the same study also revealed that adults with CVS had high Karolinska Scales of Personality (KSP) scores, which are both sensitive and specific for mitochondrial dysfunction, findings not reconciled by their study results. One possible explanation for this may be the presence of yet unidentified mitochondrial DNA polymorphisms. With the availability of next-generation sequencing, future studies examining the entire mitochondrial and nuclear

TABLE 11-1
ROME III CRITERIA FOR THE DIAGNOSIS OF CYCLIC VOMITING SYNDROME IN ADULTS
1. Stereotypical episodes of vomiting regarding onset (acute) and duration (less than 1 week)
2. Three of more discrete episodes in prior year
3. Absence of nausea and vomiting between episodes
4. No metabolic, gastrointestinal or CNS structural or biochemical disorders
* Must have for at least 3 months with onset at least 6 months previous

genome will shed light on this important question of whether mitochondrial DNA polymorphisms contribute to symptoms of CVS.

Emerging research also points to brain-gut interactions as a possible mechanism. CVS is often triggered by emotional stress, suggesting a central mechanism causing symptoms. Preliminary functional magnetic resonance imaging (MRI) studies of patients have shown significant differences in functional connectivity of the nausea network between CVS patients and healthy controls following emotional stress.[20] That stress plays a major role is also supported by recent data showing an increase in salivary cortisol levels during a CVS episode versus the asymptomatic/well phase.[21] Median salivary cortisol levels were also significantly higher during an episode compared to the well phase, with no differences between controls and the well phase in patients.[21]

There is also a considerable amount of interest in the role of marijuana in patients with this condition. A large proportion of CVS patients (approximately 40%) use marijuana for CVS symptoms. A recent survey of 437 patients who used marijuana reported improvement in nausea, vomiting, appetite, general well-being, and stress levels.[22] However, a retrospective study of 98 patients with prior marijuana use was associated with cyclic vomiting. Specific data on marijuana use were available only in 37 patients. Of this subset of patients, chronic daily marijuana use was associated with the "compulsive hot water bathing pattern." Follow-up data of 1 to 3 months were available only in 10 patients.[23] These findings need to be reconciled with the antiemetic effects of cannabinoid agonists in both animal models and use of marinol in humans. The dose of tetrahydrocannabinol (THC) and the exact mechanism of action of phytocannabinoids in nausea and vomiting need to be elucidated in future studies.

The endocannabinoid system consists of 2 endogenous ligands, N-arachidonylethanolamine and 2-arachidonoylglycerol (2-AG); 2 G-protein-coupled cannabinoid receptors (CB1 and CB2); and related synthetic and degradation enzymes. The endocannabinoid system has an important role in modulation of stress as well as nausea and vomiting.[24] Cannabinoid agonists and synthetic delta-9-THC such as nabilone and dronabinol have been used as antiemetics in the past.[25] In a pilot study of CVS, anadamide and 3 closely related compounds called N-acylethanolamines (NAEs), N-oleoylethanolamine (OEA), and N-palmitoylethanolamine (PEA) were significantly increased during an episode vs. the well phase. N-acylethanolamine concentrations were not different between patients in the well phase and controls.[21] Future studies exploring the role of the endocannabinoid system in nausea and vomiting are warranted.

> ### TABLE 11-2
> ## NASPGHAN CRITERIA FOR THE DIAGNOSIS OF CYCLIC VOMITING SYNDROME IN CHILDREN
>
> 1. At least 5 episodes, or a minimum of 3 over a 6-month period
>
> 2. Episodic attacks of intense nausea and vomiting that lasts 1 hour to 10 days, occurring at least 1 week apart
>
> 3. Stereotypical pattern and symptoms in the individual patient
>
> 4. Vomiting during episodes occurs at least 4 times an hour for at least 1 hour
>
> 5. A return to baseline health during episodes
>
> 6. Not attributed to another disorder

DIAGNOSIS

Currently, the diagnosis of CVS is based on clinical criteria. There is no specific test or biomarker that can diagnose it. A cyclic pattern of vomiting is key in the diagnosis. The Rome III working group has developed criteria for the diagnosis of CVS in adults (Table 11-1).[14] The North American Society for Pediatric Gastroenterology, Hepatology and Nutrition (NASPGHAN) guidelines for the diagnosis of CVS in children were formulated, as the Rome criteria were not appropriate in children. The NASPHAGN guidelines also emphasize a stereotypical pattern and asymptomatic interepisodic period, but they also define the episodes more specifically (Table 11-2).[26] While Rome III criteria are used in clinical practice, their diagnostic accuracy remains to be proven. For instance, the criteria specify that episodes should last less than a week when in fact patients can sometimes have much longer episodes based on experience. This underscores the need for further research into the mechanism of CVS and development of better diagnostic tools.

Most patients with CVS undergo extensive investigations for their symptoms, and the optimal workup for patients has not been evaluated. It is the practice of most experts to perform at least an upper endoscopy and a small bowel follow-through/computed tomography (CT) scan to exclude gastric and small bowel pathology that can mimic CVS. Algorithm for workup of episodic vomiting is depicted in Figure 11-2. If patients have underlying diabetes mellitus, a gastric emptying study can be useful, although the pattern of vomiting differs in these patients. NASPGHAN guidelines recommend that children with cyclic vomiting be evaluated for a possible metabolic or neurological disorder if any of the following conditions are met: presentation at less than 2 years of age, vomiting episodes associated with intercurrent illnesses, prior fasting or increased protein intake, and any neurological findings such as ataxia, dystonia, gait disturbance, mental retardation, seizure disorders, or acute encephalopathy.[26]

Patients with neurological disorders or focal neurological signs may need further evaluation with an MRI of the head to exclude structural abnormalities such as intracerebral tumors, hydrocephalus, Chiari malformation, or a subdural hematoma. Patients with CVS can also present with other intercurrent illnesses such as appendicitis or biliary disorders and must be evaluated carefully upon presentation to ensure that the episode is consistent with their usual CVS flare. If there is clinical suspicion for any other intra-abdominal emergency, workup should be pursued as indicated.

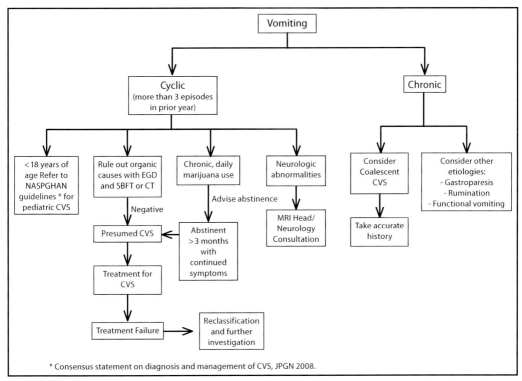

Figure 11-2. Diagnostic algorithm for CVS.

TREATMENT

A multidisciplinary approach based on a biopsychosocial model is imperative to the successful treatment of a patient with CVS. In addition to pharmacotherapy, adequate reassurance and addressing stressors that trigger episodes are crucial. Treatment of CVS can be divided into 3 categories: 1) prophylactic, 2) abortive, and 3) supportive (Table 11-3).

Prophylactic treatment is typically initiated during the interepisodic well phase. It can include lifestyle modifications aimed at avoidance of triggers, such as sleep deprivation, stress, and certain foods. Prophylactic therapy should be considered in patients with severe and frequent symptoms. TCAs are first-line therapy, although the mechanism of action is unknown. In an open-label study of 41 patients, amitriptyline resulted in an overall subjective improvement in 80% of patients. A prospective open-label study of TCAs in CVS found that 87% of CVS patients responded to therapy with a significant reduction in the number of emergency department visits and hospitalizations over 2 years.[27] Nonresponders were more likely to have a history of migraine headaches, coexisting psychological disorders, chronic marijuana use, and opiate use.[28] In a retrospective review of 101 adult patients with CVS, 86% were found to respond to a prophylactic medication regimen of amitriptyline and/or topiramate and mitochondrial supplements. Nonresponse was associated with noncompliance, chronic marijuana use, coalescence of symptoms, chronic opiate use, severity of disease, and disability, but only noncompliance was a significant factor on multivariate analysis. Doses of TCAs that are effective in CVS are typically higher than those used for other functional GI disorders, and 1mg/kg in children and 80 to 100 mg/daily in adults have been effective. Medications are typically administered at night, as daytime sedation is a frequent

Table 11-3

Medications Used in the Treatment of Cyclic Vomiting Syndrome

MEDICATION	DOSAGE	SIDE EFFECTS	SPECIAL CONSIDERATIONS
Prophylactic Therapies			
Tricyclic Antidepressants			
Amitriptyline/ Nortriptyline	80 to 100 mg/ daily	Drowsiness, weight gain	Regular monitoring of QT interval
Supplements			
Coenzyme Q10	200 mg bid	Elevated liver function tests	
L-carnitine	100/mg/kg/day divided bid	Fishy odor	
Anticonvulsants			
Topiramate	100 mg bid	Acidosis, nephrolithiasis	Basic metabolic panel every 6 months
Zonisamide	400 mg daily	Somnolence, muscle weakness	
Antihistamine			
Cyproheptadine	0.25 to 0.5mg/kg/ day tid or qhs	Drowsiness, dry mouth, weight gain	Use as first line in children <5 years
Abortive Therapies			
Triptans			
Sumatriptan	Nasal spray		Contraindicated in CAD
Zolmitriptan	Nasal spray		Contraindicated in CAD
Antiemetics			
Ondansetron	8 mg every 6 hours prn	QT prolongation	Regular monitoring of QT interval
Promethazine	25 mg every 6 hours prn	Drowsiness, dry mouth	
Aprepitant	1 kit (125 mg/80 mg/80 mg)	Fatigue	

bid: twice daily; tid: three times daily; qhs: every night at bedtime; CAD: coronary artery disease; prn: as needed.

* All of the medications are off-label uses.

side effect. Monitoring of the QT interval is also suggested in these patients given the small risk of cardiac arrhythmias. Other medications shown to be effective include anticonvulsants such as Zonegran (zonisamide), Keppra (levetiracetam), and topiramate.[29] Mitochondrial treatment such as coenzyme Q10,[30] riboflavin, and carnitine[31] was beneficial in a small retrospective study. Future double-blind, therapeutic, placebo-controlled trials are warranted in CVS to determine optimal therapy.

The antimigraine medications called triptans have been found to be effective in aborting CVS attacks. In a study of adult patients with both adult- and pediatric-onset CVS, 89% responded to intranasal administration of triptans.[32] During an episode, supportive treatment may include sedation, hydration, antiemetics, and analgesics. Sedation with lorazepam and/or diphenhydramine is frequently used. Analgesics with opioids may be necessary to control abdominal pain if present during the attack. Intravenous (IV) fluids are used to prevent dehydration. Anecdotally, IV fluids containing 10% dextrose have been thought to be more effective, although prospective data are lacking. Experts also recommend abstinence from chronic marijuana use, as this seems to be associated with nonresponse to treatment. However, the role of marijuana in CVS needs further study given that cannabinoid agonists are antiemetic, but chronic heavy marijuana appears to perpetuate vomiting episodes. A subset of CVS frequently utilizes the emergency department, and emergency medicine physicians play a critical role in their care. Appropriate referral and early recognition of the pattern of symptoms may prevent future episodes.[3]

CONCLUSION

CVS is a chronic functional disorder associated with stereotypic episodes of nausea, vomiting, and abdominal pain with a return to normalcy once an episode has been terminated. This usually afflicts children and young adults and may be more common than once thought. There is unfortunately a significant delay in diagnosis, with patients being subjected to extensive investigations and even unnecessary surgery. Prompt diagnosis and treatment with TCAs for prophylaxis are recommended. Other medications such as coenzyme Q10, carnitine, and riboflavin targeted at mitochondrial function may also be used as preventive therapy. Abortive medications such as nasal triptans and antiemetics may be used in the prodromal phase. Patients are also advised about marijuana cessation, as marijuana use appears to worsen symptoms. Other comorbid conditions such as anxiety, depression, and autonomic dysfunction need to be addressed. Cyclic vomiting syndrome takes a significant toll on both patients and families, and about 20% of patients are disabled. CVS sufferers and their families may avail of services offered by voluntary, nonprofit organizations such as the Cyclic Vomiting Syndrome Association and the International Foundation for Functional GI Disorders, which provide support for patients and families. Studies that explore the pathogenesis of this disorder should provide an avenue for the development of better treatment in the future.

REFERENCES

1. Drossman DA. The functional gastrointestinal disorders and the Rome III process. *Gastroenterology*. 2006;130:1377-1390.
2. Kumar N, Bashar Q, Reddy N, et al. Cyclic vomiting syndrome (CVS): is there a difference based on onset of symptoms: pediatric versus adult? *BMC Gastroenterol*. 2012;12:52.
3. Venkatesan T, Tarbell S, Adams K, et al. A survey of emergency department use in patients with cyclic vomiting syndrome. *BMC Emerg Med*. 2010;10:4.
4. Gee S. On fitful or recurrent vomiting. *St. Bart Hosp Rep*. 1882;18:1-6.

5. Hayman J. Charles Darwin's mitochondria. *Genetics.* 2013;194:21-25.

6. Li BU, Misiewicz L. Cyclic vomiting syndrome: a brain-gut disorder. *Gastroenterol Clin North Am.* 2003;32:997-1019.

7. Abu-Arafeh I, Russell G. Cyclical vomiting syndrome in children: a population-based study. *J Pediatr Gastroenterol Nutr.* 1995;21:454-458.

8. Kugathasan S, Judd RH, Hoffmann RG, et al. Epidemiologic and clinical characteristics of children with newly diagnosed inflammatory bowel disease in Wisconsin: a statewide population-based study. *J Pediatr.* 2003;143:525-531.

9. Venkatasubramani N, Venkatesan T, Li B. Extreme emesis: cyclic vomiting syndrome. *Practical Gastroenterol.* 2007;34:21-34.

10. Fleisher DR, Gornowicz B, Adams K, Burch R, Feldman EJ. Cyclic vomiting syndrome in 41 adults: the illness, the patients, and problems of management. *BMC Med.* 2005;3:20.

11. Prakash C, Clouse RE. Cyclic vomiting syndrome in adults: clinical features and response to tricyclic antidepressants. *Am J Gastroenterol.* 1999;94:2855-2860.

12. Prakash C, Staiano A, Rothbaum RJ, Clouse RE. Similarities in cyclic vomiting syndrome across age groups. *Am J Gastroenterol.* 2001;96:684-688.

13. Pareek N, Fleisher DR, Abell T. Cyclic vomiting syndrome: what a gastroenterologist needs to know. *Am J Gastroenterol.* 2007;102:2832-2840.

14. Sato T, Igarashi N, Minami S, et al. Recurrent attacks of vomiting, hypertension and psychotic depression: a syndrome of periodic catecholamine and prostaglandin discharge. *Acta Endocrinologica.* 1988;117:189-197.

15. Boles RG, Powers AL, Adams K. Cyclic vomiting syndrome plus. *J Child Neurol.* 2006;21:182-188.

16. Boles RG, Zaki EA, Lavenbarg T, et al. Are pediatric and adult-onset cyclic vomiting syndrome (CVS) biologically different conditions? Relationship of adult-onset CVS with the migraine and pediatric CVS-associated common mtDNA polymorphisms 16519T and 3010A. *Neurogastroenterol Motility.* 2009;21:936-e72.

17. Venkatesan T, Prieto T, Barboi A, et al. Autonomic nerve function in adults with cyclic vomiting syndrome: a prospective study. *Neurogastroenterol Motility.* 2010;22:1303-1307, e339.

18. Lawal A, Barboi A, Krasnow A, Hellman R, Jaradeh S, Massey BT. Rapid gastric emptying is more common than gastroparesis in patients with autonomic dysfunction. *Am J Gastroenterol.* 2007;102:618-623.

19. Li BU, Balint JP. Cyclic vomiting syndrome: evolution in our understanding of a brain-gut disorder. *Adv Pediatr.* 2000;47:117-60.

20. Samuel EB, Kern A, Siwiec M, Patel R, Nencka A, Hyde A, Venkatesan J, Shaker, T. Resting and guided thinking state functional connectivity of the nausea network in cyclic vomiting syndrome: the effect of emotional stress. *Gastroenterol Hepatol.* 2013;144:661.

21. Venkatesan T, Samuel E, Kumar N, et al. The endocannabinoid system and the hypothalamic-pituitary-adrenal axis in adults with cyclic vomiting syndrome. *Gastroenterol Hepatol.* 2013;144:S-924.

22. Venkatesan T LA, Sengupta J, Schroeder A. Marijuana and hot shower use in patients with cyclic vomiting syndrome. *Conference Proceedings: Biology and Control of Nausea and Vomiting.* 2013;62.

23. Simonetto DA, Oxentenko AS, Herman ML, Szostek JH. Cannabinoid hyperemesis: a case series of 98 patients. *Mayo Clinic Proceedings. Mayo Clinic.* 2012;87:114-119.

24. Strewe C, Feuerecker M, Nichiporuk I, et al. Effects of parabolic flight and spaceflight on the endocannabinoid system in humans. *Rev Neurosci.* 2012;23:673-680.

25. Parker LA, Rock EM, Limebeer CL. Regulation of nausea and vomiting by cannabinoids. *Br J Pharmacol.* 2011;163:1411-1422.

26. Li BU, Lefevre F, Chelimsky GG, et al. North American Society for Pediatric Gastroenterology, Hepatology, and Nutrition consensus statement on the diagnosis and management of cyclic vomiting syndrome. *J Pediatr Gastroenterol Nutr.* 2008;47:379-393.

27. Hejazi RA, Reddymasu SC, Namin F, Lavenbarg T, Foran P, McCallum RW. Efficacy of tricyclic antidepressant therapy in adults with cyclic vomiting syndrome: a two-year follow-up study. *J Clin Gastroenterol.* 2010;44:18-21.

28. Hejazi RA, Lavenbarg TH, Foran P, McCallum RW. Who are the nonresponders to standard treatment with tricyclic antidepressant agents for cyclic vomiting syndrome in adults? *Alimentary Pharmacol Ther.* 2010;31:295-301.

29. Clouse RE, Sayuk GS, Lustman PJ, Prakash C. Zonisamide or levetiracetam for adults with cyclic vomiting syndrome: a case series. *Clin Gastroenterol Hepatol.* 2007;5:44-48.

30. Boles RG, Lovett-Barr MR, Preston A, Li BU, Adams K. Treatment of cyclic vomiting syndrome with co-enzyme Q10 and amitriptyline, a retrospective study. *BMC Neurol.* 2010;10.

31. Van Calcar SC, Harding CO, Wolff JA. L-carnitine administration reduces number of episodes in cyclic vomiting syndrome. *Clinical Pediatr.* 2002;41:171-174.

32. Kumar N, Kumar G, Schroeder A, Hogan WJ, Venkatesan T. Efficacy of nasal triptans as abortive therapy in adults with cyclic vomiting syndrome: a tertiary care experience. *Gastroenterology.* 2011;140:S463-S463.

Rumination Syndrome

Chad J. Cooper, MD; Joseph K. Sunny, Jr, MD;
and Richard W. McCallum, MD, FACP, FRACP (AUST), FACG, AGAF

KEY POINTS

- Rome III consensus criteria for rumination syndrome in adults are used for clinical diagnosis of rumination syndrome.

- Rumination syndrome in adults can be primary, where a very stressful setting is a trigger, or conditioned vomiting, where underlying gastroparesis is present.

- Rumination syndrome is a clinical diagnosis relying on a detailed history to identify the unique timing and characteristics of the event.

- Upper gastrointestinal manometry has shown a simultaneous pressure wave (R wave) pattern associated with a rumination episode. Esophageal high-resolution/impedance can be used to demonstrate that regurgitation begins in the stomach and ascends into the esophagus and can be followed by reswallowing.

- The mainstay of therapy for adult rumination syndrome is teaching diaphragmatic breathing distraction and relaxation therapies along with reassurance, education, and diet.

- Nutrition support, fluid, electrolyte, and micronutrient needs during therapy may require an enteral tube placement.

DEFINITION

Rumination is part of the normal digestive process in animals such as goats, sheep, and cattle. Rumination syndrome is used to describe this digestive behavior in humans and is defined as the act of regurgitating partially digested food, with the outcome of either subsequent reswallowing or vomiting of the food.

Rao SSC, Parkman HP, McCallum RW, eds.
Handbook of Gastrointestinal Motility and Functional Disorders (pp 145-155).
© 2015 Taylor & Francis Group.

INTRODUCTION

Rumination syndrome was first described in the 17th century by Edouard Brown-Sequard, who acquired the condition while swallowing sponges tied to a string for evaluation of the gastric pH.[1] He therefore acquired the learned behavior of regurgitating the sponge. Eventually, he developed habitual regurgitation of food within minutes of intake. This situation more fits the entity of "conditioned" vomiting—a learned skill—and a term that is interchangeable with pure rumination, but the clinical settings where they occur are different.

According to the Rome III consensus criteria for rumination syndrome, the patient must have painless, repetitive bouts of regurgitation with either expulsion or rechewing and subsequent swallowing of the regurgitated food.[2] This act of regurgitation occurs immediately after ingestion of a meal—within 20 minutes, but sometimes less than 5 minutes. Other key characteristics are the lack of preceding nausea or retching; no occurrence during sleep; no response to therapy for gastroesophageal reflux; and no evidence of inflammatory, metabolic, anatomic, or neoplastic explanations and symptoms persisting for at least 3 to 6 months.

The typical "clinical setting," however, includes more than this idealistic "textbook" description implies. The effortless regurgitation of gastric contents begins within minutes of intake, includes liquids or solids (although solids are more predictable), and can intermittently persist for up to 1 to 2 hours. Even a glass of water can trigger this reflex. Rumination occurs every day and with every meal. The stomach is "programmed," and the patient essentially has no control over this reflex. The regurgitated material is recognizable food, and it is often preceded by a period of belching and burping of air. Nausea can be in the picture later on, but it does not generally occur before this effortless and abrupt regurgitation event. The patient can make a conscious decision as to whether to swallow or spit out the regurgitated material. The decision to swallow the food is usually influenced by the patient's social situation: reswallowing allows time to retreat to a safe setting to vomit the recently ingested contents. Patients can return and continue activities and conversations while in no apparent distress. The patient recognizes the regurgitated gastric contents, often with a pleasant taste initially, but a burning sensation from the accompanying gastric acid may develop as reswallowing begins—hence, the possible confusion with the spectrum of gastroesophageal reflux. Another common complaint is abdominal pain, and this is explained by the fact that the rectus abdominus muscles are contracting with each regurgitation. The consequences of ongoing rumination include weight loss, dehydration, electrolyte disturbances, malnutrition, halitosis, dental decay, disability, and social aversion.

EPIDEMIOLOGY

Rumination syndrome was first described in infants, children, and mentally handicapped individuals. The prevalence of rumination in mentally handicapped individuals is 6% to 10%.[3,4] However, rumination syndrome in adults with normal intelligence is now being increasingly recognized. The epidemiology of rumination syndrome in the adult population has not been determined.[5] Rumination syndrome is likely more prevalent than it appears, and adequate knowledge of this syndrome among physicians is necessary to even consider the possibility of this diagnosis and initiate early intervention.[6] The embarrassing nature of rumination can prevent patients from seeking medical attention sooner. Rumination syndrome is more prevalent in young adults, and females are more commonly affected than males. The prevalence of rumination is higher in patients diagnosed with bulimia nervosa. O'Brien et al observed that 17% of female patients with rumination syndrome also had a history of bulimia.[7] Therefore, in a minority, this entity could be further classified as an atypical eating disorder by psychiatrists, but this is not the case in the majority, where patients are of normal weight or even overweight. Therefore, confusion could exist in classifying this disorder as a variant of bulimia nervosa or an atypical eating disorder. The personality of ruminators is generally not one of obsession about food and weight control. These patients suffer a significant amount of functional disability with absence from work or school, frequent hospitalizations, and emergency department visits and are motivated to seek treatment. The weight loss is mainly related to avoiding embarrassing social settings by electing not to eat. The reliance on small liquid volumes can lead to dehydration concerns, and hypokalemia can be in the background.

PATHOPHYSIOLOGY

The etiology and pathophysiology of rumination syndrome in humans are not fully understood. No genetic association has been established. Rumination is believed to be an unconscious learned disorder involving the voluntary relaxation of the diaphragm combined with contraction of the abdominal muscles. Patients with what is termed *"primary" rumination syndrome* have a predictable "trigger" from their social/psychological setting—for example, increased stress at work, divorce, marriage, graduating or starting at a new school, new jobs, loss of job, relocations, death or illness in the family—the timing of these events and onset of rumination is key. In the subset where there is suspicion that rumination is a technique to control their weight, bulimia is an overlap. Depression has been noted in more than 25% of patients after a formal psychiatric evaluation.[19] Attri et al[8] found that 67% of patients in their study had a stressful life situation such as loss of a family member, career setback, or financial problems. One-third of patients also had psychological problems such as anxiety, depression, or obsessive-compulsive disorder.

The other subgroup—termed *"conditional" vomiting*—has a background of a gastrointestinal illness such as an established diagnosis of gastroparesis, dyspepsia, and nausea, or a cholecystectomy preceded by nausea and vomiting. In the setting of gastroparesis, which we commonly see in our practice, the vomiting initially occurred more than 1 to 2 hours postprandially. Then this pattern changes to within a few minutes of eating. In gastroparesis patients, this immediate vomiting is a learned condition in an effort to prevent or relieve their symptoms of bloating, nausea, and discomfort, which invariably have been present following meals. Immediate regurgitation literally aborts this sequence. In this "conditioned" subset, background nausea is common and may be continuous. A stressful event may also be identified as the trigger explaining the change in timing of their vomiting. In both primary ruminators and conditioned vomiting, seeing food, smelling food, and beginning to eat food are the triggers for the reflex. Their stomachs are trapped and programmed. The patient is powerless to prevent the outcome. Hence, essentially every meal every day is the story, which can include medications taken with water.

MECHANISM

Rumination is believed to be a learned adaptation of the belch reflex. The forward extension of the head is used to open the upper esophageal sphincter. Food is initially stored in the fundus and proximal stomach, a property referred to as receptive relaxation and accommodation. The requirement for the regurgitation of gastric contents during straining is a lower esophageal sphincter (LES) pressure that is lower than the generated intragastric pressure. This low LES pressure could be intrinsically present or periodically reduced during events termed *postprandial transient LES relaxation*.[9] The force of retropulsion of gastric contents, which are located immediately adjacent to the LES through the esophagus into the oropharynx, is thought to originate in the abdominal

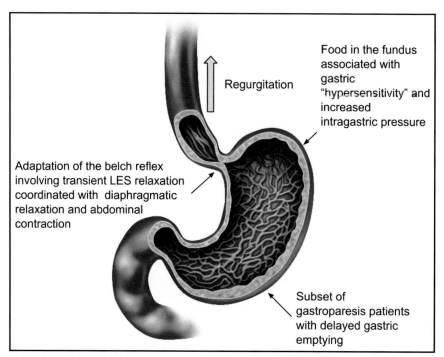

Figure 12-1. Pathophysiology.

compartment from the increased intra-abdominal and/or intragastric pressure. This could occur if there is simultaneous relaxation of the LES combined with increased intra-abdominal pressure at the same time. This allows an increase of intragastric hydrostatic pressure and normal contraction of the proximal stomach that can overcome the resistance to regurgitation at the level of the gastroesophageal junction.[10] The force and speed of the regurgitated material are enough to overcome the protective mechanism of secondary peristalsis. Another explanation is that the secondary peristalsis is inhibited through the same learned process that results in the inhibition of the LES. The patients are unaware that they are straining or contracting their abdominal muscles, although this explains their complaints of epigastric pain. The preceding belching can be regarded as a "warm-up" or rehearsal to transition from air to gastric contents. In the primary cases, there is normal gastric emptying, and after more than 30 minutes, the food has been moved into the distal body and antrum. Therefore, the "effortless, fountain-like regurgitation" when the food is located near the LES is not then possible.

Sensorimotor dysfunction of the proximal stomach has been proposed as another theory for rumination syndrome, specifically increased gastric sensitivity to mechanical stimulation (Figure 12-1). Rumination patients had greater nausea, bloating, and aggregate symptom scores, but not pain, compared to control patients after distension of a barostatically controlled gastric bag. In addition, rumination patients were noted to have a greater LES tone reduction than controls during inflation of the barostat.[28]

Diagnosis

Rumination syndrome is an underdiagnosed condition in adolescents and adults with normal intelligence. Clinicians do not usually consider rumination syndrome among the differential diagnoses of vomiting because of lack of awareness. The average time from symptom onset to confirmed diagnosis is approximately 17 months.[10] Patients visit an average of 5 physicians over 2 to 3 years before being correctly diagnosed.[11] Individuals with rumination syndrome are often misdiagnosed or undergo extensive, costly, and invasive testing before diagnosis.[12] Rumination syndrome in adults can mimic other gastroesophageal disorders and lead to inappropriate management. Patients tend to undergo invasive procedures that may not contribute much to their management. When rumination is attributed to gastroparesis as the diagnosis, they may have received botulinum injections to the pylorus, undergone gastric electrical stimulator placement, received total parenteral nutrition and/or jejunostomy tubes (j-tube) for nutrition requirements, as well as become dependent on pain medications to treat unexplained abdominal pain.

As already discussed, rumination syndrome can be confused with gastroparesis, eating disorders, gastroesophageal reflux disease (GERD), and gastrointestinal motility disorders. In gastroparesis, vomiting is a very physically demanding event in contrast to effortless regurgitation with rumination and occurs much later in the postprandial period, generally greater than 1 to 2 hours and up to 12 hours. In addition, there is a longer history of accompanying early satiety, an inability to finish a normal-sized meal, fullness, and nausea. A liquid, mechanically soft diet is often well tolerated. The symptoms of GERD are often worse in a supine position at nighttime, whereas there is no rumination at night during sleep, and heartburn is a transient symptom during the reswallowing period. Proton pump inhibitor (PPI) use will not improve postmeal regurgitation. Bulimia nervosa should be considered, and an association exists between bulimia and rumination in a subset of patients. However, bulimics tend to self-inflict the vomiting reflex, not reswallow the regurgitated food, and may develop calluses on the backs of their hands from repeated self-induced vomiting. Differential diagnosis in rumination syndrome should also include achalasia, esophageal obstruction, and gastric outlet obstruction.

Therefore, studies required to exclude other conditions include upper endoscopy, gastric emptying studies, 24-hour esophageal pH monitoring, high-resolution esophageal manometry, impedance, and gastric/small bowel motility. An upper endoscopy will rule out esophagitis, achalasia, peptic stricture, gastritis, or pyloric obstruction. Soykan et al[19] showed normal upper endoscopy and gastric emptying studies in "primary" rumination patients. Subsequent studies by this group identified a subset of delayed gastric emptying patients. Their report indicates a 60:40 ratio of normal to slow gastric emptiers.[26] In a large cohort of ruminating and conditioned vomiting patients, approximately 5% of all gastroparetics of all etiologies acquire this conditioned reflex.[27] Patients with normal gastric emptying can be considered the primary ruminators, while patients with slow gastric emptying studies can be considered conditioned vomitors, acquiring a learned reflex from the chronic meal-induced symptoms. However, performing a gastric emptying study can be a challenge, and the history of inability to complete a gastric emptying study due to immediate vomiting is a "clinical pearl" for considering the diagnosis of rumination/conditioned vomiting. In fact, these patients almost boast that a gastric emptying study cannot be done, further making this a clinician's "art of medicine" diagnosis.

Gastroduodenal manometry is invasive, but can be of diagnostic value. Under fluoroscopic guidance, an 8-lumen manometric tube is inserted over a guidewire into the small intestine. The five 1-cm-spaced proximal ports are placed across the antroduodenal junction, and the three 10-cm-spaced distal ports are placed into the small intestine. The manometric ports are connected by strain-gauge transducers and capillary tubes to a pneumohydraulic pump that contains distilled, degassed water, and contractions from the jejunum, duodenum, and antrum are recorded.[14] Another option is to simultaneously monitor the pH at 5 cm above the gastroesophageal junction. The recordings are performed in the fasting period and after a meal. Patients are also instructed to record each episode of regurgitation. Soykan et al[19] demonstrated that rumination patients had normal upper gastrointestinal motility, specifically normal fasting phase three migrating motor complexes (MMC). A characteristic pattern that could help confirm the diagnosis has been

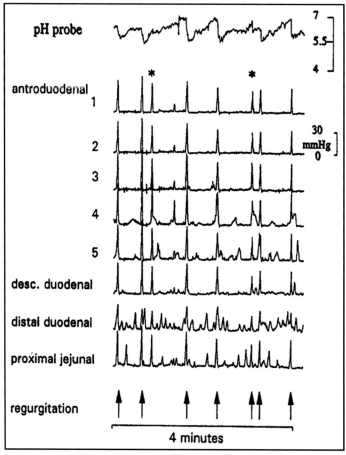

Figure 12-2. R waves during regurgitation on antroduodenal manometry. (Adapted from O'Brien MD, Bruce, BK, Camilleri M. The rumination syndrome: differentiation from psychogenic intractable vomiting. *Indian J Psychiatry.* 2012;54(3):283-285).

observed. Simultaneous pressure waves (R or rumination waves) have been noted throughout all recording levels.[15] The R wave indicates a sudden increase in intra-abdominal pressure from the contraction of abdominal wall muscles and represents a marker that coincides with the time of regurgitation.[16] These R waves have also been correlated with a sudden decrease in the esophageal pH relating to the presence of acidic gastric contents regurgitated into the esophagus (Figure 12-2). However, this is a specialized test that is only available at a limited number of tertiary medical centers. The diagnosis of rumination does not require manometry. In the rare case of diagnostic uncertainty, a manometric evaluation may confirm the diagnosis of rumination syndrome by revealing tall R waves in gastric manometry tracings[17] and normal MMC activity. This can also be necessary when families want more assurance and, hence, this level of investigation may be warranted.

The combination of esophageal impedance measurement and manometry with intragastric pressure transducers is a more recently introduced concept that can better document the sequence of events leading to regurgitation. Increased gastric pressure initiates reflux events associated with transient LES relaxation, which are then identified by impedance.[24] In a recent study, 70% of patients with rumination syndrome had gastric pressure peaks > 30 mm Hg on manometry during regurgitation, distinguishing them from patients with GERD (Figure 12-3).[21] A pH test is not recommended for rumination syndrome since reflux is a consequence and not a cause of symptoms.

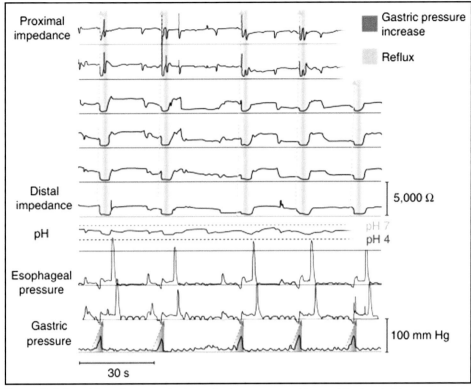

Figure 12-3. Repetitive primary rumination episodes as measured by combined ambulatory manometry and pH-impedance monitoring. (Adapted from Kessing BF, Bredenoord AJ, Smout AJ. Objective manometric criteria for the rumination syndrome. *Am J Gastroenterol.* 2014;109(1):52-59.)

Among patients who have had pH monitoring, there is no significant nocturnal or supine reflux, but there are numerous drops in pH during brief postprandial episodes.[25] Even though manometry, impedance, and pH findings have been demonstrated as having specific findings in rumination syndrome (Figure 12-4), the main prerequisites remain an accurate clinical history and the experience to know that the classic timing and setting make rumination the right fit and the only diagnosis. Therefore, these studies are used sparingly.

Algorithm for Evaluation of Suspected Rumination/Conditioned Vomiting

Treatment

Behavioral Therapy

The treatment of adult rumination syndrome consists of education, reassurance, and behavioral therapy based on breathing exercises that act as a distraction, as in the breath exercises practiced by women during labor and delivery, with a reported success of up to 80%.[19] Reassurance and education of the patient and the family are the first steps in management. This involves providing a detailed explanation of the condition and the time to fully address the physiology of the upper gastrointestinal tract, findings of past tests, and shortcomings of past therapies and to manage expectations of the patient and family. No clinical trials have been performed to assess the

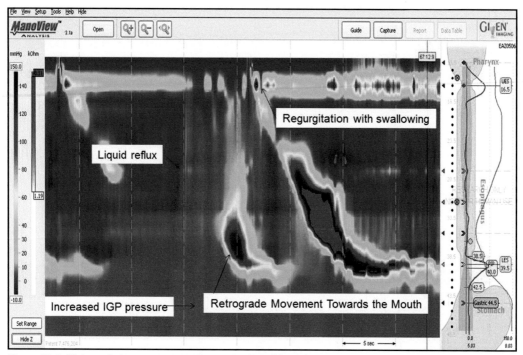

Figure 12-4. High-resolution manometry of rumination syndrome demonstrating the sequence of increased gastric pressure, LES relaxation, and regurgitation followed by reswallowing.

efficacy of the different treatment strategies. A multidisciplinary team approach is recommended to address breathing technique, relaxation, meditation, and pharmacologic approaches to augment breathing programs. Soykan et al[19] suggest that relaxation techniques utilizing tapes and instructions are helpful.

The diaphragmatic breathing technique is best taught by behavioral therapists and is the mainstay of treatment. It is based on habit reversal by using several strategies such as biofeedback, relaxation, and diaphragmatic breathing. Aversive training involves the association of the ruminating behavior with negative reinforcement and rewarding the desired behavior. For example, patients can place a bitter or sour taste on their tongue when they start to have breathing patterns or abdominal muscle contractions that precede the ruminating behavior. Supportive therapy and diaphragmatic breathing have shown improvement in 56% of cases, and total cessation of rumination in 30%.[18] These techniques will return these patients to a better, but not necessarily normal, functioning level and achieve a better quality of life. However, occasional breakthroughs can still occur but must be fully understood by the patient and family. The possibility of relapse in the future associated with stress is an aspect of discussion with the patient.

The diaphragmatic breathing works by physically preventing the contraction of the abdominal muscles required to regurgitate the gastric contents. Behavioral treatment for rumination syndrome consists of habit reversal using diaphragmatic breathing as the competing response to regurgitation. The targeted behavior can be eliminated by consistent use of the competing behavior because the targeted behavior and the competing behavior cannot occur at the same time. Therefore, if done on a consistent basis, the competing behavior will dominate and can reduce or even eliminate the occurrence of regurgitation.

Patients should be encouraged to practice diaphragmatic breathing as they begin the meal. The maneuver should also be repeated after each episode of regurgitation. The patient is told to sit in a relaxed position and place one hand on their upper chest and the other hand on the abdomen directly below the ribs at the bottom of the sternum. Patients are instructed to take a deep inspiratory breath by moving only the abdomen and simultaneously keeping the chest motionless.[19,20]

Hence, only the hand on the abdomen moves with respiration. Patients must initiate diaphragmatic breathing throughout the meal since it is assumed regurgitation will occur as it has in the past with every meal. The goal is for diaphragmatic breathing to slowly occur unconsciously and continuously to suppress the urge to precipitate regurgitation. Inhalation or exhalation should be slow and last approximately 3 seconds. Once patients have exceeded 3 minutes postprandial, this reflex does not occur since "violent" vomiting would be needed because the food is more distal in the stomach.

Once patients understand relaxation techniques, diets should be advanced slowly. First, they should demonstrate the ability to eat small snacks (eg, a cracker), accompanied before and after with relaxation. Once the success rate reaches 90%, patients can progress in a stepwise fashion to the most difficult level of eating (eg, a full steak dinner).

Pharmacological Therapy

Several options are available for supplementary medical therapy. PPIs may be briefly required to provide some improvement in the symptom of heartburn and protection of the esophageal mucosa. Backup antiemetics may also be needed. Both medications are only used in combination with the breathing and relaxation therapies. Low-dose tricyclic antidepressants (TCAs) such as nortriptyline can be started at 10 mg orally at night then increased gradually every 2 or 3 weeks up to 50 to 100 mg as tolerated. Gastric hypersensitivity, sensation of fullness, and painful abdominal muscles may be ameliorated with TCAs. Sometimes, tramadol may be briefly needed to address abdominal pain, while breathing therapy begins to reduce events. Chronic antiemetics and prokinetics will be necessary, along with dietary changes, in the subset where underlying gastroparesis has been present prior to the new vomiting pattern.

Baclofen, an agonist of the γ-aminobutyric acid B receptor, which increases LES pressure and reduces transient relaxations after eating, has been shown to be beneficial in rumination syndrome.[22] Patients taking baclofen 10 mg orally 3 times a day showed decreased postprandial flow events on high-resolution manometry-impedance recordings and decreased symptoms. In addition, baclofen reduces postprandial swallowing frequency.

Nutritional Support During Therapy

The behavioral therapy may take some time (eg, months) to be effective, and this is particularly the case when symptoms may have been present for years. Hence, there can be challenges relating to maintaining weight, addressing micronutrients, preventing severe hypokalemia, and maintaining hydration. These aspects can lead to emergency room visits, as well as hospitalizations. Therefore, we have initiated the use of temporary j-tube placement for nutritional support while awaiting response to therapy. We prefer a surgically placed j-tube, and at the time of placement, full-thickness biopsies of the gastric smooth muscle can be obtained to help prove normal or abnormal function—namely ganglia status and interstitial cells of Cajal. Over time, the j-tube can be converted to a Mic-Key button (Halyard Worldwide, Inc), which is more cosmetic, manageable, and patient friendly. The weight loss and "fragile" nature of these patients may warrant this aggressive approach to allow patients to become functional, return to work, and have more energy to devote to their behavioral therapy.

Surgery

In patients not responding to all of the previous approaches, Nissen fundoplication has been suggested. Five rumination syndrome patients who underwent Nissen fundoplication all reported complete cessation of symptoms.[23] Dysphagia can be a transient postoperative complication, as well as associations with gas, bloat, poor belching, retching, and gastroparesis. Patients at the same time must be undergoing behavioral therapy, since chronic retching against the fundoplication will eventually break and disrupt it. Overall, this is not a currently recommended next step.

Rarely, some patients may not respond to the medical measures we have reviewed. They usually have a long-term history (eg, greater than 5 years) and have failed or resisted behavioral approaches. They often believe their stomach is still the cause. Our group has performed a subtotal gastrectomy now in 2 patients meeting this description who were reduced to living on j-tube feedings and who were nonfunctional in terms of quality of life. The subtotal gastrectomy removes the patient's ability to vomit ingested material. The patient is capable of a dry heave or can still ruminate small amounts of bile from the small bowel. A j-tube will be needed for nutritional support immediately after the surgery. Slowly, the patient can adjust to oral intake after the subtotal gastrectomy when behavioral therapy is being practiced, and the j-tube can then be removed.

Rumination syndrome is a challenging condition to diagnose and treat. The hallmark of the diagnosis is the history of effortless regurgitation immediately after meals and where there is no other explanation for this specific timing. Patients improve after behavioral and relaxation therapies, but referral centers will be required to provide this kind of expertise. During this therapy, nutrient and fluid support may be needed. Rarely, patients may need a surgical intervention.

REFERENCES

1. Khan S, Hyman PE, Cocjin J, Di Lorenzo C. Rumination syndrome in adolescents. *J Pediatr.* 2000;136(4):528-531.
2. Gourcerol G, Dechelotte P, Ducrotte P, Leroi AM. Rumination syndrome: when the lower oesophageal sphincter rises. *Dig Liver Dis.* 2011;43(7):571-574.
3. Talley NJ. Rumination syndrome. *Gastroenterol Hepatol.* 2011;7(2):117-118.
4. Rajindrajith S, Devanarayana NM, Crispus Perera BJ. Rumination syndrome in children and adolescents: a school survey assessing prevalence and symptomatology. *BMC Gastroenterol.* 2012;12:163.
5. Tack J, Blondeau K, Boecxstaens V, Rommel N. Review article: the pathophysiology, differential diagnosis and management of rumination syndrome. *Aliment Pharmacol Ther.* 2011;33(7):782-788.
6. Gupta R, Kalla M, Gupta JB. Adult rumination syndrome: differentiation from psychogenic intractable vomiting. *Indian J Psychiatry.* 2012;54(3):283-285.
7. O'Brien MD, Bruce BK, Camilleri M. The rumination syndrome: clinical features rather than manometric diagnosis. *Gastroenterology.* 1995;108(4):1024-1029.
8. Attri N, Ravipati M, Agrawal P, Healy C, Feller A. Rumination syndrome: an emerging case scenario. *South Med J.* 2008;101(4):432-435.
9. Kanodia AK, Kim I, Sturmberg JP. A personalized systems medicine approach to refractory rumination. *J Eval Clin Pract.* 2011;17(3):515-519.
10. Kessing BF, Bredenoord AJ, Smout AJ. Objective manometric criteria for the rumination syndrome. *Am J Gastroenterol.* 2013. doi: 10.1038/ajg.2013.428.
11. Lee H, Rhee PL, Park EH, et al. Clinical outcome of rumination syndrome in adults without psychiatric illness: a prospective study. *J Gastroenterol Hepatol.* 2007;22(11):1741-1747.
12. Chial HJ, Camilleri M, Williams DE, Litzinger K, Perrault J. Rumination syndrome in children and adolescents: diagnosis, treatment, and prognosis. *Pediatrics.* 2003;111(1):158-162.
13. Fernandez S, Aspirot A, Kerzner B, Friedlander J, Di Lorenzo C. Do some adolescents with rumination syndrome have "supragastric vomiting"? *J Pediatr Gastroenterol Nutr.* 2010;50(1):103-105.
14. Malcolm A, Thumshirn MB, Camilleri M, Williams DE. Rumination syndrome. *Mayo Clin Proc.* 1997;72(7):646-652.
15. Kessing BF, Govaert F, Masclee AA, Conchillo JM. Impedance measurements and high-resolution manometry help to better define rumination episodes. *Scand J Gastroenterol.* 2011;46(11):1310-1315.
16. Chitkara DK, Van Tilburg M, Whitehead WE, Talley NJ. Teaching diaphragmatic breathing for rumination syndrome. *Am J Gastroenterol.* 2006;101(11):2449-2452.
17. Cooper CJ, Said S, Nunez A, Alkhateeb H, McCallum RW. Chronic vomiting and diarrhea in a young adult female. *Am J Case Rep.* 2013;14:449-452.
18. Tucker E, Knowles K, Wright J, Fox MR. Rumination variations: aetiology and classification of abnormal behavioural responses to digestive symptoms based on high-resolution manometry studies. *Aliment Pharmacol Ther.* 2013;37(2):263-274.
19. Soykan I, Chen J, Kendall BJ, McCallum RW. The rumination syndrome: clinical and manometric profile, therapy, and long-term outcome. *Dig Dis Sci.* 1997;42(9):1866-1872.
20. Papadopoulos V, Mimidis K. The rumination syndrome in adults: a review of the pathophysiology, diagnosis and treatment. *J Postgrad Med.* 2007;53(3):203-206.
21. Kessing BF, Bredenoord AJ, Smout AJ. Objective manometric criteria for the rumination syndrome. *Am J Gastroenterol.* 2014;109(1):52-59.

22. Blondeau K, Boecxstaens V, Rommel N, et al. Baclofen improves symptoms and reduces postprandial flow events in patients with rumination and supragastric belching. *Clin Gastroenterol Hepatol*. 2012;10(4):379-384.

23. Oelschlager BK, Chan MM, Eubanks TR, Pope CE 2nd, Pellegrini CA. Effective treatment of rumination with Nissen fundoplication. *J Gastrointest Surg*. 2002;6(4):638-644.

24. Bredenoord AJ, Tutuian R, Smout AJ, Castell DO. Technology review: esophageal impedance monitoring. *Am J Gastroenterol*. 2007;102(1):187-194.

25. Chial HJ, Camilleri M, Williams DE, Litzinger K, Perrault J. Rumination syndrome in children and adolescents: diagnosis, treatment, and prognosis. *Pediatrics*. 2003;111(1):158-162.

26. Miller C, Twillman R, Foran P, et al. Gastric emptying results in conditioned vomiting disorder: the concept of a primary entity as well as learned reflex. *J Investig Med*. 2008;56(1):436 (abstract 281).

27. Hejazi R, McCallum RW. Rumination syndrome: a review of current concepts and treatments. *Amer J Medical Sciences*. In press. March 2014.

28. Thumshirn M, Camilleri M, Hanson RB, Williams DE, Schei AJ, Kammer PP. Gastric mechanosensory and lower esophageal sphincter function in rumination syndrome. *Am J Physiol*. 1998;275(2 Pt 1):G314-321.

Section III

Small Intestinal Disorders

Small Intestinal Dysmotility Symptoms
Bloating, Distension, and Gas

Juan R. Malagelada, MD and Carolina Malagelada, PhD, MD

KEY POINTS

- Abdominal bloating and distension are not synonymous terms. Bloating refers to the feeling of distension of the abdomen, whereas distension describes appreciable abdominal enlargement.

- In organic forms of abdominal distension, the intra-abdominal volume is expanded, whereas in functional forms of abdominal distension, changes in abdominal shape may give the impression of distension without a real volume increase.

- Minor, transient bloating episodes do not require in-depth or extensive diagnostic testing. These should be reserved for unusually severe cases.

- In difficult cases, advanced diagnostic technologies may be applied to elucidate the mechanism of abdominal bloating/distension and to help establish the appropriate therapy.

DEFINITION OF SYMPTOMS

Bloating is a feeling of distension in the abdomen that may or may not be accompanied by visible enlargement of the waist. If there is appreciable abdominal enlargement, we refer to it as abdominal distension. However, abdominal distension may be sometimes quite apparent, as for example, in ascites, without significant sensation of bloating. Thus, abdominal bloating and abdominal distension are distinct clinical manifestations that may sometimes, but not necessarily, coincide.[1]

Gas is a term that may have different meanings for patients and for physicians. Furthermore, it may be used inconsistently as, for instance, when patients use it to describe "bloating" and/or "distension" (ie, "I am full of gas."). Not infrequently, they may use it to describe abdominal cramping and, even more often, tend to use the same term to describe what they perceive as excessive expulsion of gas: belching and/or flatulence.

Rao SSC, Parkman HP, McCallum RW, eds.
Handbook of Gastrointestinal Motility and Functional Disorders (pp 159-170).
© 2015 Taylor & Francis Group.

Figure 13-1. Plain abdominal x-ray in a patient with bloating and severe aerophagia.

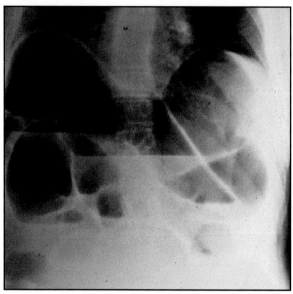

Both bloating and distension may indeed reflect excessive accumulation of gas inside the gastrointestinal tract (which is what many symptomatic patients intuitively suspect) but, most often, this is not the case. By contrast, belching and flatulence usually do reflect expulsion of excess intraluminal gas, although again, sometimes the patient overestimates the actual volume of gas expelled.

Bloating and distension may be described by patients as either diffuse or relatively well localized, usually in the upper, middle, or lower abdomen. Upper abdominal bloating may also appear as part of the dyspepsia syndrome and hence is associated with other manifestations such as pain, early satiety, and nausea. Patients with chronic aerophagia and belching who inflate their stomachs by swallowing air may also refer upper abdominal bloating (Figure 13-1). The most common and prominent variety of abdominal bloating is diffuse or in the mid/lower abdominal area. Patients complain of an uncomfortable sensation of distended abdomen and tight clothes. This type of bloating may present as an isolated symptom or, quite commonly, as a feature of irritable bowel syndrome (IBS) in association with its hallmarks: abdominal pain and altered bowel habits (Table 13-1).[2]

PREVALENCE OF SYMPTOMS

We will refer here to symptoms that develop in the context of functional bloating. Organic bloating and distension are discussed later as part of the differential diagnosis.

Many individuals experience bloating, but their level of concern and impact on quality of life are quite variable. Some otherwise healthy individuals occasionally get bloated, particularly if they overindulge in a large meal or if they consume fermentable foodstuffs. Such bloating and/or distension tends to be relatively short lasting (a few hours) and disappears with the passage of stool and/or gas. This type of self-provoked and predictable bloating rarely constitutes cause for concern or medical consultation since cultural knowledge and personal experience discount its pathological significance. An important exception, however, is individuals with unrealistic expectations of "binge" tolerance. Some patients are also self-indulgent to the point that they may seek specialized consultation requesting some form of preventive therapy that would allow them to continue their unhealthy habits without suffering the uncomfortable consequences.

| TABLE 13-1 |
| CLINICAL CONDITIONS ASSOCIATED WITH BLOATING |

CHRONIC CONSTIPATION

- Up to 80% of patients with chronic constipation complain of bloating
- Experimentally induced constipation is associated with bloating

IRRITABLE BOWEL SYNDROME

- Bloating is a prominent and frequent symptom in IBS
- Bloating is more likely in IBS-C than IBS-D
- Bloating in IBS markedly worsens quality of life

FUNCTIONAL DYSPEPSIA

- Bloating may be present in about one-third of patients with FD
- Bloating tends to localize in the upper abdomen and develops after meals

ALIMENTARY DISORDERS

- Bloating is relatively common in anorexia nervosa, bulimia, or obesity

The type of bloating that most often motivates patients to request medical consultation is diffuse and uncomfortable bloating, with or without associated abdominal distention, that is long lasting, frequent, and without obvious relation to meal ingestion. Some patients manifest associated IBS or dyspepsia features, whereas others do not (functional bloating). This kind of clinically significant bloating is influenced by a number of factors (Table 13-2) and tends to incorporate some recognizable features that help establish an accurate office diagnosis, usually without carrying on any tests. These distinctive features are as follows. First, it affects predominantly, although not exclusively, females and it tends to worsen during the premenstrual and menstrual periods, and sometimes also during ovulation. Second, bloating tends to be absent or minor in the morning and builds up progressively during the day to a peak in late afternoon/evening. Third, it bears no apparent relation to dietary composition or meal times, although some patients may complain that it increases postprandially, particularly if fatty meals are ingested. Hence, patients often manifest an inability to prevent bloating by dietary self-control or other maneuvers. Fourth, many patients readily acknowledge that stress and tension worsen their bloating, and it is not unusual to encounter patients who get bloated on workdays and feel relieved during relaxing weekends or while on vacation. Likewise, bloating exceptionally bothers the patient during the night and, as indicated earlier, the bloating sensation has usually faded away when the patient wakes up in the morning. Fifth, patients not infrequently attribute their bloating to excess gas inside the abdomen, but indicate that passing gas or stool per rectum may somewhat ameliorate the bloating, but rarely relieves it. On the other hand, social inhibition may play a contributory role, as most individuals find it inconvenient to expel flatus when in the company of other people. It is often worthwhile to inquire about such feature because experimentally, voluntarily restraining the urge to pass flatus may induce bloating and distension.[3]

Bloating and flatulence are not synonymous, although they may coexist. Experimental evidence suggests that increasing fermentable substrate in the colon—for instance, by administration of a poorly absorbable disaccharide like lactulose—will produce in most healthy individuals an

TABLE 13-2
FACTORS AND CIRCUMSTANCES WORSENING BLOATING

POSITION AND EMOTIONS

- Standing and stress/anxiety make bloating more likely and worse

MEALS

- Bloating often develops in the postprandial period
- Bloating is worsened by diets rich in fermentable substrates

CIRCADIAN RHYTHM

- Bloating tends to be less likely in the morning and progressively increases later in the day
- This clinical observation has been validated by plethysmography studies

MENSTRUAL CYCLE

- Bloating may be more prominent in IBS females during the menstrual period

increase in colonic gas production (mostly H_2) and subsequent flatulence. However, under these circumstances, bloating usually does not occur, since the normal gut efficiently disposes of the increased gas loads by rapid evacuation. Only when the rate of gas production increases beyond the maximal rate of intraluminal gas consumption or rectal expulsion, will both flatulence and bloating coexist. Some individuals (healthy or otherwise) do behave as "gas retainers" (ie, by not passing gas per rectum) and may become bloated as a result. However, even then, it will resolve after gas evacuation rates catch up with excess production or unusual retention. These considerations help explain the clinical experience that suggests that people who consult because of increased flatulence may not necessarily complain of bloating.

Commonly, the reverse situation is observed. Bloating may present as the most prominent symptom in the absence of increased flatulence. Such "pure bloaters" are often self-persuaded that expelling gas per anus or belching would make them feel better and bitterly complain that they are unable to expel gas on demand. The classic studies of Levitt et al[4] in healthy volunteers have elegantly shown the disparities between bloating and flatulence by observing the responses to oral loads of either lactulose (fermentable) or psyllium (nonfermentable).

CAUSES AND MECHANISMS OF BLOATING/ABDOMINAL DISTENSION

Organic

Increased intra-abdominal content is a major cause of bloating and/or abdominal distention. The physical nature of content varies according to the type of bloating. In organic causes of bloating, solids, fluids, or gas may accumulate inside the gut lumen or intraperitoneally. Such organic causes of bloating should always be considered first in the differential diagnosis of bloating/distension. Acute diarrheal diseases such as salmonellosis and other intestinal infections may be

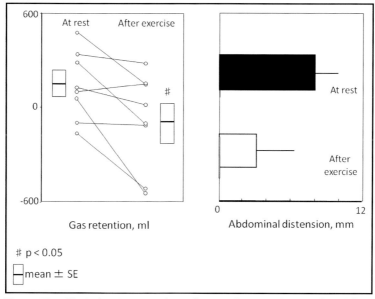

Figure 13-2. Physical activity stimulates clearing of intestinal gas. (Adapted from Dainese R, Serra J, Azpiroz F, Malagelada J-R. Effect of physical activity on intestinal gas transit and evacuation in healthy subjects. *Am J Med.* 2004;116:536-539.)

associated with severe bloating in the early stages of the clinical picture, usually starting prior to the onset of diarrhea. When the latter starts, the true nature of the process rapidly becomes apparent. Malabsorptive conditions, chiefly celiac disease and other mucosal small bowel enteropathies, may be associated with significant bloating, and in that case, the diagnosis may not be so obvious. Acute or subacute bowel ischemia from left cardiac failure or mesenteric insufficiency may present as bloating, which is often associated with visible abdominal distension caused by dilated bowel loops filled with liquid and gas. Partial or complete bowel obstruction is, of course, an important cause of bloating whether it takes place in the small bowel, in the colon, or both. Pseudoobstruction and other intestinal motor disorders (dealt with in another chapter) may also cause bloating and/or abdominal distension via excessive accumulation of luminal content. Finally, extraintestinal causes of abdominal distention, such as ascites or large tumors, may distend the abdomen, with or without the associated sensation of bloating, and need to be considered in the differential diagnosis.

Functional

Intraluminal gas is a key element in the pathogenesis of functional bloating. Sources of intraluminal gas include swallowed air, which is mostly nitrogen, chemical reactions in the small bowel that generate rapidly diffusible CO_2, and colonic fermentation that produces hydrogen and other gases.

In our laboratory, we have demonstrated the extremely high capacity of normal gut motility to clear and expel any quantity of gas present in the lumen. Exercise also stimulates gas clearance (Figure 13-2).[5] Thus, physiologically, there is only a relatively small amount of gas (< 400 mL) present in the small bowel and colon at any time. However, when gut motility disturbances interfere with the mechanism of gas clearance, accumulation occurs even with normal gas production. Such motor abnormalities are a feature of enteric dysmotilities and major gut motility disorders. More subtle but relevant alterations in gas clearance have also been shown in patients with IBS and functional bloating (Figure 13-3).[6,7]

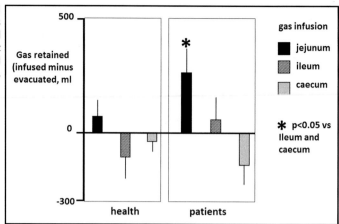

Figure 13-3. In functional bloating and IBS, there is impaired clearing of gas in the upper small bowel. (Adapted from Salvioli B, Serra J, Azpiroz F, et al. Origin of gas retention and symptoms in patients with bloating. *Gastroenterology.* 2005;128:574-579.)

To describe the sequence of events that we consider to be responsible for the development of functional bloating/distension, we will first describe the nature of the intraluminal stimuli that may act as triggers for the viscerosomatic reflex mechanism. Second, we will examine the muscular activity reflex responses that culminate in the abnormal bloating sensation and abdominal distension, and third, we examine the therapeutic approaches that may be adopted based on those pathogenetic mechanisms.

The Nature of the Intra-abdominal Stimuli

In many functional patients, we believe that the usual stimulus is intraluminal gas. Because of the diminished ability to clear gas both in the small bowel and in the colon,[6,8] small intraluminal pouches of gas develop. The source may be swallowed air or postprandial CO_2 in the small bowel or gas produced by fermentation of dietary residue in the colon. Other possible stimuli may be accumulated fluid or dietary components (original or modified by digestion or microbiota action or both).[9]

As indicated earlier, the volumes of gas responsible for abnormal gut stimulation may be small. This may explain why previous studies in bloated/distended individuals have failed to demonstrate larger quantities of intraintestinal gas relative to normal individuals in the basal state.[10] However, our own data indicate the presence of slightly larger amounts during episodes of bloating, which would be consistent with the hypothesis.

The Role of Visceral Hypersensitivity

Such small volumes of accumulated gas or other intraluminal stimuli would not produce pathological responses without a concomitant increase in visceral perception. This trait, described as visceral hypersensitivity (which may be conscious or unconscious) is a common feature of functional gut disorders. The phenomenon of "spatial summation" of many sources of stimulation along the gut potentiates the stimulus input.[11] This hypersensitivity induces afferent stimuli that become intense enough to trigger viscerovisceral and especially viscerosomatic reflexes that aggravate perception and produce abdominal distension through an aberrant accommodation mechanism that reshapes the abdominal cavity. Stress and dietary fat increase visceral hypersensitivity, the latter via a mechanism in part associated with cholecystokinin (CCK).

Abnormal Viscerosomatic Reflex Responses

We and others have shown that in patients with bloating and abdominal distension there is an aberrant accommodation response to intraluminal distending stimuli. Confronted with identical

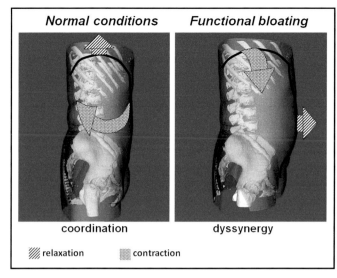

Normal conditions **Functional bloating**

coordination dyssynergy

/// relaxation ░ contraction

Figure 13-4. Functional bloating and distention are associated with dyssynergic accommodation of intra-abdominal volume expansion: lowering of the diaphragm and relaxation of oblique abdominal muscles. (Adapted from Accarino A, Perez F, Azpiroz F, Quiroga S, Malagelada JR. Abdominal distension results from caudo-ventral redistribution of contents. *Gastroenterology.* 2009;136:1544-1551.)

amounts of intraluminal intestinal gas, patients generate a paradoxical contraction of the diaphragm associated with a relaxation of the abdominal wall muscles that is opposite to the normal physiological response of diaphragmatic relaxation and abdominal muscle contraction.[12,13] Despite the different accommodation response observed in functional bloating and healthy individuals, total intra-abdominal volume remains the same; only the shape of the abdomen changes, with anterior protrusion of the abdominal wall in patients associated with an externally invisible descent and flattening of the diaphragm (Figure 13-4). This abnormal accommodation is a potentially reversible phenomenon that matches the clinical observation that distension may develop at certain times (often postprandially or in the evening), but at other times the abdomen does not appear to be distended.

DIAGNOSTIC EVALUATION OF BLOATING AND ABDOMINAL DISTENTION

The diagnostic process should be planned according to the combination of mechanisms emphasized earlier. Clinicians should first answer the question: is total intra-abdominal volume increased? The answer to this question may be sometimes evident on a simple physical exam, for instance, if there is ascites or dilated bowel. Conventional imaging, with computed tomography (CT) scan probably being the most helpful, should establish whether there is intra-abdominal volume expansion and the nature of the expansor: gas, fluid, retained stool, fat, etc. The findings determine further diagnostic evaluation according to standard clinical norms.

If no obvious evidence of increased intra-abdominal volume is obtained, then functional bloating and distention become the most likely diagnostic possibility. The next steps should be adopted after careful assessment of severity, degree of concern and uncertainty. Not every patient with suspected functional bloating and distention needs to be fully evaluated at high expense. Frequently, clinical criteria, as established by Rome III, will suffice. However, there are patients in whom it may be advisable to establish more objectively the mechanism of their bloating to allay concerns and facilitate therapeutic compliance. In that case, several advanced technical approaches may be pursued contingent on availability and priority.[14]

Breath tests for fructose and lactose intolerance are relatively unhelpful in the clinical evaluation of bloating. Fructose and lactose malabsorption tend to produce cramping and flatulence in addition to bloating when products rich in these substances are ingested. Dietary restriction and observation usually suffice to establish whether symptoms are related to disaccharide maldigestion. If uncertainty remains after dietary manipulation, the hydrogen breath test may help clarify the issue. However, more commonly, the opposite is true and breath test positivity cannot be taken as a reliable indicator that the patient's symptoms are related to fructose or lactose malabsorption. The psychological influence on clinical manifestations associated with sugar malabsorption is important and often confounding. To be noted, consumption of ≤ 12 g of lactose at once (about 1 cup of milk) does not cause symptoms even in proven lactase-deficient individuals.[15] The glucose breath test for small bowel bacterial overgrowth also tends to produce equivocal results in the context of a clinical evaluation of bloating and should not be ordered routinely, but only if there are other indicators of an organic condition predisposing to small bowel bacterial overgrowth, such as small bowel diverticulosis, blind loops, or dilated intestinal neuromyopathy. There is no current evidence that it is useful in the evaluation of functional bloating, with or without associated IBS.[15]

ADVANCED DIAGNOSTIC EVALUATION

Quantitative Imaging of the Abdominal Contour and Its Content

As indicated earlier, conventional CT scan is a useful imaging test to help differentiate the various causes of organic bloating and distension based on its power to identify intra-abdominal masses, tissue swelling, and major accumulations of gas, fluid, or solids inside or outside the bowel. However, in the evaluation of functional bloating, further refinements of the CT approach are in order. Thus, our group has developed and validated a CT application that allows accurate quantification of intraluminal gas.[13] The morphovolumetric image analysis program yields gas volumes contained in different segments of the gut, including stomach; small bowel; and right, transverse, left, and pelvic colon. At the same time, the application allows measurement of total intra-abdominal volume and dynamic variations in abdominal shape. The latter measurements are based on establishing the exact position of the diaphragm, as well as the abdominal circumference and coordinates at various levels of the abdomen. The computing process is relatively complex, but it has been automatized.

With this method we have shown that most patients with functional bloating and abdominal distension do not experience a true expansion of intra-abdominal volume due to massive gas accumulation, as patients themselves often believe. Rather, they present anterior protrusion of their abdomens due to inappropriate relaxation of the oblique abdominal wall muscles in conjunction with diaphragmatic descent.[16]

The aforementioned CT technology is best used during episodes of bloating and distention because the changes that may occur in these functional patients are often reversible and the abdomen may be completely normal outside the symptomatic periods.

Electromyography of the Diaphragm and Abdominal Muscles

This technique may provide useful complementary information to the CT assessment of the abdominal shape. It provides direct information on whether the diaphragm and abdominal wall muscles contract or relax at specific points in time. The method consists of the attachment of electromyogram (EMG) electrodes to the anterior abdominal wall and placing them over the rectus and oblique muscle groups. At the same time, EMG diaphragmatic activity is recorded via transesophagic electrodes.[17]

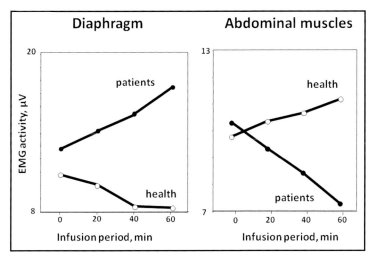

Figure 13-5. Functional bloaters and healthy individuals have different muscle activity responses of the diaphragm and abdominal wall muscles to progressive volume increments. (Adapted from Villoria A, Azpiroz F, Burri E, Cisternas D, Soldevilla A, Malagelada J-R. Abdomino-phrenic dyssynergia in patients with abdominal bloating and distension. *Am J Gastroenterol.* 2011;106:815-819.)

In response to intracolonic infusion of a predetermined gas load, patients with functional bloating and distention characteristically contract the diaphragm and relax the oblique muscles. These changes in muscular tone are detected by the EMG recordings[18,19] and support the diagnosis of functional bloating and distension (Figure 13-5).

Assessment of Intestinal Motility Patterns

This technology does not specifically evaluate bloating, like the aforementioned methods, but may be useful to identify patients with enteric dismotility and pseudoobstruction that may present as significant bloaters. Various useful methodologies may be applied.[20] Intestinal manometric recordings have been applied at specialized medical centers over the past 3 decades now. The manometric method may help identify severe contractile disturbances in the small bowel, but it is usually unable to identify abnormal patterns in functional patients with IBS and/or bloating.

Intestinal motility evaluation by endoluminal image analysis is a noninvasive technique developed and validated in our laboratory.[21] It is based on computer vision analysis of specific features of sequential intraluminal images recorded by the endoscopic capsule as it travels along the small bowel. These features, which describe contractile and noncontractile motility patterns, are quantitatively analyzed by specific mathematical models that result in numerical parameters. These numerical parameters (each one of which defines one feature) are then processed.

Using machine learning techniques, the computer ultimately determines whether a given individual has normal or abnormal intestinal motility. We have shown that endoluminal image analysis has at least the same specificity and sensitivity as intestinal manometry and it is better accepted by patients than catheter manometry, being relatively noninvasive and simple to perform.

In a recent study including 50 healthy individuals and 80 patients with functional-type intestinal symptoms, 29% of the patients showed an abnormal intestinal motility.[22] These results corroborated earlier studies by our group using gas infusion into the jejunum that also disclosed a relatively high proportion of abnormal gut motility among patients diagnosed with IBS by symptom criteria. This is further evidence that some patients currently categorized as IBS may in fact experience a subtle intestinal neuromuscular disorder potentially diagnosed by applying appropriate advanced methodologies.

Other methods used to investigate potential abnormalities in intestinal motility include measurements of intestinal transit and intraluminal fluid by scintigraphy and the wireless pressure and pH capsule. Scintigraphy may be performed by means of a nondigestible and nonabsorbable marker delivered directly to the distal small bowel/proximal colon by means of an enteric-coated capsule. The wireless capsule method provides an assessment of small bowel transit and colonic transit via its pH-sensitive sensor that detects the change from the intragastric acidic environment to the duodenal alkaline environment, signaling gastric emptying of the capsule. The interval from gastric emptying time to rectal evacuation is taken as total intestinal time.

Colonic transit by radiopaque markers is a relatively simple approach that may be useful in verifying slow transit constipation and distinguish it from normal colonic transit in patients claiming to be constipated but without objective evidence for it. A more refined and potentially useful assessment of colonic motility may be obtained by stationary laboratory measurements of colonic tone by the barostat. For this purpose, the barostat is combined with manometry to obtain both tonic and phasic colonic motility assessments. Direct measurement of colonic motility is regarded as a more reliable indicator of colonic inertia than are transit studies.

PRACTICAL CONSIDERATIONS

Once organic causes of bloating and distention have been reasonably excluded, technology-based evaluation will depend on severity and the need to demonstrate a pathophysiological basis for the symptoms. The most direct assessment is via CT shape measurement technology complemented by abdominal muscle and diaphragmatic EMG.[19] If these tests, performed during a symptomatic episode of bloating, fail to detect any changes in intra-abdominal volume or shape, we conclude that the patient experiences the sensation of being bloated but no confirmation of this subjective feeling may be obtained. We may categorize such patients as experiencing psychogenic bloating and direct attention to the underlying affective disorder. A second group of patients are those whom we may categorize as true functional bloaters, who complain of abdominal distention and show clear evidence of abnormal viscerosomatic reflex accommodation with consistent shape and EMG changes. Measurement of intestinal sensitivity to distension in these patients may provide additional useful information. A third group are bloaters who retain large amounts of intraluminal gas as verified by CT. Many patients in this category suffer from substantial intestinal motor disturbances such as enteric dysmotility and pseudoobstruction. Hence, such patients may need further evaluation to assess intestinal motor activity and intraluminal transit. Tests such as intestinal manometry and the less invasive and probably more sensitive endoluminal image analysis method would be most useful. If evidence of small bowel dysmotility is obtained, then performance of a gas infusion or a gas plus lipid test may be appropriate. Patients with abnormal intestinal motility and/or marked (> 800 mL) gas retention, particularly if associated with a low perception score (Figure 13-6),[23] are likely to suffer from a gut neuromuscular disorder and may be candidates for a full-thickness biopsy to further ascertain the nature of their bowel disease. If there is associated protracted constipation, colonic tests appear to be particularly useful to establish whether the patient also suffers from colonic inertia.

MANAGEMENT

The management of bloating and abdominal distension should be planned according to pathogenesis. Organic bloating/distension require causal treatment, and it is beyond the scope of this chapter to detail specific therapy for the diverse conditions that may produce it.

Functional bloating and distension are best managed according to a clinical priority ranking combined with pathophysiology-based approaches. Clinical priority means that most patients with mild, intermittent bloating, which patients relate to dietary overindulgence or stress, may be managed by simple reassurance and advice to adopt a healthy lifestyle. Patients with protracted,

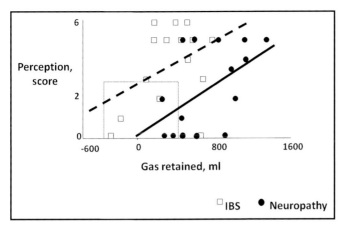

Figure 13-6. Functional bloaters and patients with severe intestinal neuropathy differ in their adaptation to intestinal gas infusion: bloaters retain less gas but manifest higher discomfort scores. (Adapted from Serra J, Villoria A, Azpiroz F, et al. Impaired intestinal gas propulsion in manometrically proven dysmotility and irritable bowel syndrome. *Neurogastroenterol Motil.* 2010;22:4-1-406.)

more severe, and uncomfortable bloating/distension who express significant concerns and low quality of life deserve a more structured approach. These bloaters may benefit from measures directed to each of the pathogenetic elements that are involved: luminal stimuli, visceral hypersensitivity, and abnormal viscerosomatic reflexes.

Luminal stimuli are generated by intestinal content whose composition depends on the nutrients ingested and the modification induced by enzymatic and microbial actions at various levels of the gut. The gas and active molecules that are generated interact with gut sensors and mucosal immune and metabolic activity. Diet modification is, therefore, an important first step in the treatment of bloating. The key objectives are 1) to reduce lipid content, as we know that absorbable lipids in the intestine augment visceral hypersensitivity;[24] and 2) to reduce fermentable substrates that generate excess gas and elicit unwanted viscerovisceral and viscerosomatic reflexes.[25,26] This is usually accomplished by decreasing the unabsorbable residue (low flatulogenic diet) or via a fermentable oligosaccharides, disaccharides, monosaccharides, and polyols (FODMAP) diet. Exercise also helps to clear gas from the bowels (see Figure 13-2). Other objectives include identifying and excluding dietary components susceptible of generating immunological inflammatory responses in the gut and preventing the accumulation of feces in the colon by promoting normal transit and relieving constipation.

Visceral hypersensitivity may be augmented by emotions, personality traits, and environmental influences. Thus, acting on anxiety/depression, if identified; encouraging positive attitudes with the help of family and friends; and improving conditions at home and work may have an important therapeutic role. Likewise, the use of anxiety-relieving techniques such as physical measures, behavioral modification, and hypnotherapy may be quite helpful. Psychopharmacology may also have a useful role at this management level.

As explained earlier, abnormal viscerosomatic reflexes are the basis for the abdominal reshaping that promotes abdominal distension in functional bloating. Some patients become extremely concerned about the protrusion of their abdomens and focus obsessively on their appearance. Through the diagnostic approaches described earlier, it is often possible to help patients understand that their abdominal distension is produced by abdominal reshaping. On that basis, we have found it useful to then apply a biofeedback technique. The approach requires continuous measurement of EMG activity of the anterior abdominal muscles and the diaphragm, which is displayed in front of the patient on a screen. Patients are instructed to relax the diaphragm and increase anterolateral abdominal muscle contraction under visual control. Early results indicate that biofeedback achieves a gratifying amelioration of the sensation of abdominal distension and a reduction in abdominal perimeter.

REFERENCES

1. Azpiroz F, Malagelada J-R. Abdominal bloating. *Gastroenterology*. 2005;129:1060-1078.
2. Malagelada J-R. Why is bloating such a problem in IBS patients? In: Lacy BE, ed. *Curbside Consultation in IBS: Clinical Questions*. SLACK, Thorofare, NJ: 2011;Question 14.
3. Serra J, Azpiroz F, Malagelada J-R. Mechanisms of intestinal gas retention in humans: impaired propulsion versus obstructed evacuation. *Am J Physiol*. 2001;281:G138-G143.
4. Levitt MD, Furne J, Olsson S. The relation of passage of gas and abdominal bloating to colonic gas production. *Ann Intern Med*. 1996;124:422-424.
5. Dainese R, Serra J, Azpiroz F, Malagelada J-R. Effect of physical activity on intestinal gas transit and evacuation in healthy subjects. *Am J Med*. 2004;116:536-539.
6. Salvioli B, Serra J, Azpiroz F, et al. Origin of gas retention and symptoms in patients with bloating. *Gastroenterology*. 2005;128:574-579.
7. Passos MC, Tremolaterra F, Serra J, Azpiroz F, Malagelada J-R. Impaired reflex control of intestinal gas transit in patients with abdominal bloating. *Gut*. 2005;54:344-348.
8. Hernando-Harder AC, Serra J, Azpiroz F, et al. Colonic responses to gas loads in subgroups of patients with abdominal bloating. *Am J Gastroenterol*. 2010;105:876-882.
9. Burri E, Barba E, Huaman JW, et al. Mechanisms of postprandial abdominal bloating and distension in functional dyspepsia. *Gut*. 2014;63:395-400.
10. Accarino A, Perez F, Azpiroz F, Quiroga S, Malagelada J-R. Intestinal gas and bloating: effect of prokinetic stimulation. *Am J Gastroenterol*. 2008;103:2036-2042.
11. Serra J, Azpiroz F, Malagelada J-R. Modulation of gut perception by spatial summation phenomena. *J Physiol*. 1998;506(2):579-587.
12. Villoria A, Azpiroz F, Soldevilla A, Perez F, Malagelada J-R. Abdominal accommodation: a coordinated adaptation of the abdominal walls to its content. *Am J Gastroenterol*. 2008;103:2807-2815.
13. Accarino A, Perez F, Azpiroz F, Quiroga S, Malagelada JR. Abdominal distension results from caudo-ventral redistribution of contents. *Gastroenterology*. 2009;136:1544-1551.
14. Malagelada J-R, Malagelada J-R. The dysfunctional gut. *Curr Gastroenterol Rep*. 2010;12:242-248.
15. Gasbarrini A, Corazza GR, Gasbarrini G, et al. 1st Rome H2-Breath Testing Consensus Conference Working Group. Methodology and indications of H2-breath testing in gastrointestinal diseases: the Rome Consensus Conference. *Aliment Pharmacol Ther*. 2009 Mar 30;29(Suppl)1:1-49.
16. Villoria A, Azpiroz F, Burri E, Cisternas D, Soldevilla A, Malagelada J-R. Abdomino-phrenic dyssynergia in patients with abdominal bloating and distension. *Am J Gastroenterol*. 2011;106:815-819.
17. Burri E, Cisternas D, Villoria A, et al. Abdominal accommodation induced by meal ingestion: differential responses to gastric and colonic volume loads. *Neurogastroenterol Motil*. 2013;Jan 29. doi: 10.1111/nmo.12068 [Epub ahead of print].
18. Burri E, Cisternas D, Villoria A, et al. Accommodation of the abdomen to its content: integrated abdomino-thoracic response. *Neurogastroenterol Motil*. 2012;24:312-e-162.
19. Barba E, Quiroga S, Accarino A, et al. Mechanisms of abdominal distension in severe intestinal dysmotility: abdomino-thoracic response to gut retention. *Neurogastroenterol Motil*. 2013.
20. Malagelada J-R, Malagelada C. Gut motility related symptoms. In: Emmanuel A, Quigley EMM, eds. *Irritable Bowel Syndrome, Diagnosis and Clinical Management*. London, UK: Wiley Blackwell; 2013:215-226.
21. Malagelada C, De Iorio F, Azpiroz F, et al. New insight into intestinal motor function via non-invasive endo-luminal image analysis. *Gastroenterology*. 2008;135:1155-1162.
22. Malagelada C, De Iorio F, Segui S, et al. Functional gut disorders or disordered gut function? Small bowel dysmotility evidenced by an original technique. *Neurogastroenterol Motil*. 2012;24:223-e-105.
23. Serra J, Villoria A, Azpiroz F, et al. Impaired intestinal gas propulsion in manometrically proven dysmotility and in irritable bowel syndrome. *Neurogastroenterol Motil*. 2010;22:401-406.
24. Caldarella MP, Azpiroz F, Malagelada J-R. Selective effects of nutrients on gut sensitivity and reflexes. *Gut*. 2007;56:37-42.
25. Manichanh C, Eck A, Varela E, et al. Anal gas evacuation and colonic microbiota in patients with flatulence: effect of diet. *Gut*. 2014;63:401-408.
26. Azpiroz F, Hernandez C, Guyonnet D, et al. Dietary treatment of gas-related symptoms. *Neurogastroenterol Motil*. 2014;in press.

14

Chronic Intestinal Pseudo-obstruction

Robert M. Siwiec, MD and John M. Wo, MD

KEY POINTS

- Chronic intestinal pseudo-obstruction (CIPO) is a small bowel motility disorder characterized by symptoms of intestinal obstruction with radiologic evidence of small bowel dilation but in the absence of mechanical obstruction.
- Primary forms of CIPO are either familial or sporadic in nature.
- Secondary forms of CIPO arise from various systemic disorders that affect gastrointestinal (GI) tract motility.
- The main treatment goals include nutritional support, promotion of GI motility, and treatment of associated complications.
- A multidisciplinary team approach is the best management strategy for patients with CIPO.

INTRODUCTION AND DEFINITION

Small bowel motility disorders represent a disease spectrum ranging from enteric dysmotility without luminal dilation to chronic intestinal pseudo-obstruction (CIPO). Chronic intestinal pseudoobstruction is a syndrome characterized by recurrent symptoms of intestinal obstruction with associated radiographic evidence of small bowel dilatation but in the absence of obvious mechanical obstruction. It is associated with significant morbidity and mortality. Although CIPO is primarily a disorder of the small bowel, it can occur anywhere along the gastrointestinal (GI) tract. Clinical manifestations of CIPO are variable and highly dependent on the underlying etiology. It is essential to make a timely and accurate diagnosis and to identify the cause. The treatment goals of CIPO are to restore proper nutrition and fluid balance, relieve symptoms, improve intestinal motility, and treat associated complications.

Rao SSC, Parkman HP, McCallum RW, eds.
Handbook of Gastrointestinal Motility and Functional Disorders (pp 171-185).
© 2015 Taylor & Francis Group.

ETIOLOGY

CIPO can be classified as either primary or secondary (Table 14-1). Primary CIPO can be categorized as either familial or sporadic. It is associated with visceral myopathy of the smooth muscle or visceral neuropathy of the enteric nervous system. Underlying genetic defects have been identified for several inheritable syndromes causing CIPO (see Table 14-1). Children and adults can be affected by mitochondrial diseases, which can result in CIPO and enteric dysmotility. Sporadic cases of visceral neuropathies, such as localized Hirschsprung disease or diffuse intestinal dysplasia, occur mostly in infants and children.[1]

Systemic disorders affecting the control of small bowel motility can cause secondary or acquired CIPO (see Table 14-1). Scleroderma, a generalized connective tissue disorder of the small arteries with associated fibrosis, can affect multiple organs. Esophageal aperistalsis, gastroparesis, and CIPO have been described in patients with scleroderma, mixed connective tissue disorders, polymyositis, dermatomyositis, and systemic lupus. Neuromuscular disorders can affect the motor neurons, peripheral nerves, neuromuscular junctions, and muscles. Central and peripheral autonomic disorders may cause gastroparesis and small bowel dysmotility, but there is no clear evidence that they cause CIPO. Paraneoplastic syndrome refers to the remote effects of cancers that express antigens mimicking the neuronal tissues, thus producing an immune-mediated inflammatory response that can affect the small bowel and lead to secondary CIPO. Amyloidosis is caused by the deposition of insoluble fibrin proteins that are resistant to proteolysis. Amyloid protein has been found in the mucosa, submucosa, and smooth muscle. The small bowel myenteric plexus itself is usually intact histologically, but can be involved in some cases. Myotonic, Duchenne, and oculopharyngeal muscular dystrophies are progressive hereditary disorders involving the skeletal muscle, but atrophy and dysfunction of the smooth muscle can also occur in the GI tract, including the small bowel, resulting in CIPO.

In some patients, the underlying cause of CIPO is unknown. An idiopathic inflammatory neuropathy has been described with neuronal and axonal degeneration associated with lymphocytic ganglionitis with neuronal degeneration.[2]

DIAGNOSIS

Nausea, vomiting, early satiety, abdominal pain, and bloating are common in patients with functional GI disorders and small bowel motility disorders. However, patients with CIPO develop recurrent episodes of retching, emesis, abdominal pain, and distention associated with a paucity of flatus and bowel movements. At first, patients are suspected of having either partial or complete small bowel obstruction because of their presenting symptoms; however, mechanical obstruction cannot be identified on radiologic testing. Symptoms are quite variable, ranging from mild postprandial distress to persistent abdominal distension associated with abdominal pain, malnutrition, and an inability to eat. Diarrhea may be present due to small intestinal bacterial overgrowth (SIBO). Weight loss is multifactorial from small bowel peristalsis failure, malabsorption due to underlying SIBO, and inadequate nutritional and caloric intake due to patient's fear of symptom exacerbation.

A high index of suspicion is essential to make a timely and accurate diagnosis of CIPO to avoid unnecessary abdominal surgeries. However, a diagnosis of CIPO is difficult to establish in patients with multiple GI surgeries and/or adhesions. Patients who have undergone a subtotal colectomy or whose ileocecal valve has been resected can present with abdominal distension due to ascending coliform bacteria, but the presence of diffusely dilated small bowel likely represents an unrecognized diffuse motility disorder prior to surgery. A detailed review of systems can identify symptoms of central nervous system (CNS) involvement, autonomic and/or peripheral neuropathies, and urologic complaints that are present in primary CIPO (see Table 14-1). Raynaud, arthralgia,

TABLE 14-1

CLASSIFICATION OF CHRONIC INTESTINAL PSEUDO-OBSTRUCTION BASED ON ETIOLOGY

I. Primary CIPO
  A. Familial
   1. Familial visceral myopathies
      a. Megaduodenum and urinary tract involvement: autosomal dominant, hereditary hollow visceral myopathy
      b. Mitochondrial dysfunction
         (a) Mitochondrial encephalopathy with lactic acidosis and stroke-like episodes (MELAS): maternally inherited, mitochondrial DNA mutation
         (b) Mitochondrial neurogastrointestinal encephalopathy (MNGIE): autosomal recessive, mutations of gene encoding thymidine phosphorylase
      c. Smooth muscle actin gene mutation
   2. Familial visceral neuropathies
      a. Familial intestinal degenerative neuropathy (autosomal dominant)
  B. Sporadic
   1. Visceral myopathies
   2. Visceral neuropathies
      a. Hirschsprung disease

II. Secondary CIPO (acquired)
  A. Connective tissue disorders
   1. Scleroderma
   2. Mixed connective tissue disorder
   3. Polymyositis
   4. Dermatomyositis
   5. Systemic lupus erythematosus
  B. Neuromuscular disorders
   1. Paraneoplastic syndrome
      a. Small cell lung cancer, multiple myeloma, breast cancer, lymphoma, thymoma
   2. Amyloidosis (monoclonal immunoglobulin light chain AL deposition)
      a. Multiple myeloma, non-Hodgkin lymphoma
   3. Myasthenia gravis
   4. Muscular dystrophies
      a. Myotonic, Duchenne, and oculopharyngeal muscular dystrophies
  c. Infections
   1. *Trypanosoma cruzi* (Chagas disease)
   2. Viral
      a. Cytomegalovirus, Epstein Barr virus, varicella zoster

(continued)

TABLE 14-1 (CONTINUED)
CLASSIFICATION OF CHRONIC INTESTINAL PSEUDO-OBSTRUCTION BASED ON ETIOLOGY

D. Endocrine
   1. Hypothyroid
   2. Pheochromocytoma
   3. Paraganglioma
E. Others
   1. Ehlers-Danlos syndrome, jejunal diverticulosis, radiation enteritis
III. Idiopathic CIPO
  A. Inflammatory neuropathy
    1. Lymphocytic ganglionitis with neuronal degeneration
  B. Inflammatory myopathy

digit swelling, muscle pain, and proximal muscle weakness may identify patients with an underlying connective tissue disorder. A history of smoking and weight loss may indicate a paraneoplastic syndrome. Back pain, proteinuria, and an elevated globulin-to-albumin ratio occur in secondary amyloidosis associated with multiple myeloma. A family history of GI motility disorders raises concern for primary hereditary CIPO. Main physical examination findings typically include abdominal distention with tenderness and a succession splash.

The diagnosis of CIPO is based on recurrent symptoms of small bowel obstruction, radiographic evidence of dilated small bowel, and no identifiable anatomic obstruction. Enteric dysmotility describes a subgroup of patients without evidence of dilated lumen. However, patients with CIPO have more severe GI dysfunction, poorer prognosis, and a greater likelihood to require total parenteral nutritional (TPN) than patients with enteric dysmotility.[3] There is no standard diagnostic strategy for CIPO. The goals of diagnostic testing are to make an early and accurate diagnosis, look for the underlying cause, and identify complications of CIPO to guide therapy.

EPIDEMIOLOGY

CIPO is a rare disorder affecting children and adults, with unknown prevalence and incidence. Available epidemiologic data primarily come from tertiary referral centers. A recent survey of targeted university and general hospitals in Japan estimated the country's prevalence of CIPO to be 0.80 to 1.0/100,000, and the incidence to be 0.21 to 0.24/100,000 with a mean age at diagnosis for males and females of 63.1 years and 59.2 years, respectively.[4]

EVALUATION

Laboratory Studies

Laboratory testing can be helpful in identifying secondary forms of CIPO related to treatable diseases. A complete metabolic panel, along with thyroid-stimulating hormone, vitamin B_{12}, complete blood count, and inflammatory markers (eg, erythrocyte sedimentation rate and C-reactive protein), should be obtained. If connective tissue disease is suspected, then antinuclear antibody, SCl-70, and aldolase should be checked. Identification of antineuronal nuclear antibodies (eg, anti-Hu, anti-Ri, anti-Purkinje cell) should be pursued in patients at risk for paraneoplastic syndrome. Other autoantibodies have been identified, but they are often absent in most patients.[5] Serum and urine protein electrophoresis are helpful if multiple myeloma is suspected. Testing for lactic acid, thymidine phosphorylase levels, nucleotide concentrations, and genetic analysis can be obtained in patients with systemic manifestations of mitochondrial disorders.[6] Serology testing for *Trypanosoma cruzi* (Chagas disease) can be obtained in patients with profound dysphagia, especially if they are from endemic areas of Central and South America.[7]

Radiologic Studies

Evaluation with radiographic testing helps to identify classic signs of intestinal obstruction (eg, dilated small bowel, air-fluid levels) (Figure 14-1). Physical obstruction must be excluded with the use of either computed tomography (CT) or magnetic resonance enterography (MRE). Presence of small intestinal diverticulosis and pneumotosis intestinalis should be identified. Recently, cine-magnetic resonance imaging (cine-MRI) was shown to be useful in assessing small bowel motility by computing small intestinal luminal diameter; however, further studies are needed to validate these findings.[8] Plain radiographs and/or CT of the chest should be obtained to exclude small cell lung cancer in patients with suspected paraneoplastic syndrome. In patients with symptoms of CNS involvement, brain imaging is helpful in identifying leukoencephalopathy associated with MNGIE.[9]

Endoscopic Studies

Upper enteroscopy to the level of the proximal jejunum should be performed in patients suspected of having CIPO. Intraluminal or extraluminal occlusion may be identified, especially in patients with duodenal and proximal jejunal dilation. Mucosal biopsies of the proximal small bowel may detect amyloidosis by Congo red stain, but rectal biopsy and fat pad aspiration are more sensitive for amyloidosis. Although endoscopic mucosal biopsies are insufficient to sample the smooth muscles and enteric neurons, future approaches like natural orifice transluminal endoscopic surgery (NOTES) may help to increase the diagnostic role of endoscopy. Viral cultures should be obtained in individuals at risk for cytomegalovirus and herpes simplex virus. During upper enteroscopy, proximal jejunal aspiration can be performed, allowing for quantitative aerobic and anaerobic bacteria cultures to look for SIBO (Table 14-2).[10] The precise diagnostic criteria for SIBO by quantitative threshold and/or type of isolated bacteria are unclear. Some authors have suggested a yield of >105 colony forming units (CFU)/mL of any aerodigestive or coliform bacteria for a diagnosis of SIBO. We recommend a growth of >104 CFU/mL of coliform bacteria (eg, *Escherichia, Klebsiella, Proteus, Acinetobacter, Enterobacter, Neisseiria, Citrobacter,*

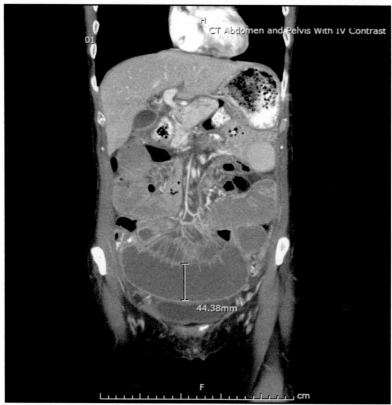

Figure 14-1. Abdominal CT of a patient with CIPO. The small bowel appears diffusely dilated, and retained food is seen in the stomach.

Bacteroides, or *Clostridium* species) for diagnosing SIBO. Overgrowth of coliform bacteria is an indication of small bowel peristaltic failure. Culture-independent 16S RNA-based amplification and high-throughput sequencing are being used to study the composition of the small bowel microbiome; however, their clinical utilization is still considered investigational.

Motility Studies

Although not available in most centers, scintigraphy allows for the evaluation of gastric, small bowel, and colonic transit. However, it is important to consider segmental GI transit before concluding that small bowel transit is abnormal. Delayed colonic transit itself may lead to delayed small bowel transit. Wireless motility capsule measures small bowel transit based on changes in pH when entering the duodenum (rise in pH) and when traversing the ileocecal junction (fall in pH).[11] Contraction frequency and amplitude of small bowel can be quantified by the wireless motility capsule, but the risk of obstruction and the severity of dysmotility generally limit its use in CIPO.

Abnormal esophageal manometry has been suggested as a surrogate marker for small bowel dysmotility. In a large retrospective series of adult patients with CIPO, about two-thirds were found to have ineffective esophageal peristalsis, including many with esophageal aperistalsis.[12] Delayed gastric scintigraphy was found in 60% of patients.[12] However, normal esophageal manometry and gastric emptying does not exclude the diagnosis of enteric dysmotility or CIPO. The pressure profile within the small bowel can be evaluated using either standard or 24-hour ambulatory antroduodenal manometry. The normal 3 phases during the fasting period should be identified based on the frequency and amplitude of contractions. Phase I is a

	TABLE 14-2 **SUGGESTED APPROACH TO UPPER ENTEROSCOPY WITH JEJUNAL ASPIRATION TO IDENTIFY SMALL INTESTINAL BACTERIAL OVERGROWTH**
	PROCEDURE DETAILS
Preparation before test	1. No colon cleansing prep for 1 month. 2. No antibiotics or probiotics for 2 weeks. 3. Stop prokinetics and opiates for 48 hours. 4. Fast for 12 hours before test. 5. Rinse patient's mouth with about 30 cc of antiseptic mouthwash before endoscopy to minimize oral flora contamination. 6. If patient is on proton pump inhibitors, patient can continue. 7. If patient has gastroparesis, patient should be on full liquid diet for 3 days before test to avoid gastric food bezoars during endoscopy.
Test methods	1. Upper enteroscopy is performed with a pediatric colonoscope or small bowel enteroscope. 2. Endoscope is advanced to proximal jejunum without attaching the suction tubing to minimize contaminating suction channel. 3. Aspiration catheter (at least 180 cm) is inserted through the endoscope into the proximal jejunum. 4. Aspiration catheter is attached to a suction trap, which is attached to wall suction, to collect at least 2 cc of luminal liquids in the suction trap.
Laboratory handling	1. Aspiration sample is placed immediately into an anaerobic transport device (free of oxygen) for quantitative anaerobic bacteria culture. 2. Remaining sample is sent for quantitative aerobic bacteria culture. 3. Samples are delivered to the microbiology lab to be plated for culture within 1 hour of collection.
Criteria for SIBO	1. Growth of > 10^4 colony forming units/mL of coliform bacteria in 48 hrs, such as *Escherichia*, *Klebsiella*, *Proteus*, *Acinetobacter*, *Enterobacter*, *Neisseiria*, *Citrobacter*, *Bacteroides*, or *Clostridium* species.

quiescent phase with only minimal spontaneous contractile activity. Phase II is variable with irregular contraction frequency and amplitude. Phase III generates the migrating motor complex (MMC) coordinated contractions that allow for the downstream propagation of luminal content (Figure 14-2).

Abnormal antroduodenal and small bowel manometric patterns lack the specificity to diagnose CIPO. However, it is helpful when the underlying cause of CIPO is unclear. Visceral myopathy is typically associated with hypomotility with low-amplitude contractions (< 10 mm Hg) in the small bowel. On the other hand, visceral neuropathy has normal contraction strength, but is identified

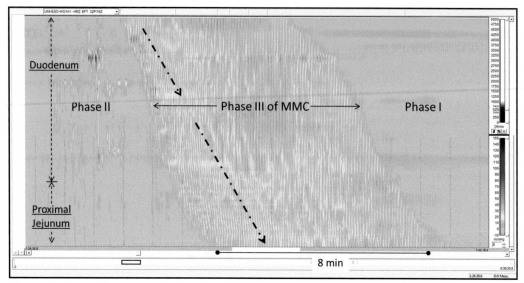

Figure 14-2. Normal fasting MMC pattern depicted using high-resolution small bowel manometry. There is normal progression from phase II (intermittent, irregular contractions) to phase III (coordinated, directional contractions at 12x per minute) to phase I (quiescent phase).

by abnormal propagation and/or configuration of the phase III of the MMC, bursts (>2 min) of nonpropagated phasic activity, and sustained periods (>30 min) of intense uncoordinated phasic activity (Figure 14-3).[3] Antroduodenal or small bowel manometry is necessary to identify patients with enteric dysmotility but without a dilated lumen, a clinical phenotype that may represent a milder form of CIPO. Autonomic testing should be considered if there is evidence of a vagal neuropathy with abnormal postprandial response on antroduodenal manometry and there is no known underlying neurologic disorder.

Histologic Evaluation

Full-thickness biopsy of the small bowel is often necessary in patients with refractory symptoms or unknown etiology to characterize the enteric neurons, smooth muscle, and interstitial cells of Cajal (ICC). Advances in minimally invasive surgical approaches make surgical biopsy an acceptable approach. Patients with CIPO often undergo exploratory surgery for recurrent small bowel obstruction episodes. For these cases, it is essential to obtain a full-thickness biopsy during surgery in patients without an identifiable mechanical obstruction.

Our recommendations for histologic and immunohistochemical evaluation are provided in Tables 14-3 and 14-4. Findings can be reported for the outer and inner smooth muscle layers and for the myenteric plexus. Pathologic findings seen in CIPO are provided in Table 14-5, adopted from the London classification of GI neuromuscular pathology of the Gastro 2009 International Working Group.[13] Many patients with CIPO have more than one pathologic feature.[12] Adult patients with CIPO are more likely to have pathologic enteric abnormalities when compared to patients with enteric dysmotility.[14] Quantification of ICC and neural elements has been advocated for severe gastroparesis,[15] but the utility in CIPO has yet to be determined.[16] Inflammatory enteric neuropathy represents an important entity with inflammatory infiltration of the enteric nervous system anywhere in the GI tract, a finding that has been described in achalasia, gastroparesis, CIPO, and megacolon. In CIPO, a myenteric ganglionitis is associated with lymphocytic invasion of the myenteric neurons with neuronal degeneration (Figure 14-4).[17] The diagnosis of myenteric ganglionitis is supported by detection of circulating antineuronal antibodies against Hu and Yo proteins, neurotransmitter receptors, and ion channels.[5]

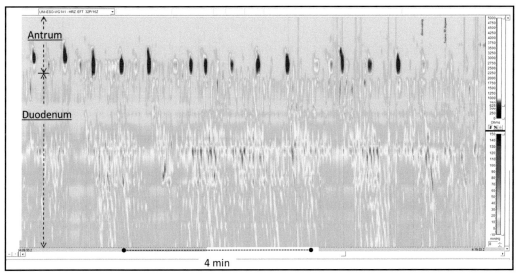

Figure 14-3. Abnormal fasting pattern depicted using high-resolution antroduodenal manometry in a patient with CIPO from visceral neuropathy. Persistent bursts of nonpropagated phasic activity are shown with a poorly developed phase III of the MMC.

TABLE 14-3
HISTOLOGIC STAINS FOR PATHOLOGIC EVALUATION OF CHRONIC INTESTINAL PSEUDO-OBSTRUCTION

STAIN	TARGET
1. H&E	• Light microscopy tissue evaluation
2. Trichrome	• Smooth muscle and fibrous tissue
3. Congo red	• Amyloid
4. PAS (Periodic Acid-Schiff) with and without diastase	• Carbohydrates and mucins; looking for polyglucosan, lipofuscin granules (secondary autophagic lysosomes), and glycogen • PAS combined with diastase treatment can differentiate between glycogen and other structures

TREATMENT

The therapeutic goals in the treatment of CIPO are the following: (1) maintain adequate nutrition, caloric intake, and fluid balance; (2) promote coordinated GI motility; and (3) address the complications of CIPO (eg, SIBO, abdominal pain) or the underlying disease process. Although current therapeutic approaches are suboptimal, recent refinements in nutritional support, pharmacological therapy, and transplant options have helped improve the management of the disease. Patients should be managed by a multidisciplinary team including a neurogastroenterologist, nutritionist, and transplant surgeon. A diagnosis of CIPO carries significant morbidity and

TABLE 14-4

IMMUNOHISTOCHEMICAL STAINS FOR PATHOLOGIC EVALUATION OF CHRONIC INTESTINAL PSEUDO-OBSTRUCTION

IMMUNOHISTOCHEMISTRY	TARGET
1. PGP (Protein Gene Product) 9.5	• Neuronal cell soma, nerve cell processes
2. C-Kit	• Tyrosine kinase receptor on ICC
3. CD45	• General immune cells
4. CD3	• T-lymphocytes
5. CD68	• Macrophages
6. Alpha-smooth muscle actin	• Myocyte contractile protein, smooth muscle cells

TABLE 14-5

CLASSIFICATION OF CHRONIC INTESTINAL PSEUDO-OBSTRUCTION BASED ON GASTROINTESTINAL NEUROMUSCULAR PATHOLOGY

I. Enteric Neuropathies
    A. Aganglionosis
    B. Hypoganglionosis
    C. Intestinal neuronal dysplasia
    D. Degenerative neuropathy
    E. Inflammatory neuropathy (myenteric ganglionitis)
        1. Lymphocytic ganglionitis
        2. Eosinophilic ganglionitis
II. Enteric Myopathies
    A. Muscularis propria malformations
    B. Inflammatory myopathy
        1. Lymphocytic myositis
        2. Eosinophilic myositis
    C. Alpha-actin myopathy
III. Enteric Mesenchymopathy
    A. Interstitial cell of Cajal abnormalities

mortality. In adults, 49% to 72% of patients will require TPN, and 84% will undergo surgical intervention.[3,18] The overall survival in adults is 65% to 69%, with a mean follow-up of 8 to 10 years, in retrospective studies.[3,18] Clinical features associated with longer survival include the ability to restore oral feedings and symptom onset before 20 years of age. Patients with scleroderma

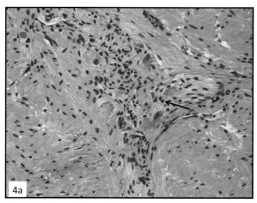 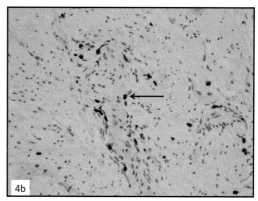

Figure 14-4. Lymphocytic ganglionitis in a patient with CIPO. (A) Lymphocytes (arrow) clustering around and infiltrating a ganglion within the small bowel myenteric plexus (H&E, magnification 400X). (B) T-lymphocytes (arrow) that have been stained with CD3 immunohistochemical stain (magnification 400X). (Reprinted with permission from Dr. Muhammad Idrees, Department of Pathology, Indiana University School of Medicine.)

typically have a poorer prognosis.[18] In a survey of 17 academic centers for children in France, 75% of children with CIPO will require TPN and 67% will undergo surgery.[19]

Nutritional Support

Patients with CIPO are often malnourished from malabsorption and inadequate food intake related to recurrent vomiting, abdominal pain, and distension. Small and frequent meals consisting of liquid or homogenized foods that are low fat and low residue are better tolerated than solids in those with adequate intestinal absorption. Fat-soluble vitamins A, D, E, and K, as well as B_{12} and folic acid, should be checked and, if necessary, supplemented. Enteral nutrition should be attempted. A nasojejunal feeding trial can be performed in malnourished patients to test the ability of the small bowel to tolerate direct nutritional supplementation. A vent-feeding percutaneous gastrojejunostomy tube should be considered in most patients with CIPO. Low-flow enteral feedings (eg, 25 to 50 mL/hr) with higher caloric concentrations (eg, 2 cal/mL) can be utilized. Furthermore, medication administration can be accomplished through the jejunostomy tube. Unfortunately, many patients with CIPO will not tolerate enteric feeding and will require TPN to maintain nutrition and adequate hydration. Complications of TPN include pancreatitis, glomerulonephritis, progressive liver disease, thrombosis, and line infection. Patients who are unable to tolerate oral or enteral feedings and rely solely on TPN should be monitored for fluid and electrolyte imbalances, liver enzyme abnormalities, and deficiencies in essential elements.

Pharmacological Interventions

The main goals of pharmacologic therapy are to stimulate and promote GI motility. This may lead to improved oral feedings and reduced risk of SIBO arising from intestinal stasis. However, efficacy of prokinetics in CIPO is generally limited. All of these agents are considered off-label for use in CIPO; thus, a discussion regarding risks and benefits should be held with the patient. Metoclopramide, a centrally acting dopamine antagonist, in doses up to 10 mg 4 times daily can promote gastric motility; however, CNS adverse effects are common, and potential extrapyramidal reactions severely limit its long-term use. Unlike metoclopramide, domperidone is a peripheral dopamine antagonist with minimal CNS side effects. Doses of domperidone can be increased if necessary. However, it is not available in the United States. Its use should be avoided in patients with a prolonged cardiac QT interval, patients receiving drugs that inhibit the CYP3A4 enzyme, and patients with frequent electrolyte abnormalities. Of note, neither metoclopramide nor domperidone affect intestinal motility beyond the proximal jejunum. Hence, the efficacy of metoclopramide and domperidone in patients with CIPO may be limited.

In a small, open-label study, erythromycin, a motilin agonist, was shown to be effective during acute exacerbations of intestinal pseudoobstruction.[20] However, long-term efficacy is limited due to the development of drug tolerance. Lower doses of erythromycin in liquid formulation (50 to 125 mg 3 times per day) may help to minimize tachyphylaxis. Azithromycin, also in liquid formulation (100 mg at night), has been utilized instead of erythromycin, but the efficacy of azithromycin for CIPO is unknown. Cisapride at doses of up to 20 mg 3 times daily has been shown to improve gastric emptying without providing any symptomatic relief in patients with CIPO.[21] Its association with drug interactions and cardiac arrhythmias, however, has limited its availability in the United States. Prucalopride, a highly selective 5-HT4 receptor agonist, has been shown to improve CIPO-related symptoms of pain, nausea, vomiting, and bloating.[22] Unlike cisapride, prucalopride has a much lower risk of cardiac arrhythmias; however, it is only available in Europe at this time.

Neostigmine is a reversible acetylcholinesterase inhibitor that stimulates muscarinic parasympathetic receptors, resulting in increased colonic motor activity. Case reports have suggested its efficacy in managing acute exacerbations of intestinal pseudoobstruction (0.5 mg intravenously [IV] over 5 minutes with cardiac monitoring).[23] Pyridostigmine, a longer-acting acetylcholinesterase inhibitor used in myasthenia gravis, can be tried in place of short-acting neostigmine. However, efficacy of pyridostigmine for small bowel motility disorders is unknown.

The use of opioid medications for abdominal pain is common in patients with CIPO. Narcotic bowel syndrome is a spectrum of opioid-induced GI dysfunction, including the development of small bowel dysmotility and dilation. It is difficult to differentiate opioid-induced small bowel dysmotility from an underlying visceral neuromuscular disorder, especially when the patient is receiving IV opiates in the hospital setting. Methylnaltrexone selectively targets peripheral μ-opioid receptors (0.15 mg/kg subcutaneously) without interfering with analgesia. Patients who receive μ-opiates may benefit from subcutaneous methylnaltrexone. However, long-term efficacy of methylnaltrexone in CIPO is unknown.

An empiric short-term trial of antibiotics should be considered in patients with CIPO, especially in patients with the complications of SIBO, indicated by the presence of diarrhea, steatorrhea, weight loss, vitamin B_{12} deficiency, and fat vitamin malabsorption. Chronic SIBO produces luminal distention and inflammatory mucosal changes, both of which heighten the sensitivity to abdominal pain in patients with CIPO. Nonabsorbable antibiotics like rifaximin can be given for 10 to 14 days, but the excessive cost commonly limits their use. Other options are metronidazole, ciprofloxacin, neomycin, tetracycline, and doxycycline. If symptoms do not improve with empiric antibiotics or require retreatment, direct jejunal aspiration cultures should be obtained to identify the coliform bacteria associated with CIPO (see Table 14-2). Coliform SIBO, an indication of small bowel motility failure, is a treatable complication of CIPO and can be aggressively treated with alternating antibiotics. To keep the regimen simple for the patient, a selected antibiotic can be used for 2 weeks on the first day of the month, followed by an antibiotic-free interval for the rest of the month. A different antibiotic is used on the first day of next month for 2 weeks and again followed by an antibiotic-free interval. This cycle repeats on the first day of the third month. However, it is important to note that the long-term efficacy of alternating antibiotics in CIPO is unclear. Furthermore, the risk of developing antibiotic-resistant infections, especially in patients with central venous access with TPN, should be considered.

Immunosuppressive therapies (eg, prednisone, rituximab, cyclophosphamide) have been shown in a few case reports to be beneficial in patients demonstrating an inflammatory enteric neuropathy or myopathy. However, these medications should be used with caution, since many patients with CIPO already have multisystem organ impairment and are at risk of TPN-related infection.

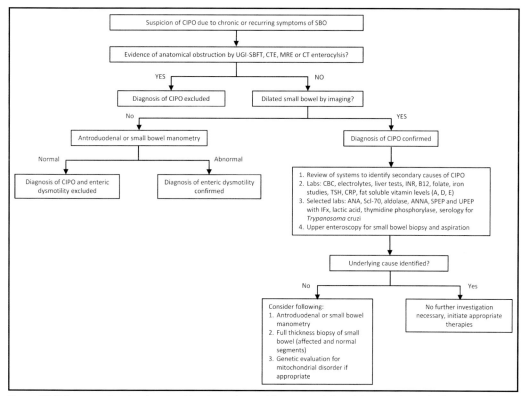

Figure 14-5. Suggested evaluation algorithm for patients with suspected chronic intestinal pseudoobstruction (CIPO). SBO (small bowel obstruction); UGI-SBFT (upper gastrointestinal-small bowel follow-through) barium radiograph; CTE (computerized tomography enterography); MRE (magnetic resonance enterography); CRP (c-reactive protein); ANA (antinuclear antibody); (Scl-70 [topoisomerase-1], ANNA (antineuronal nuclear antibodies); SPEP (serum protein electrophoresis); UPEP (urine protein electrophoresis); IFx (immunofixation).

Surgical Therapy

In general, surgery has a limited role in the management of CIPO. Small case series have shown benefit in a select group of patients undergoing surgical bypass or resection of a dysfunctional GI segment. However, the efficacy of surgery is limited due to the progressive nature of the underlying gut dysfunction. Morbidity and mortality of abdominal surgeries are high.[24] Creation of a gastrostomy or enterostomy can relieve debilitating symptoms of vomiting and abdominal distention in selected patients. Surgery is often required if patients develop acute volvulus of the small bowel and cecum due to a dilated lumen. Electrical stimulation of the stomach in patients with CIPO has been reported, but it should be considered experimental at this time.

Intestinal Transplantation

Isolated or multivisceral intestinal transplantation is a last-resort option for patients with recurrent line sepsis, loss of vascular access, TPN-associated hepatotoxicity, or disease-related poor quality of life.[25,26] The 5-year graft and patient survival in adults with CIPO are reported to be 60% and 70%, respectively, but the number of patients is small.[24] Given the inherent morbidity and mortality associated with intestinal transplantation, along with the long-term complications of immunosuppression, transplantation should be considered when all other medical and nutritional interventions have failed.

CONCLUSION

Chronic intestinal pseudoobstruction is a rare, disabling, and potentially life-threatening disorder characterized by recurrent symptoms of intestinal obstruction, radiographic evidence of dilated small bowel, and no identifiable mechanical obstruction. Both children and adults are affected; however, the true prevalence and incidence are unknown. Although abdominal pain and distention are the most common complaints, clinical manifestation of CIPO can be variable and dependent on the underlying etiology. Figure 14-5 provides a suggested evaluation algorithm for patients with suspected CIPO. The main goals of diagnostic testing are to make an early and accurate diagnosis, look for underlying secondary causes, and identify complications of CIPO in order to guide therapy. Full-thickness biopsies can help to identify and characterize pathologies of the enteric neurons, smooth muscle, and ICC. Nutritional support is essential in patients with frequent vomiting and suboptimal oral intake. Enteral or parenteral nutrition is often needed. Selective use of prokinetic agents and antibiotics for SIBO may provide symptomatic relief. Surgical interventions should be avoided. Isolated or multivisceral transplantation is reserved for patients who are unable to tolerate long-term parenteral nutrition. Although the past few decades have seen an increase in awareness of CIPO with improvements in diagnosis and treatment, continued clinical and basic research is still needed before CIPO is fully understood.

REFERENCES

1. Rudolph CD, Hyman PE, Altschuler SM, et al. Diagnosis and treatment of chronic intestinal pseudo-obstruction in children: report of consensus workshop. *J Ped Gastroenterol Nutrit.* 1997;24:102-112.
2. De Giorgio R., Barbara G, Stanghellini V, et al. Clinical and morphofunctional features of idiopathic myenteric ganglionitis underlying severe intestinal motor dysfunction: a study of three cases. *Am J Gastroenterol.* 2002;97:2454-2459.
3. Lindberg G, Iwarzon M, Tornblom H. Clinical features and long-term survival in chronic intestinal pseudo-obstruction and enteric dysmotility. *Scand J Gastroenterol.* 2009;44:692-699.
4. Iida H, Ohkubo H, Inamori M, Nakajima A, Sato H. Epidemiology and clinical experience of chronic intestinal pseudo-obstruction in Japan: a nationwide epidemiologic survey. *J Epidemiol.* 2013;23:288-294.
5. Tornblom H, Lang B, Clover L, Knowles CH, Vincent A, Lindberg G. Autoantibodies in patients with gut motility disorders and enteric neuropathy. *Scand J Gastroenterol.* 2007;42:1289-1293.
6. Lara MC, Valentino ML, Torres-Torronteras J, Hirano M, Marti R. Mitochondrial neurogastrointestinal encephalomyopathy (MNGIE): biochemical features and therapeutic approaches. *Biosci Rep.* 2007;27:151-163.
7. Prata A. Chagas disease. *Inf Dis Clin North Am.* 1994;8:61-76.
8. Ohkubo H, Kessoku T, Fuyuki A, et al. Assessment of small bowel motility in patients with chronic intestinal pseudo-obstruction using cine-MRI. *Am J Gastroenterol.* 2013;108:1130-1139.
9. Scarpelli M, Ricciardi GK, Beltramello A, et al. The role of brain MRI in mitochondrial neurogastrointestinal encephalomyopathy. *Neuroradiol J.* 2013;26:520-530.
10. Bohm M, Siwiec RM, Wo JM. Diagnosis and management of small intestinal bacterial overgrowth. *Nutr Clin Pract.* 2013;28:289-299.
11. Kuo B, Maneerattanaporn M, Lee AA, et al. Generalized transit delay on wireless motility capsule testing in patients with clinical suspicion of gastroparesis, small intestinal dysmotility, or slow transit constipation. *Dig Dis Sci.* 2011;56:2928-2938
12. Amiot A, Joly F, Cazals-Hatem D, et al. Prognostic yield of esophageal manometry in chronic intestinal pseudo-obstruction: a retrospective cohort of 116 adult patients. *Neurogastroenterol Motil.* 2012;24:1008-e542.
13. Knowles CH, De GR, Kapur RP, et al. The London Classification of gastrointestinal neuromuscular pathology: report on behalf of the Gastro 2009 International Working Group. *Gut.* 2010;59:882-887.
14. Lindberg G, Tornblom H, Iwarzon M, Nyberg B, Martin JE, Veress B. Full-thickness biopsy findings in chronic intestinal pseudo-obstruction and enteric dysmotility. *Gut.* 2009;58:1084-1090.
15. Grover M, Bernard CE, Pasricha PJ, et al. Clinical-histological associations in gastroparesis: results from the Gastroparesis Clinical Research Consortium. *Neurogastroenterol Motil.* 2012.
16. Knowles CH, Veress B, Kapur RP, et al. Quantitation of cellular components of the enteric nervous system in the normal human gastrointestinal tract: report on behalf of the Gastro 2009 International Working Group. *Neurogastroenterol Motil.* 2011;23:115-124.

17. De Giorgio R, Guerrini S, Barbara G, et al. Inflammatory neuropathies of the enteric nervous system. *Gastroenterology.* 2004;126:1872-1883.

18. Amiot A, Joly F, Alves A, Panis Y, Bouhnik Y, Messing B. Long-term outcome of chronic intestinal pseudo-obstruction adult patients requiring home parenteral nutrition. *Am J Gastroenterol.* 2009;104:1262-1270.

19. Faure C, Goulet O, Ategbo S, et al. Chronic intestinal pseudoobstruction syndrome: clinical analysis, outcome, and prognosis in 105 children. French-Speaking Group of Pediatric Gastroenterology. *Dig Dis Sci.* 1999;44:953-959.

20. Emmanuel AV, Shand AG, Kamm MA. Erythromycin for the treatment of chronic intestinal pseudo-obstruction: description of six cases with a positive response. *Aliment Pharmacol Ther.* 2004;19:687-694.

21. Camilleri M, Malagelada JR, Abell TL, Brown ML, Hench V, Zinsmeister AR. Effect of six weeks of treatment with cisapride in gastroparesis and intestinal pseudoobstruction. *Gastroenterology.* 1989;96:704-712.

22. Emmanuel AV, Kamm MA, Roy AJ, Kerstens R, Vandeplassche L. Randomised clinical trial: the efficacy of prucalopride in patients with chronic intestinal pseudo-obstruction: a double-blind, placebo-controlled, cross-over, multiple n=1 study. *Aliment Pharmacol Ther.* 2012;35:48-55.

23. Borgaonkar MR, Lumb B. Acute or chronic intestinal pseudoobstruction responds to neostigmine. *Dig Dis Sci.* 2000;45:1644-1647.

24. Sabbagh C, Amiot A, Maggiori L, Corcos O, Joly F, Panis Y. Non-transplantation surgical approach for chronic intestinal pseudo-obstruction: analysis of 63 adult consecutive cases. *Neurogastroenterol Motil.* 2013;25:e680-e686.

25. Lauro A, Zanfi C, Dazzi A, et al. Disease-related intestinal transplant in adults: results from a single center. *Transplant Proc.* 2014;46:245-248.

26. Lauro A, Zanfi C, Pellegrini S, et al. Isolated intestinal transplant for chronic intestinal pseudo-obstruction in adults: long-term outcome. *Transplant Proc.* 2013;45:3351-3355.

Small Intestinal Bacterial Overgrowth

Baha Moshiree, MD and Yehuda Ringel, MD, AGAF, FACG

KEY POINTS

- Small intestinal bacterial overgrowth (SIBO) is an important consideration in many other gastrointestinal (GI) diseases with refractory symptoms such as diarrhea and weight loss.
- Diagnosis can be made by use of breath testing or by small bowel aspirates.
- SIBO is usually treated by empiric antibiotics, with or without prokinetics, and with appropriate dietary measures to correct nutritional deficits.

DEFINITION

SIBO has been traditionally defined as "clinical and/or laboratory evidence of maldigestion and/or malabsorption related to increased numbers of small bowel bacteria."[1] This definition includes two components: an increase in the number of bacteria in the small bowel and associated clinical and/or laboratory abnormalities indicating altered physiology. However, recent research on the role and function of intestinal bacteria (also referred to as intestinal microbiota) suggests additional aspects that may be relevant to the definition of SIBO. First, it is recognized that both quantitative (eg, increase in total numbers) and qualitative (eg, alterations in type and/or function of specific bacterial groups) changes in intestinal microbiota can lead to altered physiology and clinical SIBO-like manifestations. Second, alterations in small bowel microbiota may have clinical and physiological manifestations beyond maldigestion and malabsorption. These may include alterations in metabolic functions secondary to abnormal intraluminal fermentation, intestinal barrier, and immune functions. Thus, emerging data from intensive microbiome research are likely to soon expand the traditional definition of SIBO. On the other hand, although there may be a need to expand the definition of SIBO to reflect emerging evidence on the role of intestinal microbiota in altering bowel physiology and associated clinical manifestations, there is also a need to avoid using the term SIBO to explain clinical symptoms associated with clinical conditions

Rao SSC, Parkman HP, McCallum RW, eds.
Handbook of Gastrointestinal Motility and Functional Disorders (pp 187-199).

(eg, irritable bowel syndrome [IBS]) in which there is no evidence for defined pathophysiological mechanisms that are directly related to observed alterations in small bowel bacteria.

To avoid confusion with current published literature, the definition of SIBO in this chapter is limited to conditions in which there exists "clinical and/or laboratory evidence of altered intestinal physiology related to increased numbers of bacteria in the small bowel."[1] Increased number of bacteria includes commensal and/or noncommensal bacteria, and altered intestinal physiology includes malabsorption and maldigestion (consistent with the traditional definition), as well as abnormalities in intestinal fermentation, barrier functions, immune functions, and sensory-motor functions.

PATHOPHYSIOLOGY

Overview of the Intestinal Microbiota

The intestinal microbiota of the GI tract is represented by a wide variety of bacteria, archaea, viruses, and eukarya. When discussing these, it is important to recognize that the GI tract is not a homogenous environment and that there are substantial differences in the bacterial load and composition of the microbial communities along the GI tract. Thus, while the bacterial load is relatively low at the proximal small bowel (~ 100 to 103), it increases significantly at the distal jejunum and ileum (~ 106 to 109) and particularly in the large intestine (~ 1010 to 1012). Furthermore, the composition of the bacterial communities also changes from mainly aerobic bacteria in the proximal small bowel to a mix of aerobes and anaerobes in the distal segments of the small bowel and to primarily anaerobes in the large intestine.[2]

In addition to longitudinal (proximal-to-distal segments) differences in the intestinal microbiota, there are significant axial (mucosal mucous layer to lumen) differences in bacterial composition. Our current understanding of the intestinal microbiota is based on data generated from studies done primarily on luminal content (eg, fecal samples or duodenal aspirates). However, it is important to recognize that this approach provides a limited perspective and that our current knowledge on the microbial composition, function, and clinical relevance of the luminal versus mucosal mucous microbial microenvironments is still under intensive investigation.[3]

Specifically, in regard to the small bowel, due to technical difficulties in collecting samples that accurately represent the intestinal bacterial communities in this relatively remote segment of the GI tract, few studies have directly investigated the composition of the intestinal microbiota in the small bowel. Furthermore, the few studies that have sampled the proximal small bowel to diagnose SIBO (in association with IBS) have been limited by the use of bacterial culture[4] and real-time polymerase chain reaction (PCR) techniques.[5] It is well recognized that these methods target only a limited number of bacteria and do not provide accurate and sufficiently comprehensive information on changes in the small bowel microbiota in this condition.

Physiological Protecting Mechanisms and Predisposing Factors

Several physiological mechanisms help prevent overgrowth of bacteria in the small bowel. The stomach has a protecting barrier role against intestinal invasion of bacteria from the outside environment, since, with the exception of *Helicobacter pylori* and a few other acid-resistant bacterial strains, its highly acidic environment is not favorable for bacterial colonization.

Other factors that help to minimize bacterial colonization in the proximal GI tract include effective propagating peristalsis that reduces stagnation of luminal content in the small bowel; the protective characteristics of the inner mucus layer produced by stomach and duodenum columnar epithelial cells; the antigen-specific immunoglobulin (Ig) A, IgG, and IgM that are secreted in both the stomach and duodenum; and the variety of antimicrobial molecules secreted by Paneth cells, including α and β defensins, collectins, and lectins.

In addition, the presence of conjugated bile acids and certain fatty acids in the duodenum helps further inhibit bacterial colonization and overgrowth in the small bowel.[6] Finally, a competent and well-functioning ileocecal valve helps to limit the reflux of colonic contents rich in anaerobic bacteria back into the ileum.

PATHOPHYSIOLOGY

The presence of bacteria in the small bowel results in intraluminal intestinal fermentation with the production of gases and several metabolic by-products that contribute to altered physiology and/or the clinical manifestations associated with the disorder. The degradation of carbohydrates by intestinal bacteria produces gases (eg, carbon dioxide, hydrogen, and methane) and short-chain fatty acids, leading to increased stool acidity, abnormal small bowel motility, abdominal bloating, distension, and flatulence. Bacterial deconjugation of bile acids can lead to the production of free and toxic bile acids, which irritate the intestinal mucosa and stimulate the secretion of water and electrolytes, leading to loose stools and diarrhea. SIBO associated with gram-negative organisms can elaborate endotoxins, which can lead not only to mucosal inflammation, but also to systemic effects (eg, arthritis and possible liver injury through activation of proinflammatory cytokines). In patients with increased intestinal permeability and hepatic impairment, degradation of protein and urea by intestinal bacteria can produce ammonia, resulting in the development or worsening of hepatic encephalopathy.

Predisposing Factors

Several predisposing conditions and risk factors have been associated with SIBO. A retrospective study of 675 patients who underwent duodenal aspirate culture for various clinical indications, including diarrhea (42%), weight loss (36%), dyspepsia (35%), abdominal pain (33%), IBS (9%), and malabsorption (8%), revealed that only a small portion (8%) of the patients investigated had abnormal duodenal aspirates (defined as intestinal bacterial counts of more than 105 cfu /mL), while the vast majority (83%) had negative cultures.[7] Several factors were found to be significantly associated with positive aspirate cultures, including older age, history of abdominal surgery, inflammatory bowel disease, pancreatitis, small bowel diverticula, steatorrhea, and use of narcotic medications. Other external factors such as alcohol consumption have also been associated with SIBO.[8]

EPIDEMIOLOGY

While a number of conditions have been associated with SIBO, its true prevalence is unknown due to the heterogeneity of its definition, lack of accurate diagnostic measures, and its overlapping symptoms with various functional and organic GI disorders with abdominal symptoms similar to those in SIBO (Table 15-1). Nevertheless, no study to date has evaluated the prevalence of SIBO in a healthy population without coexisting GI disease using the current available diagnostic measures.

Evidence does suggest that some populations may be at increased risk for SIBO, including the elderly and obese. In one study of 328 residents in nursing homes, 11% tested positive for SIBO, although only some of these seniors exhibited diarrhea or weight loss, suggesting that the elderly may have increased risk of SIBO.[9] Other studies suggest higher rates of a positive glucose

TABLE 15-1
COMMON CLINICAL CONDITIONS PREDISPOSING TO SMALL INTESTINAL BACTERIAL OVERGROWTH
CLINICAL DIAGNOSIS (*DENOTES CONFLICTING EVIDENCE)
Celiac disease
Chronic pancreatitis
Cirrhosis
Connective tissue diseases (scleroderma/lupus)
Diabetes (gastroparesis/enteropathy)
Diverticulosis (small bowel)
Gastroparesis
IBD (with or without fistulae)
*IBS
Medications (*PPIs, narcotics)
Old age
*Obesity
Parkinson disease
Prior surgery (such as for peptic ulcer disease)

breath test in the obese asymptomatic population (17%) compared to healthy nonobese subjects (2.5%, *p* value 0.031).[10] In obese patients, the presence of SIBO and metabolic syndrome were independent risk factors for hepatic steatosis.

Other conditions may also have an association with SIBO, including cirrhosis and systemic and neurological conditions affecting small bowel motility or pancreatic and biliary secretions. In several clinical studies, patients with cirrhosis were at significant (as high as 49%) risk for SIBO compared to controls.[11] However, these studies relied strictly on breath testing, while other studies of patients with cirrhosis, using qualitative cultures of jejunal aspirates, failed to establish significant associations with SIBO.[12] In addition, disorders that affect the physiological protection mechanisms such as chronic pancreatitis, small bowel diverticulosis, cystic fibrosis, connective tissue diseases such as systemic sclerosis, and Parkinson disease may be associated with SIBO.

Diseases associated with intestinal inflammation can disrupt the normal intestinal physiology and luminal ecology and increase the risk for SIBO. These include celiac sprue (66% of subjects), ulcerative colitis (15%), and Crohn's disease (28%).[13-15] Patients with both Crohn's disease and SIBO have lower weights and increased rates of abdominal pain. Given that the ileocecal valve restricts anaerobic bacteria to the colon, this association of inflammatory bowel disorders with SIBO is clear in patients having resection of the ileocecal valve.

Surgeries that lead to decreased gastric secretion, including vagotomy and surgery for peptic ulcer, can also predispose patients to SIBO.[16] Surprisingly, a prior history of cholecystectomy may protect against SIBO.[8] SIBO is common in patients with gastroparesis, especially in patients with a longer duration of gastroparesis, with 40% of patients testing positive for SIBO based on glucose breath testing.[17] This finding may relate to impaired migrating motor complex (MMC) activity and altered intestinal motility beyond the stomach similar to what is seen in small intestinal pseudoobstruction or postvagotomy syndromes.

Widespread use of proton pump inhibitors (PPIs) has also been implicated in the development of SIBO and even fungal overgrowth.[18] PPI therapy may lead to hypochlorhydria and an increase in stomach pH, resulting in elimination of the gastric acid barrier and an increase in the stomach bacteria, most of which are gram-negative bacteria. Most studies suggest an association between PPI use and increased odds for larger bacterial colonies in the proximal small intestine based on small bowel aspirates even if insufficient quantities for diagnosis of SIBO are found.[18-20] However, this association remains a matter of controversy, as conflicting evidence exists, with some studies of relatively small patient populations linking SIBO with PPI therapy[19] and other, larger population studies finding no statistically significant association.[7,20]

Several studies over the past decade have established IBS as the most prevalent condition associated with SIBO. Nevertheless, its exact prevalence remains difficult to pin down, due to overlapping symptoms and lack of a diagnostic biomarker for IBS. Furthermore, depending on the type of diagnostic testing for SIBO—breath testing versus jejunal aspirates and cultures—the reported prevalence of SIBO ranges from 54% with lactulose and 31% with glucose breath testing to only 4% with "gold standard" jejunal aspirates and cultures.[21] Others have combined scintigraphy with breath testing and based on this stricter diagnostic criterion, found that 39% of IBS patients had SIBO versus only 8% of controls.[22] In contrast, none of the other clinically used breath-testing criteria showed an increased risk of SIBO in the study's IBS patients. As a result, some controversy remains over the true prevalence of SIBO in IBS and whether patients with IBS should be tested for SIBO. Currently, breath testing is not a part of the diagnostic criteria for IBS. However, in IBS patients with pronounced symptoms of abdominal bloating, distention, and gas, breath testing can be considered, as the two conditions may coexist and treatment of concomitant SIBO may improve patients' symptoms.

DIAGNOSIS

Clinical Manifestations

The clinical presentation of a patient with SIBO may be similar to other GI diseases. Functional bowel diseases such as IBS, diseases with organ pathology such as the inflammatory bowel diseases, and even partial mechanical obstruction can all present with symptoms resembling those of SIBO. In addition, various GI diseases may coexist with SIBO and the two can be clinically indistinguishable. Clinical symptoms may include abdominal fullness, excess flatulence, bloating, upper periumbilical or epigastric abdominal pain, borborygmi (abdominal noises), diarrhea with steatorrhea, and/or nausea with vomiting and weight loss.

Clinical signs of SIBO may include abdominal distension, tympany, abnormal bowel sounds, and weight loss in severe cases. (See Table 15-2 for a description of physical exam findings in patients with SIBO.)

Laboratory Tests

There are no sensitive and specific diagnostic laboratory tests for SIBO. The majority of patients with SIBO have normal laboratory tests. However, in severe cases or when SIBO is associated with significant systemic diseases or underlying anatomical or physiological abnormalities, laboratory findings may be abnormal. In these conditions, the abnormal laboratory tests may reflect associated malabsorption of nutrients and vitamins, including vitamin B_{12} deficiency with associated

TABLE 15-2
TYPICAL PHYSICAL EXAM FINDINGS WITH SMALL INTESTINAL BACTERIAL OVERGROWTH

EXAM LOCATION	FINDING	CAUSE
Vitals	Low body mass index (BMI) < 25	Malabsorption
Skin	Rosacea Rash Pigmented nevi Café au lait spots, neurofibromas	Connective tissue diseases (CTDs) Zinc deficiency/CTD Visceral myopathies Neurofibromatosis
HEENT (head, eyes, ears, nose, throat)	Ophthalmoplegia Mydryasis Ptosis Conjunctival pallor	Multiple sclerosis (MS) or neuropathy, myopathy Anemia (B_{12} or iron deficiency)
Abdomen	Distension and tympanic Scarring Succussion splash Organomegaly	Pseudoobstruction (any cause) or obstruction Adhesions from prior surgeries Gastroparesis Infiltrative process (sarcoidosis)
Neurological exam	Autonomic dysfunction Peripheral neuropathy Other neurologic signs	Diabetes, CTD, or neuropathies MS, Parkinson's, B_{12} deficiency Parkinson's, MS, neurofibromatosis, paraneoplastic syndrome
Musculoskeletal	Muscle weakness/atrophy Tetany	Muscular dystrophy, MS Calcium deficiency

macrocytic anemia and neurologic side effects, and low levels of vitamin B_1 (thiamine) and B_3 (nicotinamide).[23]

Bacterial deconjugation of bile acids may result in fat malabsorption with associated steatorrhea and deficiencies of fat-soluble vitamins (A, D, E, and K), while intraluminal degradation of protein precursors by bacteria may lead to decreased absorption of amino acids with associated hypoalbuminemia and protein-losing enteropathy in severe cases. Nevertheless, in the presence of SIBO, folate and vitamin K may present with normal or high levels, as they can be produced by intestinal bacteria.

Radiological findings with computed tomography (CT), magnetic resonance imaging (MRI), or x-ray may show dilated loops of bowel and air-fluid levels without any specific narrowing at any transition points. In the presence of these symptoms or laboratory and/or radiological findings, clinicians should seek a detailed personal history and family history that can reveal underlying

TABLE 15-3 CAUSES OF SMALL INTESTINAL PSEUDOOBSTRUCTION PREDISPOSING TO SMALL INTESTINAL BACTERIAL OVERGROWTH		
MYOPATHIC AND NEUROPATHIC CAUSES OF PSEUDOOBSTRUCTION	**CAUSES**	**DISEASES**
Primary visceral myopathy and neuropathy	Autosomal recessive Autosomal dominant	Familial visceral myopathy
	Autosomal recessive Autosomal dominant	Nonfamilial visceral myopathy
Secondary visceral myopathies	Connective tissue disease	CREST (calcinosis, Raynaud phenomenon, esophageal dysmotility, sclerodactyly, and telangiectasia), progressive systemic sclerosis, dermatomyositis, lupus, mixed connective tissue diseases
	Infiltrative diseases	Sarcoidosis, diffuse lymphoid infiltration, amyloidosis
	Muscular dystrophies	Duchene dystrophy, myotonic dystrophy
Secondary visceral neuropathies	Neurologic diseases	Parkinson disease, multiple sclerosis, diabetic neuroenteropathy (also myopathic), postinfectious (viral infections such as Cytomegalovirus, EBV, herpes, other enteroviruses), Chagas disease, Shy-Drager, neurofibromatosis, spinal muscle atrophy, paraneoplastic disease (malignancy)

associated diseases and autosomal-dominant visceral myopathies or neuropathies related to chronic intestinal pseudoobstruction (Table 15-3).

Endoscopy: Aspiration and Culture

The traditional gold standard for SIBO is based on direct testing of duodenal or jejunal aspirates. The presence of $> 10^5$ cfu/mL of colonic-type bacteria is commonly considered a cutoff threshold for the definition of the condition. However, this gold standard diagnostic measure for SIBO has several limitations. First, it requires an invasive and costly endoscopic procedure. Second, appropriate collection of the samples may be technically challenging and difficult, as samples can easily be contaminated by oral flora. Third, aspiration of content only from the proximal small bowel may not be informative enough in conditions related to SIBO in the distal segments of the small bowel (eg, in colonic bacterial migration into distal ileum). Fourth, using a threshold of $>10^5$ cfu/mL may not be sensitive enough in early SIBO and/or certain clinical conditions (eg, IBS) in which lower threshold levels have been recently suggested.[4,21,24] Fifth, as already mentioned, the majority of intestinal bacteria cannot be cultured. Thus, these culture-based methods do not reveal the full magnitude of changes in small bowel microbiota that may contribute to the physiological abnormalities and clinical presentation of SIBO.

Breath Tests

Hydrogen breath tests are widely used in clinical practice as alternative approaches for the diagnosis of SIBO. In contrast to sampling and quantitative culture of proximal small bowel aspirates, hydrogen breath tests are noninvasive, technically simple, and relatively inexpensive. These tests are based on the principle that certain gases (eg, hydrogen and methane) are produced endogenously only through bacterial fermentation of intraluminal intestinal carbohydrates. Thus, detection of these gases in exhaled breath indicates intraluminal fermentation and the presence of intestinal bacteria. The timing and magnitude of the excreted hydrogen and/or methane in breath serve as surrogate markers for the location and level of bacterial fermentation along the GI tract.

Breath tests for the diagnosis of SIBO involve oral administration of lactulose or glucose, which serve as substrates for intraluminal bacterial fermentation, and measurement of exhaled gases in breath samples collected every 20 to 30 minutes for 2 to 4 hours. The most commonly used protocol for the lactulose breath test involves ingestion of 10 grams of lactulose in 200 mL of water. A positive test is defined as >20 parts per million (ppm) breath hydrogen level at fasting, and/or an early increase in breath hydrogen concentration of >20 ppm over baseline within 90 minutes of lactulose ingestion, and/or a sustained increase of >10 ppm on consecutive samples. The detection of high baseline levels or the early increase of excreted breath hydrogen is interpreted as indication for the presence of bacteria in the small bowel, while the appearance of a second late (>90 minutes of ingestion) increase corresponds with the substrate (ie, lactulose) reaching the proximal colon and its fermentation by colonic bacteria. However, this classical "double peak" pattern of lactulose breath test is not usually seen in clinical practice. For the glucose breath test, most centers use 50 to 100 grams of glucose in 200 mL of water. A positive test is defined as a baseline of hydrogen level >20 ppm and/or increase in breath hydrogen level of >12 to 15 ppm over baseline.[25,26]

Production of methane gas is also associated with intestinal carbohydrate fermentation, which, similar to hydrogen, is also excreted and can be detected in exhaled breath. Since methane is the main gas produced by intestinal bacteria in up to 30% of the population, the addition of methane to the hydrogen measurement can increase the accuracy of the carbohydrate-based breath test in diagnosing SIBO. A positive test is defined as an increase of >10 ppm in breath methane level when baseline is <10 ppm. Despite the relatively widespread use of hydrogen and methane breath testing for the diagnosis of SIBO in clinical settings, the results may vary between laboratories due to a lack of standardization, with differences in patient preparation, test protocols, and results interpretation.[27]

Thus, clinicians should be aware of the different protocols and the possible factors that may affect the interpretation of the results. The important points are the selection of carbohydrate substrate (eg, lactulose vs glucose), which affects carbohydrate bioavailability for bacterial fermentation in different segments of the GI tract. Lactulose is a synthetic, nonabsorbable disaccharide and therefore can be available for bacterial fermentation throughout the small intestine and colon. The use of lactulose can increase the sensitivity of detecting SIBO in the distal small bowel. However, because lactulose is an osmotic laxative, it can accelerate intestinal transit, resulting in rapid arrival of the substrate to the cecum and right colon, and in early (<90 min) fermentation by colonic bacteria. In this scenario, which is of particular concern in patients with diarrhea, the interpretation of the test may be difficult since the early rise in hydrogen or methane breath levels can reflect a short intestinal transit time and gas production by colonic fermentation

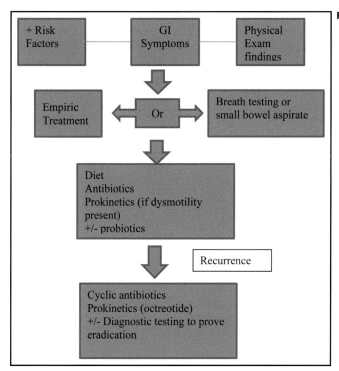

Figure 15-1. Treatment algorithm for SIBO.

rather than SIBO. Unlike lactulose, glucose is rapidly absorbed in the proximal small intestine and under normal circumstances is not expected to reach the distal small bowel or colon. This increases the specificity of the glucose hydrogen breath test; however, because glucose may not reach the distal parts of the small bowel, the sensitivity of the glucose breath test in detecting SIBO in the distal bowel is reduced. Additional carbon dioxide (CO_2)-based breath tests for the diagnosis of SIBO have been reported in the literature. These tests use a poorly absorbed monosaccharide (D-xylose) or a bile acid (glycocholic acid) as substrates with isotopically labeled (13C) or radioactively labeled (o14C) CO_2. However, use of isotopes adds significantly to the complexity and cost of these tests, and so has fallen out of use.

TREATMENT

The treatment of SIBO should be based on reducing or eliminating predisposing factors and correcting underlying diseases whenever possible. One of these easily reversed predisposing factors is narcotic use, which should be discontinued in patients with both gastroparesis and SIBO.[7] Unfortunately, treatments for these conditions are often suboptimal and may lend to only palliative and symptomatic treatments. Treatment should also depend on the degree of malnutrition and vitamin deficiency, both of which correlate with the severity of SIBO. Figure 15-1 illustrates a proposed algorithm for the management of patients with suspected SIBO, taking into account that one should either test and treat, or treat empirically.

Dietary Management

Patients experiencing abdominal pain, bloating, and excess gas could benefit from a diet that is low in carbohydrates, that is low residue/low fiber, and that avoids nonabsorbable sugars, including commonly used artificial sweeteners like aspartame, saccharine, or sorbitol. In addition, encouraging patients to avoid dairy products in the initial stages of treatment may help control diarrhea, which can be exacerbated by lactose.

Depending on the severity and chronicity of the disorder, clinicians should check for micronutrient deficiency and supplement with fat-soluble vitamins to redress deficiencies. Vitamin B_{12} deficiency can be treated with oral supplements or via intramuscular injection once monthly. In addition, patients with steatorrhea could benefit from pancreatic enzyme replacement to improve absorption of fat, protein, and starch.

In severe cases of SIBO with significant weight loss, enteral feedings may be considered. In some cases, patients with both SIBO and short bowel syndrome or intestinal failure may require total parenteral nutrition (TPN).

Antibiotics

The goal of antibiotic therapy in SIBO is to reduce intestinal fermentation and achieve symptomatic improvement. Despite increased research on SIBO, antibiotic therapy is still widely empiric, given the number and variety of microbiota species and the limited understanding of their contribution to the clinical manifestation.

The choice of antibiotic regimen requires assessment of patient history of tolerance, risk of *Clostridium difficile* infection, systemic absorption, potential for or history of resistance to treatment, and cost of the drug. Unfortunately, clinicians lack clear evidence for which antibiotic might prove most appropriate for the length of time required for antibiotics to prove efficacious in the management of SIBO. To date, existing data mainly feature small sample sizes, in addition to issues stemming from the reliability of different breath tests to identify both SIBO and clinical outcomes. In general, clinicians aim at antibiotic coverage for gram-negative and anaerobic organisms to reduce patients' gas and lessen diarrhea and malnutrition stemming from SIBO. Although in many studies, a target of effectiveness of treatment is the normalization of breath testing, achieving meaningful relief of SIBO-associated symptoms may be a more appropriate goal in the clinical setting.

Commonly used antibiotics for the treatment of SIBO include rifaximin, tetracycline, amoxicillin-clavulanic acid, norfloxacin, ciprofloxacin, neomycin, and metronidazole. Rifaximin, a nonsystemically absorbed antibiotic, is the most widely studied of the antibiotics and has success rates as high as 82% in the treatment of SIBO.[28] Rifaximin covers the spectrum of pathogens commonly implicated in SIBO—both gram-positive and gram-negative organisms, aerobes, and, more importantly, anaerobes. Nevertheless, repetitive therapy is often necessary to successfully treat SIBO. Using in vitro studies, rifaximin has a demonstrated potent effect on specific small bowel flora, including *Escherichia coli*, *Enterococcus faecalis*, and *Staphylococcus aureus*. One study that used a subset of diarrhea-predominant IBS patients found that rifaximin 600 mg for 10 days improved symptoms of stool frequency and consistency in patients with diagnosed SIBO but not in those without positive breath testing.[22] Besides rifaximin, ciprofloxacin and metronidazole have been often used for the treatment of SIBO in symptomatic patients with underlying GI disorders, including chronic intestinal pseudoobstruction and Crohn's disease.[29]

In the sole meta-analysis performed on antibiotic therapy for SIBO, the authors identified 10 publications based on diagnosis of SIBO on breath testing done prospectively.[30] Based on this meta-analysis, the nonabsorbable antibiotic rifaximin was most commonly studied antibiotic, followed by ciprofloxacin, metronidazole, neomycin, and chlortetracycline. Duration of treatment varied from 7 to 14 days. Compared to placebo, normalization of breath testing was seen in 51% of patients given antibiotics vs 9.8% in the placebo group. Although rifaximin (based on 2 well-designed studies) led to symptom improvement posttreatment, the antibiotic still failed to achieve statistical improvement (effectiveness ratio 1.97; 0.93 to 4.17 for 95% CI). In contrast, for all 10 studies evaluated, the effectiveness ratio was ultimately statistically significant when data were pooled (effectiveness ratio 2.55; 95% CI 1.29 to 5.04). Ranges of normalization of breath testing were 21.7% (rifaximin ;600/800 mg/d) to 100% (ciprofloxacin).

For pediatric patients, rifaximin, trimethoprim-sulfamethoxazole, and metronidazole are effective treatments. Trials in children with IBS on rifaximin at 600 mg a day for 7 days have shown normalization of lactulose breath test in 64% of patients and improvement of GI symptoms based on the visual analog scale (VAS) scoring system.[31] Other studies have tried trimethoprim-sulfamethoxazole and metronidazole to treat SIBO with normalization of breath testing in 95% of subjects after a 14-day course of treatment.[32]

As with adult patients, studies to date have failed to establish the efficacy of cyclic therapy in pediatric patients diagnosed with SIBO, especially important given their high recurrence rates after antibiotic therapy[33] and the potential for antibiotic-associated diarrhea and *C difficile* infections. SIBO can recur in up to 40% of all patients, as measured by glucose breath testing, even after confirmed successful eradication. Since recurrence of symptoms usually follows, most patients should be retreated with antibiotics accordingly. However, no randomized controlled trials have yet focused on the efficacy of treatments in preventing SIBO recurrence. Currently, continuous or cyclic therapy for the first 5 to 10 days of each month may be advocated in those patients with intestinal failure and refractory symptoms.[34] At present, larger randomized controlled trials are necessary to establish any antibiotic as primary treatment and to find its optimal dose and duration of therapy.

Probiotics

Probiotics are live bacterial organisms that, when administered in adequate amounts, confer a health benefit on the host. Probiotics can reduce pathogenic bacterial colonization, enhance mucosal barrier function, and improve intestinal motility, thus theoretically benefiting patients with SIBO. Unfortunately, scant data exist regarding their benefit in SIBO. Data from one human study did show *Lactobacillus plantarum* 299v to be effective in children for prevention of SIBO or for delaying recurrence.[35] Other studies have used probiotics in patients on PPI therapy and showed reduction of intestinal bacterial overgrowth by bacterial cell counts after treatment.[36] Well-designed studies must be conducted before probiotics can be part of any therapeutic algorithm.

Prokinetics

Although a few prospective randomized controlled trials have documented the efficacy of prokinetic use in SIBO, prokinetics may have therapeutic potential in cases of SIBO associated with gastroparesis, intestinal dysmotility, or chronic intestinal pseudo-obstruction. Since not all patients with SIBO have dysmotility of the small bowel, clinicians should assess intestinal transit when considering adding treatment with prokinetics. In patients with intestinal dysmotility, one approach may be to add prokinetics to the antibiotic regimen. The most studied prokinetic agents for the treatment of SIBO are cisapride, erythromycin, azithromycin, and octreotide, all of which have potentially negative side effects.[37-39] Of these agents, cisapride is no longer available in the United States due to its cardiac risk profile. Octreotide is the most potent agent, promoting small bowel motility by inducing MMCs in the small bowel at lower doses of 25 to 50 mcg in patients with dysmotility and even scleroderma, but can delay small bowel activity in higher doses.[38] Both macrolides erythromycin and azithromycin promote gastric antral activity, but azithromycin also induces small bowel MMCs, although not to the degree induced by octreotide when administered intravenously.[39] The macrolides also cause cardiac arrhythmias, however, are limited owing to tachyphylaxis with prolonged use.

Acid Suppression and Small Intestinal Bacterial Overgrowth

Although current data are inconclusive as to the linkage between PPIs and SIBO, clinicians should discuss decreasing or outright cessation of acid suppression therapy in patients at risk for SIBO, especially when no clear-cut reason for prolonged PPI use exists. Furthermore, PPI therapy alters bile acid metabolism and may predispose patients to development of SIBO, as well as deficiencies of fat-soluble vitamins [40]

REFERENCES

1. Quigley EMM. Small intestinal bacterial overgrowth: what it is and what it is not. *Curr Opin Gastroenterol.* 2014;30(2):141-146.
2. Flint HJ, Scott KP, Louis P, Duncan, SH. The role of the gut microbiota in nutrition and health. *Nat Rev Gastroenterol Hepatol.* 2012;9:577-589.
3. Carroll IM, Ringel-Kulka T, Keku TO, et al. Molecular analysis of the luminal and mucosal-associated intestinal microbiota in diarrhea-predominant irritable bowel syndrome. *Am J Physiol Gastrointest Liver Physiol.* 2011;301(5):G799-807.
4. Posserud I, Stotzer PO, Björnsson ES, Abrahamsson H, Simrén M. Small intestinal bacterial overgrowth in patients with irritable bowel syndrome. *Gut.* 2007;56:802-808.
5. Kerckhoffs AP, Samsom M, van der Rest ME, et al. Lower Bifidobacteria counts in both duodenal mucosa associated and fecal microbiota in irritable bowel syndrome patients. *World J Gastroenterol.* 2009;15:2887-2892.
6. Hofmann AF, Eckmann L. How bile acids confer gut mucosal protection against bacteria. *Proc Natl Acad Sci USA.* 2006;103:4333-4334.
7. Choung RS, Ruff KC, Malhotra A, et al. Clinical predictors of small intestinal bacterial overgrowth by duodenal aspirate culture. *Aliment Pharmacol Ther.* 2011;33:1059.
8. Gabbard SL, Lacy BE, Levine GM, Crowell MD. The impact of alcohol consumption and cholecystectomy on small bowel bacterial overgrowth. *Dig Dis Sci.* 2014;59:638-644.
9. Parlesak A, Klein B, Schecher K, et al. Prevalence of small bowel bacterial overgrowth and its associations with nutrition intake in nonhospitalized older adults. *J Am Geriatr Soc.* 2003;51:768-773.
10. Sabate J-M, Jouet P, Harnois F, et al. High prevalence of small intestinal bacterial overgrowth in patients with morbid obesity: a contributor to severe hepatic steatosis. *Obes Surg.* 2008;18:371-377.
11. Pande C, Kumar A, Sarin S. Small intestinal bacterial overgrowth in cirrhosis is related to the severity of liver disease. *Aliment Pharmacol Ther.* 2009;29:1273-1281.
12. Bauer TM, Schwacha H, Steinbruckner B, et al. Diagnosis of small intestinal bacterial overgrowth in patient with cirrhosis of the liver; poor performance of glucose breath hydrogen test. *J Hepatol.* 2000;33:382-386.
13. Tursi A, Brandimarte G, Giorgetti G. High prevalence of small intestinal bacterial overgrowth in celiac patients with persistence of gastrointestinal symptoms after gluten withdrawal. *Am J Gastroenterol.* 2003;98:839-843.
14. Rana SV, Sharma S, Kaur J, et al. Relationship of cytokines, oxidative stress and GI motility with bacterial overgrowth in ulcerative colitis patients. *J Crohn's Colitis.* 2014;Jan 20;PMID:24456736.
15. Klaus J, Spandiol U, Adler G, et al. Small intestinal bacterial overgrowth mimicking acute flare as a pitfall in patient with Crohn's disease. *BMC Gastroenterol.* 2009;9:61.
16. Paik CN, Choi MG, Park JM, et al. The role of small intestinal bacterial overgrowth syndrome in postgastrectomy patients. *Neurogastroenterol Motil.* 2011;23(5):e191-196.
17. Reddymasu SC, McCallum RW. Small intestinal bacterial overgrowth in gastroparesis: are there any predictors? *J Clin Gastroenterol.* 2010;44(1):e8-13.
18. Jacobs C, Adame EC, Attaluri A, et al. Dysmotility and proton pump inhibitor use are independent risk factors for small intestinal bacterial and/or fungal overgrowth. *Aliment Pharmacol Ther.* 2013;37:1103-1111.
19. Lombardo L, Foti M, Ruggia O, Chiecchio A. Increased incidence of small intestinal bacterial overgrowth during proton pump inhibitor therapy. *Clin Gastroenterol Hepatol.* 2010;8:504-508.
20. Ratuapli SK, Ellington TG, O'Neil MT, et al. Proton pump inhibitor therapy use does not predispose to small intestinal bacterial overgrowth. *Am J Gastroenterol.* 2010;107:730-735.
21. Ford AC, Spiegel BM, Talley NJ, Moayyedi P. Small intestinal bacterial overgrowth in irritable bowel syndrome: systematic review and meta-analysis. *Clin Gastroenterol Hepatol.* 2009;7(12):1279-1286.
22. Zhao J, Zheng X, Chu H, et al. A study of the methodological and clinical validity of the combined lactulose hydrogen breath test with scintigraphic oro-cecal transit test for diagnosing small intestinal bacterial overgrowth in IBS patients. *Neurogastroenterol Motil.* 2014;26:794-802.
23. Tabaqchali S, Pallis C. Reversible nicotinamide-deficiency encephalopathy in a patient with jejunal diverticulosis. *Gut.* 1970;11:1024.

24. Spiegel BM. Questioning the bacterial overgrowth hypothesis of irritable bowel syndrome: an epidemiologic and evolutionary perspective. *Clin Gastroenterol Hepatol.* 2011;9:461-469.

25. Saad RJ, Chey WD. Breath tests for gastrointestinal disease: the real deal or just a lot of hot air? *Gastroenterology.* 2007;133:1763-1766.

26. Saad RJ, Chey WD. Breath testing for small intestinal bacterial overgrowth: maximizing test accuracy. *Clin Gastroenterol Hepatol.* 2013; S1542-3565.

27. Gasbarrini A, Corazza GR, Gasbarrini G, et al. Methodology and indications of H2-breath testing in gastrointestinal diseases: the Rome Consensus Conference. *Aliment Pharmacol Ther.* 2009;29(Suppl 1):1-49.

28. Pistiki A, Galani I, Pyleris E, et al. In vitro activity of rifaximin against isolates from patients with small intestinal bacterial overgrowth. *Int J Antimicrob Agents.* 2014;43:236-241.

29. Castiglione F, Rispo A, Di Girolamo E, et al. Antibiotic treatment of small bowel bacterial overgrowth in patients with Crohn's disease. *Aliment Pharmacol Ther.* 2003;18:1107-1112.

30. Shah SC, Day LW, Somsouk M, Sewell JL. Meta-analysis: antibiotic therapy for small intestinal bacterial overgrowth. *Aliment Pharmacol Ther.* 2013;38:925-934.

31. Scarpellini E, Giorgio V, Gabrielli M, et al. Rifaximin treatment for small intestinal bacterial overgrowth in children with irritable bowel syndrome: a preliminary study. *Eur Rev Med Pharmacol Sci.* 2013;17:1314-1320.

32. Tahan S, Melli LC, Mello CS, et al. Effectiveness of trimethoprim-sulfamethoxazole and metronidazole in the treatment of small intestinal bacterial overgrowth in children living in a slum. *JPGN.* 2013;57:316-318.

33. Lauritano EC, Gabrielli M, Scarpellini E, et al. Small intestinal bacterial overgrowth recurrence after antibiotic therapy. *Am J Gastroenterol.* 2008;103:2031-2035.

34. Kumar A, Forsmark CE, Toskes PP. The response of small bowel bacterial overgrowth to treatment: effects of coexisting conditions. *Gastroenterology.* 1996;110-A340.

35. Young RJ, Vanderhoof JA. Probiotic therapy in children with short bowel syndrome and bacterial overgrowth. *Gastroenterology.* 1997;112:A916.

36. Piano MD, Anderloni A, Balzarini M, et al. The innovative potential of Lactobacillus rhamnosus LR06, Lactobacillus pentosus LPS01, Lactobacillus plantarum LP01, and Lactobacillus delbrueckii Subsp. Delbrueckii LDD01 to restore the "gastric barrier effect" in patients chronically treated with PPI: a pilot study. *J Clin Gastroenterol.* 2012;44:S1.

37. Di Lorenzo C, Reddy SN, Villanueva-Meyer J, et al. Cisapride in children with chronic intestinal pseudo-obstruction. An acute, double-blind, crossover, placebo-controlled trial. *Gastroenterology.* 1991;101:1564-1570.

38. Verne GN, Eaker EY, Hardy E, Sninskey CA. Effect of octreotide and erythromycin on idiopathic and scleroderma-associated intestinal pseudo-obstruction. *Dig Dis Sci.* 1995;40:1892-1901.

39. Chini P, Toskes PP, Waseem S, Hou W, McDonald R, Moshiree B. Effect of azithromycin on small bowel motility in patients with gastrointestinal dysmotility. *Scand J Gastroenterol.* 2012;47(4):422-427.

40. Shindo K, Machida M, Fukumura, et al. Omeprazole induces altered bile acid metabolism. *Gut.* 1998;42:266-271.

16

Food Intolerance and Dietary Concepts in Functional Bowel Disorders

Abimbola O. Aderinto-Adike, MD and
Eamonn M.M. Quigley, MD, FRCP, FACP, FACG, FRCPI

KEY POINTS

- Food-related symptoms are common in all functional gastrointestinal disorders (FGID).
- The precise mechanisms whereby food items trigger symptoms in FGIDs are, for the most part, unclear.
- Classical IgE-mediated food allergy is not a major factor in the induction of food-related symptoms in FGIDs.
- Many food modifications have been recommended for FGID patients; few have any evidence base.
- Weight loss is effective in gastroesophageal reflux disease (GERD).
- Fiber is effective in chronic constipation.
- Low fermentable oligosaccharides, disaccharides, monosacharides, and polyols (FODMAPs) diets show promise in irritable bowel syndrome (IBS).

Given the pivotal role of all parts of the gastrointestinal (GI) tract in the ingestion, distribution, digestion, and assimilation of the food that we eat and in its elimination, it should come as little surprise that eating is a major trigger of many GI symptoms. Thus, for most sufferers, heartburn is a postprandial phenomenon, and dyspepsia, or its lay equivalent, indigestion, directly implies a food-related phenomenon. In the lower gut, eating is a major trigger of irritable bowel syndrome symptoms. The high prevalence of constipation in the West can be attributed to our low intake of dietary fiber. Although these close relationships between eating and a host of GI ills have been recognized for centuries (*vide supra*), serious scientific interest in relationships between food, dietary constituents, and functional GI problems has been much more recent. The adoption by many of our patients of a host of dietary changes and supplements to prevent or ameliorate symptoms, and

Rao SSC, Parkman HP, McCallum RW, eds.
Handbook of Gastrointestinal Motility and Functional Disorders (pp 201-208).
© 2015 Taylor & Francis Group.

TABLE 16-1
AN APPRAISAL OF THE DIETARY MANAGEMENT OF GASTROESOPHAGEAL REFLUX DISEASE

EVIDENCE-BASED	PROPOSED BUT STATUS UNCERTAIN
Weight loss, if overweight or obese	Eliminate carbonated beverages, caffeine, chocolate, spearmint, citrus fruits, spice
Avoid eating shortly before lying down	Low-fat diet

usually without any scientific basis, renders this issue of central and pressing importance to the clinician and clinical researcher alike.

GASTROESOPHAGEAL REFLUX DISEASE

Globally, heartburn is among the most common of all symptoms, and its underlying disorder, GERD, is one of the most common diseases of the upper GI tract (Table 16-1). Although the manifestations of GERD range from symptoms alone to Barrett's esophagus and even adenocarcinoma, the fundamental issue is the reflux of gastric contents (and especially acid) into the esophagus. The global burden of GERD continues to rise—a phenomenon that is being observed at the same time as the epidemic that is food-related is obesity.

The traditional, if unproven, lifestyle modifications recommended for GERD reflect the focus of food in its pathogenesis. Thus, patients are counseled to avoid eating large meals and, especially, lying down immediately after eating, with elevation of the bed being recommended to mitigate the latter.[1] While these instructions owe more to tradition than to evidence, obesity has been shown to be an important, independent risk factor for the development of GERD and its progression.

With regard to meal characteristics and contents, there are data from human physiological experiments to incriminate large meals, alcohol, fatty foods, chocolate, peppermint, coffee, tea, and tomato and citrus products in the pathophysiology of GERD through increasing gastric distention, promoting transient relaxation of the lower esophageal sphincter (LES), stimulating gastric acid production, and/or delaying gastric emptying, which worsen reflux disease.[1] Although time honored in its recommendation, there is little evidence to support efficacy for avoiding these foods in improving the symptoms of reflux. Citrus foods, although commonly cited as aggravating heartburn, have not been identified to improve symptoms of GERD when avoided. Carbonated drinks have been shown to increase reflux and increase transient LES relaxation, but there is no convincing evidence that carbonated beverages worsen GERD.[2] There are conflicting findings on the effect of caffeine on reflux, and there is also no consistent evidence to suggest that caffeine consumption is a risk factor for reflux disease.[3] In addition, while chocolate has been found to increase acid exposure and decrease transient LES pressure,[4] again, there is an absence of studies showing that chocolate consumption worsens GERD symptoms. There is no convincing evidence that mint, including spearmint and peppermint, has a negative effect on GERD symptomatology.[5] Neither is there evidence to suggest that consumption of spicy or fatty meals exacerbates reflux, although patients who notice that their symptoms worsen with consumption of such meals should abstain from them. Alcohol is associated with increased acid production and impaired gastric emptying, but there is insufficient evidence to suggest an improvement in reflux symptoms with abstinence.

TABLE 16-2
AN APPRAISAL OF THE DIETARY MANAGEMENT OF FUNCTIONAL DYSPEPSIA

EVIDENCE-BASED	PROPOSED BUT STATUS UNCERTAIN
Food diary to identify trigger symptoms Low-fat diet	Food allergy

Weight loss, however, has been associated with improvement in symptoms of GERD. In a prospective cohort study, Singh et al[6] found that weight loss was associated with resolution of reflux symptoms in up to 65% of patients who lost weight (n = 124). Ness-Jensen et al[7] found that the association was dose dependent, with patients with the highest body mass index (BMI) loss having the most significant reduction in reflux symptoms as well as response to treatment.

FUNCTIONAL DYSPEPSIA

Functional dyspepsia (FD) comprises a heterogeneous group of symptoms, loosely described as "indigestion" by the lay public, which includes such complaints as postprandial fullness, early satiety, epigastric pain/discomfort, nausea, and vomiting (Table 16-2). By definition, no organic cause for these common symptoms is evident, and anxiety and depression are common comorbidities. Some affected individuals report the sudden onset of their dyspeptic symptoms following an enteric infection, including food-borne gastroenteritis. In the third iteration of the Rome criteria for the functional GI disorders, Rome III, two syndromes were identified within FD: the postprandial distress syndrome and the epigastric pain syndrome. Since the former is more likely to be associated with delayed gastric emptying, dietary strategies that are employed in gastroparesis, such as smaller, low-fat, low-fiber meals may be appropriate; this approach has not, however, been formally tested.

Most patients report symptoms after meals[8]; however, the precise mechanisms whereby food may initiate or perpetuate symptoms in FD are largely unknown. FD patients often exhibit an exaggerated response to food ingestion, demonstrating a hypersensitivity to food components that is not perceived by healthy subjects.[9] This hypersensitivity appears to be most acute in relation to fat intake, as glucose did not elicit the same exaggerated response.[10] Meals with a high fat content have indeed been implicated in the induction of symptoms in FD.[11] Pilichiewicz et al[10] found that fatty meals, in comparison to carbohydrates, induced more symptoms of bloating, nausea, and abdominal pain. Fats induce symptoms at lower nutrient loads in patients with FD when compared with healthy subjects.[10,11] However, the role fat plays in FD needs to be further elucidated, as a number of population-based dietary surveys have provided conflicting results on fat intake in FD.[12,13] The documentation of increased numbers of eosinophils in the duodenal mucosa raised the possibility of a specific food allergy in FD, and especially among those with epigastric pain syndrome, although none, as yet, have been convincingly documented. Given the paucity of data, dietary recommendations in FD remain rudimentary and include keeping a food diary to facilitate the identification of food items that trigger symptoms, eating smaller but more frequent meals, and reducing fat intake.[8] FD commonly overlaps with irritable bowel syndrome (IBS), and symptoms such as bloating, distention, and "gas" are therefore common; dietary strategies that are used to address these symptoms in IBS (see later) may, accordingly, be considered.

TABLE 16-3	
AN APPRAISAL OF THE DIETARY MANAGEMENT OF CHRONIC CONSTIPATION	
EVIDENCE-BASED	PROPOSED BUT STATUS UNCERTAIN
Fiber	Increased fluid intake
	Exercise

CONSTIPATION

Chronic idiopathic (or functional) constipation (CIC) encompasses not just infrequent defecation, but also several symptoms that reflect some difficulty with the act of defecation, as well as some commonly associated symptoms such as bloating (Table 16-3). Constipation is a common symptom, affecting up to 10% to 20% of the general population and increases in prevalence with increasing age, affecting up to one-third of individuals over the age of 60. While constipation may be secondary to a long list of medications or underlying medical disorders, the focus in this discussion will be on functional constipation.

Lifestyle and dietary changes have been first-line recommendations in the management of constipation. Although exercise and an adequate fluid intake (typically in excess of 1500 mL/day of water) are typically recommended, the evidence base for both is slim. In summary, there is no evidence that increased fluid intake (unless dehydrated) or regular physical activity will alleviate chronic constipation.[14]

Those who experience constipation incriminate various foods (chocolate, bananas, and black tea) as causative and others (prunes, coffee, wine, and beer) as therapeutic[26]; prospective assessments of dietary interventions based on these perceptions are lacking.

The relationship between fiber intake and constipation rests on a firmer footing. Thus, epidemiological evidence supports a relationship between constipation and inadequate intake of dietary fiber, and an increase in dietary fiber and/or fiber-containing supplements has been shown to ameliorate symptoms.[15] Sufferers are encouraged to consume at least 25 to 30 g of fiber daily. High-fiber foods include bananas, prunes, kiwis, whole grains, bran, and vegetables. Fiber acts to increase the water content in the stool and stimulates the growth of bacterial populations in the colon. Insoluble fiber, such as bran, is nondegradable and retains more water than soluble fiber. Soluble fibers include methylcellulose and psyllium. The evidence for use of soluble fiber to relieve chronic constipation is more consistent than that for insoluble fibers. In a meta-analysis of six trials, use of soluble fiber (psyllium, inulin, and maltodextrin) in doses of 10 to 20 g/day improved stool frequency, decreased defecation time, and reduced the sensation of incomplete evacuation.[16] In contrast, studies of insoluble fiber, including bran in a dose of 20 g/day and rye bread at 320 g/day, provided conflicting results, with one trial reporting improvement in stool frequency and another trial showing no difference.[16] Adverse effects of the use of soluble fiber include abdominal pain. Bloating, abdominal pain, and flatulence are commonly reported with insoluble fiber. Despite the paucity of high-quality trials and the inconclusive nature of their results, there is evidence that fiber is cost-effective in the management of constipation.[17]

TABLE 16-4	
AN APPRAISAL OF THE DIETARY MANAGEMENT OF IRRITABLE BOWEL SYNDROME	
EVIDENCE-BASED	PROPOSED BUT STATUS UNCERTAIN
Food diary to identify trigger symptoms Soluble fiber Low FODMAPs	Food allergy Gluten-free diet Insoluble fiber Lactose-free diet Low-sucrose and low-sorbitol diet Low-fat diet Mediterranean diet

IRRITABLE BOWEL SYNDROME

IBS is a poorly understood functional GI disorder that is estimated to affect between 10% and 20% of the general adult population in Europe and North America (Table 16-4). The cardinal clinical features of IBS are recurrent/episodic abdominal pain in association with an altered bowel habit; bloating and distension are common additional complaints. Since, by definition, IBS has no identifiable organic cause and no reliable diagnostic biomarker has been identified, the diagnosis rests on clinical features alone. Various stool patterns may predominate in a given individual: constipation (IBS-C), diarrhea (IBS-D), or an alternating or mixed pattern (IBS-M). While IBS types may overlap, there is some evidence to suggest that IBS-C and IBS-D are distinct phenotypes. The pathophysiology of IBS is unknown, with a variety of factors such as dysmotility, visceral hypersensitivity, aberrant brain processing of visceral events, psychopathology, immune activation, and an altered gut microbiome being variously proposed.

While diet has, traditionally, been assigned a relatively minor role in the pathogenesis of IBS, this is in contrast to the experience of patients, who often report exacerbations of their IBS symptoms as either a direct or deferred reaction to certain foods.[18] Indeed, diet along with stress and the menstrual cycle are by far the most common precipitating or exacerbating factors in IBS, and recent studies have demonstrated the diagnostic value of the induction of symptoms by food in IBS.[19,20]

Surveys of GI clinic patients found that 30% to 50% believed that their symptoms represented food allergy or food intolerance.[18,21,22] Most food-related IBS symptoms appear to represent food intolerance, although only 11% to 27% of patients can accurately identify the presumed offending food when rechallenged in a double-blind manner. It should come as no surprise, therefore, that formal dietary surveys have not identified a consistent pattern of food avoidance among IBS patients. Based on their own experiences with food, and despite a lack of objective evidence to incriminate a specific food, studies have shown that a majority of IBS patients institute dietary changes, sometimes to an extent that may compromise their nutrition.[21]

The use of fiber in the management of IBS is controversial, as systematic reviews have revealed conflicting findings on the impact of fiber in general.[15] While one recent meta-analysis found no support for the use of bulking agents in the management of IBS,[23] another showed that soluble fibers, such as psyllium, are beneficial in IBS.[24] Studies on the use of dietary fibers such as fruits, cereals, and vegetables in management of IBS are limited. Such foods, however, may aggravate symptoms of IBS, as they contain a high content of FODMAPs.[15] Like FD, patients with IBS have an exaggerated physiological response to lipid ingestion. Again, although a significant number of patients with IBS identify fatty meals as a trigger of symptoms, it is not clearly established that exclusion of fats alleviates IBS.[11]

Currently, in both the lay press and the medical literature, the two dietary interventions that have attracted the most attention are the low-FODMAPs and gluten-free diets. The FODMAP concept was introduced in the early 2000s and proposes that specific non- or poorly digested carbohydrates contribute to common IBS symptoms through the induction of alterations in gut motility and secretion. Symptoms associated with a high-FODMAP diet include pain, bloating, distension, flatulence, and diarrhea. Low-FODMAP diets have been shown to reduce GI symptoms when compared with high-FODMAP diets and unrestricted diets.[25,26] A low-FODMAP diet is quite restrictive—patients should work with an experienced dietician to ensure that they are able to derive essential nutrients from other dietary sources.

Gluten intolerance or sensitivity, including nonceliac gluten sensitivity (NCGS), in functional bowel disorders has been the focus of much lay interest, with the gluten-free food industry now a billion-dollar industry. Though patients report resolution of GI symptoms on a gluten-free diet,[27] and studies demonstrate the precipitation of symptoms on exposure to gluten-containing diets,[28,29] the mechanisms by which gluten induces GI symptoms in functional bowel disorders remain unclear. On the one hand, some studies suggest the existence of a specific, perhaps immunologically mediated, effect of gluten[29,30]; others suggest that any effect of a wheat-free diet is related to the exclusion of the FODMAPs and fructans, and that the addition of gluten restriction to a low-FODMAP diet offers little additional benefit.[31]

Patients often report reproducible symptoms with certain foods, with resolution after such exposures are discontinued, leading them to conclude that they have a food allergy. It needs to be stressed that a food allergy refers to a specific immunologically mediated reaction to a food, and may be IgE mediated or non-IgE mediated. Food intolerance or sensitivities, on the other hand, are nonimmunologically mediated reactions to food that may encompass a broad range of disorders or complaints, ranging from lactose intolerance to idiosyncratic reactions to certain proteins such as gluten and cow's milk, taste aversion, eating disorders, and other psychologically mediated food sensitivities.

There is little evidence for a role for classical IgE-mediated food allergy in IBS,[32] although there has been a suggestion that elimination diets based on IgG-mediated antibody tests may provide some benefit.[27] The status of IgG antibodies to food components remains disputed, and allergy testing cannot be recommended at this time. Food intolerance, in contrast, may be more relevant; the role of FODMAPs and gluten has already been discussed; other evidence suggests a role for other potentially to poorly absorbed carbohydrates, such as fructose, lactose, sorbitol, and other sugar alcohols in IBS.[33] Many of these are incorporated under the umbrella of FODMAPs; the benefits of exclusion of just one of these carbohydrates are less certain.

It must also be stressed that psychological factors may interact with other phenomena to exaggerate or perpetuate food-related symptoms in IBS and other functional GI disorders.[34]

Finally, a further entity deserves mention: the microbiome. Alterations in the colonic microbiome have been demonstrated in IBS, though the primacy of these abnormalities in the pathogenesis of IBS remains to be defined. Nevertheless, diet is a major modifier, both in the short and the long term, of the microbiota,[35] and it remains distinctly possible that interactions between diet and the microbiota (be it normal or disturbed) could play a role in the genesis of food-related symptoms in IBS.

REFERENCES

1. Dore MP, Maragkoudakis E, Fraley K, et al. Diet, lifestyle and gender in gastro-esophageal reflux disease. *Dig Dis Sci.* 2008;53:2027-2032.

2. Johnson T, Gerson L, Hershcovici T, Stave C, Fass R. Systematic review: the effects of carbonated beverages on gastro-oesophageal reflux disease. *Aliment Pharmacol Ther.* 2010;31:607-614.

3. Nilsson M, Johnsen R, Ye W, Hveem K, Lagergren J. Lifestyle related risk factors in the aetiology of gastro-oesophageal reflux. *Gut.* 2004;53:1730-1735.

4. Murphy DW, Castell DO. Chocolate and heartburn: evidence of increased esophageal acid exposure after chocolate ingestion. *Am J Gastroenterol.* 1988;83:633-636.

5. Bulat R, Fachnie E, Chauhan U, Chen Y, Tougas G. Lack of effect of spearmint on lower oesophageal sphincter function and acid reflux in healthy volunteers. *Aliment Pharmacol Ther.* 1999;13:805-812.

6. Singh M, Lee J, Gupta N, et al. Weight loss can lead to resolution of gastroesophageal reflux disease symptoms: a prospective intervention trial. *Obesity.* 2013;21:284-290.

7. Ness-Jensen E, Lindam A, Lagergren J, Hveem K. Weight loss and reduction in gastroesophageal reflux. A prospective population-based cohort study: the HUNT study. *Am J Gastroenterol.* 2013;108:376-382.

8. Lacy BE, Talley NJ, Locke GR 3rd, et al. Review article: current treatment options and management of functional dyspepsia. *Aliment Pharmacol Ther.* 2012;36:3-15.

9. Feinle-Bisset C, Azpiroz F. Dietary and lifestyle factors in functional dyspepsia. *Nat Rev Gastroenterol Hepatol.* 2013;10:150-157.

10. Pilichiewicz AN, Feltrin KL, Horowitz M, et al. Functional dyspepsia is associated with a greater symptomatic response to fat but not carbohydrate, increased fasting and postprandial CCK, and diminished PYY. *Am J Gastroenterol.* 2008;103:2613-2623.

11. Feinle-Bisset C, Azpiroz F. Dietary lipids and functional gastrointestinal disorders. *Am J Gastroenterol.* 2013;108:737-747.

12. Saito YA, Locke GR 3rd, Weaver AL, Zinsmeister AR, Talley NJ. Diet and functional gastrointestinal disorders: a population-based case-control study. *Am J Gastroenterol.* 2005;100:2743-2748.

13. Carvalho RV, Lorena SL, Almeida JR, Mesquita MA. Food intolerance, diet composition, and eating patterns in functional dyspepsia patients. *Dig Dis Sci.* 2010;55:60-65.

14. Bove A, Bellini M, Battaglia E, et al. Consensus statement AIGO/SICCR diagnosis and treatment of chronic constipation and obstructed defecation (part II: treatment). *World J Gastroenterol.* 2012;18:4994-5013.

15. Eswaran S, Muir J, Chey WD. Fiber and functional gastrointestinal disorders. *Am J Gastroenterol.* 2013;108:718-727.

16. Suares NC, Ford AC. Systematic review: the effects of fibre in the management of chronic idiopathic constipation. *Aliment Pharmacol Ther.* 2011;33:895-901.

17. Schmier JK, Miller PE, Levine JA, et al. Cost savings of reduced constipation rates attributed to increased dietary fiber intakes: a decision-analytic model. *BMC Public Health.* 2014;14:374.

18. Simren M, Mansson A, Langkilde AM, et al. Food-related gastrointestinal symptoms in the irritable bowel syndrome. *Digestion.* 2001;63:108-115.

19. Posserud I, Strid H, Störsrud S, et al. Symptom pattern following a meal challenge test in patients with irritable bowel syndrome and healthy controls. *United Eur Gastroenterol J.* 2013;1:358-367.

20. Le Nevé B, Posserud I, Böhn L, et al. A combined nutrient and lactulose challenge test allows symptom-based clustering of patients with irritable bowel syndrome. *Am J Gastroenterol.* 2013;108:786-795.

21. Hayes P, Corish C, O'Mahony E, et al. A dietary survey of patients with irritable bowel syndrome. *J Hum Nutr Diet.* 2013;2014;27(Suppl 2):36-47.

22. Bohn L, Storsrud S, Tornblom H, et al. Self-reported food-related gastrointestinal symptoms in IBS are common and associated with more severe symptoms and reduced quality of life. *Am J Gastroenterol.* 2013;108:634-641.

23. Ruepert L, Quartero AO, de Wit NJ, van der Heijden GJ, Rubin G, Muris JW. Bulking agents, antispasmodics and antidepressants for the treatment of irritable bowel syndrome. *Cochrane Database Syst Rev.* 2011; CD003460.

24. Ford AC, Quigley EM, Lacy BE, et al. American College of Gastroenterology monograph on the management of irritable bowel syndrome and chronic idiopathic constipation. *Am J Gastroenterol.* 2014 (in press).

25. Halmos EP, Power VA, Shepherd SJ, et al. A diet low in FODMAPs reduces symptoms of irritable bowel syndrome. *Gastroenterology.* 2013.

26. Staudacher HM, Lomer MC, Anderson JL, et al. Fermentable carbohydrate restriction reduces luminal bifidobacteria and gastrointestinal symptoms in patients with irritable bowel syndrome. *J Nutr.* 2012;142:1510-1518.

27. Boettcher E, Crowe SE. Dietary proteins and functional gastrointestinal disorders. *Am J Gastroenterol.* 2013;108:728-736.

28. Biesiekierski JR, Newnham ED, Irving PM, et al. Gluten causes gastrointestinal symptoms in subjects without celiac disease: A double-blind randomized placebo-controlled trial. *Am J Gastroenterol.* 2011;106:508-514.

29. Vazquez Roque MI, Camilleri M, Smyrk T, et al. A controlled trial of gluten-free diet in patients with irritable bowel syndrome-diarrhea: effects on bowel frequency and intestinal function. *Gastroenterology.* 2013;144:903-911.

30. Carroccio A, Mansueto P, D'Almcamo A, Iacono G. Non-celiac wheat sensitivity as an allergic condition: personal experience and narrative review. *Am J Gastroenterol.* 2013;108:1845-1852.

31. Biesiekierski JR, Peters SL, Newnham ED, et al. No effects of gluten in patients with self-reported non-celiac gluten sensitivity after dietary reduction of fermentable, poorly absorbed, short-chain carbohydrates. *Gastroenterology.* 2013;145:320-328.

32. Park MI, Camilleri M. Is there a role of food allergy in irritable bowel syndrome and functional dyspepsia? A systematic review. *Neurogastroenterol Motil.* 2006;18:595-607.

33. Shepherd SJ, Lomer MC, Gibson PR. Short-chain carbohydrates and functional gastrointestinal disorders. *Am J Gastroenterol.* 2013;108:707-717.

34. Farre R, Tack J. Food and symptom generation in functional gastrointestinal disorders: physiological aspects. *Am J Gastroenterol.* 2013;108:698-706.

35. David LA, Maurice CF, Carmody RN, et al. Diet rapidly and reproducibly alters the human gut microbiome. *Nature.* 2014;505:559-563.

Section IV

Colonic and Anorectal Disorders

Colonic Symptoms
Constipation, Diarrhea, and Fecal Incontinence

Lawrence R. Schiller, MD

KEY POINTS

- The colon is responsible for reclaiming most of the water, electrolytes, and nutrients that pass into it from the small intestine. This process involves the interaction of motility, mucosal function, luminal contents, and the microbiome contained within the colon.

- Constipation develops 1) when slow transit allows more time for mucosal absorption and bacterial fermentation to reduce the amount of luminal contents presented to the rectum, or 2) when the rectum and continence mechanisms malfunction, producing ineffective defecation. Diagnosis is usually straightforward, and therapies are effective.

- Diarrhea may develop if transit through the colon is too rapid or if the mucosa does not absorb sufficient water before material gets to the rectum because of mucosal dysfunction or the presence of osmotically active materials in the colon that retain water. Evaluation of these patients may be difficult due to the number of potential causes, but can be aided by identifying the diarrhea as being watery, inflammatory, or fatty. Nonspecific therapy can help if a specific diagnosis is not realized.

- Fecal incontinence is a troubling symptom that indicates a problem with the continence mechanisms (rectum, pelvic floor, anal sphincters and associated innervation). Assessment with physical examination and simple tests can identify the pathophysiology in most cases. A variety of treatments are available, ranging from modifying stool habits and biofeedback to complex surgeries.

NORMAL FUNCTIONS OF THE COLON AND RECTUM

Each day the colon receives 1 to 1.5 L of material from the small intestine.[1] This material is largely salt water and undigested ingested substances, such as fiber and incompletely absorbed carbohydrates. The colon mucosa is able to absorb water and salt quite efficiently, and typically all

Rao SSC, Parkman HP, McCallum RW, eds.
Handbook of Gastrointestinal Motility and Functional Disorders (pp 211-219).
© 2015 Taylor & Francis Group.

but 80 mL of water and almost all of the sodium chloride is removed from luminal contents daily. Under intestinal perfusion conditions, steady-state absorption rates can reach 3 to 4 L/24 h; thus, there is potential capacity to compensate for increased delivery of fluid to the colon that might occur if the small intestine is diseased. Under ordinary circumstances, steady-state conditions are not present and net absorption depends on motility, which determines the delivery and distribution of fluid to the absorptive surface. Rapid transit through the colon dramatically reduces the time available for absorption and can cause diarrhea. Conversely, slow transit through the colon can lead to more complete absorption of water and salt and delivery of less material to the rectum each day.[2]

The composition of the fluid entering the colon also modulates water absorption.[3] Some poorly absorbable substances, such as magnesium salts, obligate water retention in the lumen osmotically, limiting water absorption and potentially producing diarrhea (thereby making them effective laxatives). Big organic polymers, such as fiber and polyethylene glycol, complex with water molecules, effectively removing them from solution and increasing the chemical activity of other solutes, thus reducing net water absorption by the colon. This water-holding capacity of solids in luminal contents is a major determinant of stool consistency.[4] For example, fat is much less capable of binding water than carbohydrates, and for any given stool water content, fatty stools will have a looser consistency than less fatty stools.

The other factor modulating colonic physiology is the microbiome contained within the colon. The colon houses a rich ecosystem of microorganisms that can ferment carbohydrates that find their way into the colon. This bacterial metabolism has several effects. Fermentation produces short-chain fatty acids that can be absorbed by the colon mucosa, providing nutrition to the epithelial cells, increasing sodium and fluid absorption, and modulating colonic motility. If produced in excess to the amount that can be absorbed by the mucosa, short-chain fatty acids can cause osmotic diarrhea. Fermentation also results in production of CO_2, H_2, and CH_4, which can contribute to bloating and excess flatus. Bacterial metabolism also produces diffusible bioactive gases, such as nitric oxide, methane, and hydrogen sulfide, which can modulate smooth muscle function and affect colon motility.[5]

Thus, delivery of contents to the rectum involves the interaction of four factors: (1) mucosal absorption, (2) motility, (3) the composition of luminal contents, and (4) the colonic microbiome. These factors interact to determine the amount of material entering the rectum. The pattern of defecation depends on four additional factors: (1) the reservoir capacity of the rectum, (2) the ability of the rectum to expel stool, (3) the ability of the pelvic floor and sphincter muscles to prevent leakage, and 4) the ability of those muscles to relax and allow for defecation.[6]

Luminal contents are retained in the sigmoid colon, and absorption of a critical last few percent of water allows luminal contents to change from a viscous liquid to a soft solid. This material is usually retained in the sigmoid colon until the gastrocolonic response stimulates emptying into the rectum. Distention of the rectum activates the rectoanal inhibitory reflex, which causes internal anal sphincter relaxation. In infants before toilet training, this is followed by rectal contraction and automatic defecation as part of the peristaltic reflex. After toilet training, contraction of the puborectalis muscle and external anal sphincter blocks defecation long enough for rectal accommodation to occur. It takes about 30 seconds for relaxation of the rectal wall to reduce intrarectal pressure enough to avoid defecation. This process depends on processing of sensory information from the anal canal and rectum and allows for deferring evacuation until voluntary, elective defecation is appropriate.[7]

The rectum is distinguished from the more proximal colon by the presence of a continuous, circumferential, longitudinal muscle coat (instead of the discontinuous taenia of the more proximal colon). This allows for shortening of the rectum, more effective "splinting" of the smooth muscle, and development of more powerfully propulsive peristaltic contractions in the circular muscle layer. Under normal circumstances, defecation is initiated by increasing intra-abdominal pressure by a Valsalva maneuver and relaxing the pelvic floor muscles and external anal sphincter.

This allows stool to come in contact with the anal canal, which is densely innervated by nerves that sense pressure. This in turn triggers rectal contractions that push stool through the anus.[8]

As mentioned, the pelvic floor and external anal sphincter muscles play a critical role in maintaining continence (by contracting and preventing evacuation) and allowing defecation (by relaxing and "getting out of the way"). The puborectalis muscle is a specialized part of the pelvic floor that loops from the pubic arch anteriorly around the rectum posteriorly and then back to the pubic arch anteriorly. It is composed of skeletal muscle with a preponderance of type I (slow twitch) fibers capable of continuous contraction. (These muscle fibers are the same type as the "antigravity" muscles of the legs and back, which remain contracted for long periods when we are standing.) When the puborectalis muscle is contracted, it pulls the rectoanal junction anteriorly, kinking the rectal outlet and preventing the passage of solid stool.[7]

CHRONIC CONSTIPATION

Clinical Symptoms

For many clinicians, constipation is synonymous with infrequent defecation (<3 bowel movements/week). Patients more often mean something else by the complaint of constipation; only 1 in 3 constipated patients experiences infrequency. The most common complaints in constipated patients are straining with evacuation (81%), passage of hard or lumpy stools (72%), and incomplete emptying (54%). Other complaints include the inability to pass stool, fullness or bloating, and use of fingers to facilitate defecation. It is incumbent upon the physician to understand exactly what the patient means by the complaint of "constipation."[9]

Pathophysiology of Chronic Constipation

In theory, an increased rate of absorption by the colonic mucosa might result in constipation by reducing the amount of material reaching the rectum each day, but this has never been demonstrated in patients with constipation. Instead, constipation is typically related to other mechanisms.[10,11]

The first group of mechanisms involves the reduced flow through the colon. Dietary considerations include reduction of overall intake, reduction of fiber intake, and modified diets, such as gluten-free diets (which also are low in fructans and other poorly absorbed carbohydrates). These reduce the volume of luminal contents entering the colon. Overall food intake may be more predictive of constipation than fiber intake. Medications may be constipating, including agents that modify luminal contents, such as aluminum and calcium salts and bile acid binders. These likely produce constipation by reducing intracolonic bile acid concentrations, which ordinarily modulate colon motility and absorption. Other drugs with direct effects on smooth muscle or nerves may inhibit colonic motility, such as anticholinergic drugs and opiates. These drugs slow motility, thereby allowing more time for the absorption of water and salt by the mucosa and more time for bacterial fermentation to metabolize luminal solids, resulting in less luminal contents reaching the colon and infrequent evacuation. In two relatively rare conditions—Hirschsprung disease and Chagas disease—abnormalities of the enteric nervous system inhibit normal motility and are responsible for constipation. The factors behind more common, idiopathic, slow-transit constipation are less well understood, but advanced cases often show evidence of loss of nerve cells in the enteric nervous system. It has been suggested that the presence of methanogenic bacteria in the colonic microbiome may produce constipation by releasing methane that diffuses into the colonic wall and affect nerves and muscles that influence motility and slow flow through the colon. Constipation may be secondary to other conditions, such as pregnancy, diabetes, hypothyroidism, neuromuscular disorders, and mechanical obstruction.[10]

A second group of mechanisms is best characterized as anorectal outlet dysfunction.[11] In these conditions, evacuation of stool from the rectum is inhibited by poor rectal expulsion or transient obstruction of the rectal outlet by untimely contraction of the puborectalis muscle and external anal sphincter ("dyssynergia") or by transient anatomic blockage. Poor expulsion may be seen in some patients with neuromuscular diseases, megarectum, or large rectoceles. Dyssynergia appears to be an acquired or learned problem that can be treated with biofeedback training. Transient mechanical obstruction may be due to rectal mucosal intussusception, anterior rectal wall rectal ulcer syndrome, enteroceles, or perineal descent. Anorectal outlet obstruction may be responsible for complaints of excessive straining on defecation or incomplete evacuation. The hallmark symptom of this problem is the patient's use of her fingers to splint the perineal or posterior vaginal wall (rectovaginal septum) to facilitate defecation.

Evaluation of Patients With Chronic Constipation

For most patients initially presenting with constipation, a thorough history and thoughtful physical examination, including a digital rectal examination, are sufficient to formulate a differential diagnosis, to exclude findings that might mandate a more extensive evaluation, and to begin therapy. This is because the majority of patients presenting with constipation do not have serious systemic or life-threatening diseases and will respond to simple measures (eg, lifestyle changes, fiber, and laxatives). For those patients who have not responded to simple therapies or who have evidence of anorectal outlet obstruction, further evaluation may be needed to exclude underlying problems and to direct therapy.

The history should cover the onset, evolution of symptoms, previous evaluation, and therapies (including home remedies), and should include review of alarm features ("red flags") that might require further evaluation. These include evidence of rectal bleeding or anemia, weight loss, family history of colorectal cancer or inflammatory bowel disease, persistent constipation that has been refractory to treatment, and the new onset of constipation in an elderly patient. Physical examination may reveal evidence of a systematic disease, but the key element is the rectal examination. The perineum should be inspected carefully with good illumination to check for hemorrhoids and anal fissures. The anal canal should be probed gently with a well-lubricated finger to assess sphincter tenderness, anal tone at rest and with squeeze, and the condition of the puborectalis muscle. This muscle is a transverse bar best appreciated posteriorly just inferior to the rectoanal junction. Note should be made of tenderness and tone at rest and when the patient is asked to squeeze to prevent evacuation. The patient also should be asked to bear down as if to evacuate: the puborectalis muscle should relax, and the outlet should change in shape from a cylinder surrounding the examining finger to a funnel that is open superiorly. The rectal vault should be examined for the presence of stool, the consistency of that stool, and its overall size. Attention should be paid to the contour of the anterior wall of the rectum: if it extends far anteriorly, a rectocele may be present.

When a patient has constipation symptoms that are refractory to treatment or if confirmation of anorectal outlet dysfunction is desired, several tests can be used.[11] Anorectal manometry is useful in assessing anal sphincter strength and innervation, rectal sensation, and the presence of pelvic floor dyssynergia. In this test a balloon-tipped probe is placed in the rectum and pressure measurements are made in the anal canal while the patient relaxes and then squeezes. The presence of dyssynergia is evaluated when the patient is asked to evacuate the partially filled balloon while anal canal pressure is monitored. During this maneuver, the anal canal should relax as the balloon is expelled. Any increase in anal canal pressure indicates the presence of dyssynergia. A simplified "balloon expulsion test" can be used as an office test. Another test that is used to assess outlet function is defecography. The presence of rectoceles and enteroceles, adequate opening of the rectoanal angle when the puborectalis muscle relaxes, excessive perineal descent, and mucosal prolapse can be evaluated. Technical issues with fluoroscopic defecography have largely been resolved, but interobserver variation and radiation exposure remain problematic. Magnetic resonance imaging can mitigate the latter concern.

The other "advanced" tests for chronic constipation measure colon transit.[9] Historically, radiopaque markers (Sitzmarks [Konsyl Pharmaceuticals]) were ingested and daily abdominal radiographs were made over 1 week to demonstrate passage of the markers through the colon. Several different protocols were validated, but concern about radiation exposure limited use of this test in its fully developed form. Currently used protocols typically involve making one radiograph 5 days after marker ingestion, with normal defined as clearance of all markers at that time. An alternative test uses a radiotelemetry capsule that is ingested and sends data regarding intraluminal pH, pressure, and temperature, which can be used to estimate transit through the stomach, small intestine, and colon. Some clinicians prefer to measure colon transit early in the evaluation of patients with refractory constipation. They claim that this identifies those patients with slow transit early in their course. It is possible to identify patients with "factitious constipation" who clear all of the markers despite claiming to have no bowel movements during the test period. There is general agreement that a colon transit study should be done before referring patients for colectomy as treatment for slow-transit constipation.

Treatment of Chronic Constipation

This is discussed in detail in another chapter. In brief, the foundation of all treatments for constipation is lifestyle change. Diet should be assessed, preferably with a prospectively obtained diet diary: an appropriate calorie intake is essential. Fiber intake also should be evaluated: if the patient is already consuming 20 to 25 g of fiber daily, further supplementation is unlikely to be helpful. The type of fiber consumed may be important as well: soluble fiber is more effective for treating constipation than insoluble fiber (eg, bran).[12] Water intake needs to be adequate to avoid dehydration; there is little evidence that taking more water by itself is helpful, since the intestine can absorb 24 or more liters of water daily, leaving little ingested water to add to stool volume. Physical activity seems to be important as well; bedbound patients have fewer stools than ambulatory subjects. It is less clear that increased physical exercise is helpful.

Laxatives and stool softeners provide relief of constipation for most patients.[9,13] They fall into four categories: bulking agents, stool softeners, osmotic agents, and stimulant laxatives. Polyethylene glycol (PEG) is a large polymer that should not produce much osmotic activity in solution because of its high molecular weight. It exerts anomalous osmotic activity,[14] however, and is a safe and effective agent.

When simple measures fail, several prescription drugs are available for the management of chronic constipation, including lubiprostone, linaclotide, and prucalopride.[15,16] Patients with anorectal outlet dysfunction due to dyssynergic defecation may benefit from biofeedback training.[17] Colectomy for slow-transit constipation should be undertaken with caution and only after extensive evaluation.[18] Any coexisting outlet problem needs to be discovered and resolved before surgery; colectomy will be an unsuccessful treatment if outlet problems persist. Patients with preexisting abdominal pain, depression, or other psychiatric disturbances have more complications postoperatively, such as bowel obstruction; surgery should be avoided in those patients.

DIARRHEA

Clinical Symptoms

For many clinicians, diarrhea is synonymous with increased stool frequency. However, patients tend to concentrate on loose stool consistency rather than just increased frequency as the primary manifestation of diarrhea. Some physicians concentrate on increased stool weight as characteristic of diarrhea, with 200 g/day as the upper limit of normal. It is not clear whether there is any essential difference in pathophysiology in patients with loose stools between those with stool weights greater than 200 g/day and those with stool weights less than that.[19,20]

For the purposes of differential diagnosis, it is useful to distinguish between acute diarrhea lasting less than 1 month and chronic diarrhea, which lasts more than 1 month. Acute diarrheas tend to be infectious in origin, whereas chronic diarrheas typically are not infectious. It has also proven to be useful to distinguish among watery, inflammatory, and fatty diarrhea based on stool characteristics.

Pathophysiology of Diarrhea

The pathophysiology of diarrhea is multifactorial in most cases.[19] Historically, increased motility and rapid transit were cited as causes of diarrhea. This mechanism would cause diarrhea by reducing the amount of time for absorption of luminal contents by the mucosa. For the past 40 years, there has been great emphasis on altered mucosal absorption rate as a cause for diarrhea. Bacterial toxins, cytokines and peptide hormones, bile acid malabsorption, altered neural regulation, and immunological factors have all been cited as reasons for alteration in mucosal absorptive function. In addition, malabsorption and maldigestion of ingested materials may contribute to luminal retention of water and altered stool consistency. The current synthesis of the pathophysiology of diarrhea implicates all of these factors. Impaired mucosal absorption rate is only part of the picture in most patients, and rapid transit plays an important role in many individuals.

The colon plays a key role in the development of diarrhea. In conditions in which small bowel function is compromised and the flow of luminal contents into the colon increases, the absorptive capacity of the colon may mitigate the increase in stool weight that might otherwise occur. In theory, the colon can absorb up to 3 to 4 L of fluid daily and so if colonic absorptive capacity is unaffected by the disease process, stool weight can be substantially reduced. This presupposes that increased flow into the colon will not stimulate colonic transit. The colon can also mitigate malabsorption of nutrients, particularly carbohydrates, by providing a place for bacterial fermentation to occur. Absorption of the products of fermentation would tend to reduce the osmotic contribution to stool weight. Of course, if the colon is involved with the disease process and if its absorptive function is reduced or transit is speeded, it may actually increase stool weight.

Evaluation of Patients With Diarrhea

Diarrhea is a symptom with many causes, and the evaluation of any patient with diarrhea begins with a thorough history and careful physical examination.[19] Often, the cause of diarrhea can be inferred from the temporal development of symptoms. For example, a patient developing diarrhea after a cholecystectomy may well have diarrhea induced by bile acid malabsorption. Some patients may have diarrhea as part of irritable bowel syndrome, a condition that is best diagnosed by history alone. In such individuals, a therapeutic trial may be indicated rather than further diagnostic evaluation.

When the likely cause of diarrhea is not apparent, deciding whether the diarrhea is acute or chronic and is categorized as watery, inflammatory, or fatty can help to direct the further evaluation of the patient. Stool analysis (including fecal electrolytes, pH, test for occult blood, test for white blood cells or white blood cell markers, and fecal fat) may be of use in distinguishing among these categories and may provide important clues to the etiology of diarrhea.[20] Further testing may include imaging of the absorptive surface of the intestine with radiography and/or endoscopy. Biopsy of the small intestine and colon may also be indicated. Tests of transit through the intestine have generally been of little use and are seldom done to evaluate diarrhea.[19]

Treatment of Diarrhea

The best treatments for diarrhea are to make a specific diagnosis and to provide specific treatment for that condition. Unlike constipation, in which idiopathic constipation is the diagnosis for a substantial proportion of patients, diarrhea is usually a symptom of a specific condition, and thus substantial efforts should be made to find a specific diagnosis when the patient presents with diarrhea.

When symptomatic therapy is required (eg, while a diagnostic evaluation is underway or if there is no specific treatment for the diagnosis that has been made), treatment with an opiate antidiarrheal drug is usually effective.[21] Many patients respond to low-potency antidiarrheals, such as diphenoxylate or loperamide. In patients with chronic diarrhea, the key is to give these drugs expectantly, typically before meals and at bedtime. Some patients require more potent opiates, such as codeine, morphine, or opium. These agents have the potential for abuse and sedation. The keys to using these drugs for chronic diarrhea are to start with low doses, titrate the dose up gradually, and monitor usage closely.

The major threat to life with diarrhea is due to volume depletion and renal insufficiency. Provision of adequate fluid replacement, either intravenously or with oral rehydration solution, can be life-saving. In some individuals, nutritional depletion is also a problem that requires attention.

FECAL INCONTINENCE

Clinical Symptoms

Fecal incontinence is the great unvoiced symptom in gastroenterology.[6] Patients often misinterpret incontinence as being due to particularly severe diarrhea and will report it as such. Doctors may not ask patients specifically about "soiling," "leakage," "accidents," or urgency, and thus may miss the opportunity to help with this embarrassing and disabling symptom. Incontinence can occur with both formed and loose stools. When it occurs with loose stools, it may improve with treatment of diarrhea. Some clinicians distinguish between various grades of incontinence, differentiating smearing from gross incontinence, but it is unclear whether this has any pathophysiologic import.

Pathophysiology of Fecal Incontinence

Incontinence occurs when there has been a compromise of rectal sensation, the reservoir capacity of the rectum, or the mechanisms that prevent defecation, such as pelvic floor and anal sphincter function.[6] If patients are unaware of the entry of luminal contents into the rectum, they may not take precautions to prevent evacuation. If the rectum is too stiff and cannot relax properly to accommodate incoming luminal contents, intraluminal pressure can rise to high levels and threaten continence. Finally, if the muscles that have to contract to prevent evacuation (puborectalis muscle and external anal sphincter) are weak, defecation may proceed without intention. A variety of problems can produce these defects and can be responsible for fecal incontinence.

Evaluation of Patients with Fecal Incontinence

The single most useful diagnostic test in patients with fecal incontinence is a thoughtful rectal examination. This should include assessment of the perianal skin, specifically looking for evidence of irritation. Digital examination should include assessment of baseline sphincter tone, the increase in pressure associated with squeezing, muscle bulk including both the anal sphincters and puborectalis muscle, and the ability of the puborectalis muscle to contract when the patient attempts to prevent evacuation. In addition, the extent of perineal descent with straining should be assessed. This descent should not be more than a few centimeters; greater degrees of perineal descent suggest pelvic floor weakness. The rectum should be assessed for its overall size and the presence of an anterior rectocele.[6]

Anorectal manometry plays an important role in the quantitative assessment of sphincter strength, rectal sensation, and the rectoanal inhibitory reflex and contractile response. It is useful to perform anorectal manometry before any biofeedback or invasive therapy, such as surgery. This allows the clinician to establish a baseline and to assess the feasibility of these interventions.

Other diagnostic studies that can be done include defecography, electromyography, and imaging studies. Defecography is not as useful in the assessment of fecal incontinence as it is in the evaluation of chronic constipation. Electromyography is of limited value and is used rarely. Imaging studies, such as endoscopic ultrasound and magnetic resonance imaging, are of value in assessing the integrity of the anal sphincters and can be of help in planning surgical repair of sphincter lacerations.

Treatment of Fecal Incontinence

The simplest approach to managing fecal incontinence is modification of bowel habits. For those patients with diarrhea, measures to mitigate diarrhea often will result in restoration of continence. In some patients, modifying stool consistency with the use of fiber products can bulk up the stool sufficiently to allow compromised continence mechanisms to prevent accidents. In other patients, using a constipating drug such as loperamide can reduce the impact of the gastrocolic reflex and reduce threats to continence.[22] The downside of this approach is the possibility of producing frank constipation, which might be difficult for the patient. Sometimes it is useful to use a constipating drug and then to stimulate evacuation at intervals with suppositories or enemas to avoid problems with constipation.

For patients who have some rectal sensation and some ability to contract the pelvic floor and external anal sphincter, biofeedback training can improve incontinence.[23] Another therapeutic option is sacral nerve stimulation.[24] Another minimally invasive approach to incontinence is injection of materials around the anal canal to stiffen it and increase resistance to flow of feces through the anal canal.[25] A surgical analog of this procedure is anal encirclement with either mesh or other materials. While the surgery itself is straightforward, placement of foreign material in this area may be complicated by infection.[26] The most effective surgical intervention—when it is feasible—is direct surgical repair of a sphincter injury, which sometimes occurs after vaginal delivery.[26] Suturing the loose ends of the lacerated sphincter together produces an intact ring of muscle, which can effectively block the anal canal. Sometimes concurrent nerve damage reduces the effectiveness of this approach.

CONCLUSION

Symptoms involving the colon, including constipation, diarrhea, and fecal incontinence, are common. They are frequently due to disruption of the normal physiology of the colon and can be mitigated by treatments that affect colon function. Because each of these symptoms may be secondary to underlying diseases, it is important to evaluate the patient comprehensively. When no specific cause is identified, symptomatic management can be very effective and may restore quality of life for these individuals.

REFERENCES

1. Rao MC, Sarathy J, Sellin JH. Intestinal electrolyte absorption and secretion. In: Feldman M, Friedman L, Brandt LJ, eds. *Sleisenger & Fordtran's Gastrointestinal and Liver Disease* 10th ed. Elsevier Saunders; 2016:1713-1735.

2. Quigley EM. What we have learned about colonic motility: normal and disturbed. *Curr Opin Gastroenterol.* 2010;26(1):53-60.

3. Hammer H, Santa Ana C, Schiller L, Fordtran J. Studies of osmotic diarrhea induced in normal subjects by ingestion of polyethylene glycol and lactulose. *J Clin Invest.* 1989;84(4):1056-1062.

4. Wenzl HH, Fine KD, Schiller LR, Fordtran JS. Determinants of decreased fecal consistency in patients with diarrhea. *Gastroenterology.* 1995;108(6):1729-1738.

5. Carbonero F, Benefiel AC, Gaskins HR. Contributions of the microbial hydrogen economy to colonic homeostasis. *Nat Rev Gastroenterol Hepatol.* 2012;9(9):504-518.

6. Bharucha AE, Rao SS. An update on anorectal disorders for gastroenterologists. *Gastroenterology.* 2014;146(1): 37-45.e2.

7. Rao SSC. Fecal incontinence. In: Feldman M, Friedman L, Brandt LJ, eds. *Sleisenger & Fordtran's Gastrointestinal and Liver Diseases* 10th ed. Elsevier Saunders; 2016:251-269.

8. Palit S, Lunniss PJ, Scott SM. The physiology of human defecation. *Dig Dis Sci.* 2012;57(6):1445-1464.

9. Bharucha AE, Pemberton JH, Locke GR, 3rd. American Gastroenterological Association technical review on constipation. *Gastroenterology.* 2013;144(1):218-238.

10. Andrews CN, Storr M. The pathophysiology of chronic constipation. *Can J Gastroenterol.* 2011;25(Suppl B):16b-21b.

11. Wald A. Motility disorders of the colon and rectum. *Curr Opin Gastroenterol.* 2012;28(1):52-56.

12. Eswaran S, Muir J, Chey WD. Fiber and functional gastrointestinal disorders. *Am J Gastroenterol.* 2013;108(5):718-727.

13. Ford AC, Talley NJ. Laxatives for chronic constipation in adults. *BMJ Clinical Res Ed.* 2012;345:e6168.

14. Schiller LR, Emmett M, Santa Ana CA, Fordtran JS. Osmotic effects of polyethylene glycol. *Gastroenterology.* 1988;94(4):933-941.

15. Camilleri M. New treatment options for chronic constipation: mechanisms, efficacy and safety. *Can J Gastroenterol.* 2011;25 Suppl B:29b-35b.

16. Gershon MD, Tack J. The serotonin signaling system: from basic understanding to drug development for functional GI disorders. *Gastroenterology.* 2007;132(1):397-414.

17. Rao SS. Biofeedback therapy for constipation in adults. *Best Pract Res Clin Gastroenterol.* 2011;25(1):159-166.

18. Knowles CH, Dinning PG, Pescatori M, Rintala R, Rosen H. Surgical management of constipation. *Neurogastroenterol Motil.* 2009;21 Suppl 2:62-71.

19. Schiller LR PD, Spiller R, Semrad CE, et al. Gastro 2013 APDW/WCOG Shanghai Working Party Report: Chronic diarrhea: definition, classification, diagnosis. *J Gastroenterol Hepatol.* 2014;296:6-25.

20. Steffer KJ, Santa Ana CA, Cole JA, Fordtran JS. The practical value of comprehensive stool analysis in detecting the cause of idiopathic chronic diarrhea. *Gastroenterol Clin North Am.* 2012;41(3):539-560.

21. Li Z, Vaziri H. Treatment of chronic diarrhoea. *Best Pract Res Clin Gastroenterol.* 2012;26(5):677-687.

22. Omar MI, Alexander CE. Drug treatment for faecal incontinence in adults. Cochrane Database Sys Rev. 2013;6:Cd002116.

23. Norton C, Cody JD. Biofeedback and/or sphincter exercises for the treatment of faecal incontinence in adults. *Cochrane Database Sys Rev.* 2012;7:Cd002111.

24. Thin NN, Horrocks EJ, Hotouras A, et al. Systematic review of the clinical effectiveness of neuromodulation in the treatment of faecal incontinence. *Br J Surg.* 2013;100(11):1430-1447.

25. Maeda Y, Laurberg S, Norton C. Perianal injectable bulking agents as treatment for faecal incontinence in adults. *Cochrane Database Sys Rev.* 2013;2:Cd007959.

26. Brown SR, Wadhawan H, Nelson RL. Surgery for faecal incontinence in adults. *Cochrane Database Sys Rev.* 2013;7:Cd001757.

18

Irritable Bowel Syndrome

Elizabeth J. Videlock, MD and Lin Chang, MD

KEY POINTS

- Irritable bowel syndrome (IBS) is a highly prevalent disorder associated with significant morbidity and cost.

- Pathophysiology involves both peripheral and central mechanisms.

- Diagnosis is based on symptoms, and the absence of alarm features; extensive diagnostic evaluation to exclude organic disease is not necessary.

- Establishing a good patient–provider relationship is a cornerstone of treatment.

- Several novel therapies are available to treat IBS including Linaclotide and Lubiprostone for IBS-C, Alosetron and Rifaximin for IBS-D, low dose antidepressants, antispasmodic and psychological therapies for all IBS.

DEFINITION

IBS is a functional gastrointestinal disorder (FGID) that is characterized by abdominal pain associated with altered bowel habits with changes in stool frequency and/or form.[1] IBS is considered a "functional" disorder due to the lack of a defining anatomic or biochemical abnormality. However, IBS could be viewed as multiple "organic" diseases.[2] IBS may be more accurately defined as a disorder of brain–gut interactions associated with alterations in gastrointestinal (GI) motility, visceral perception, mucosal and immune function, gut microbiota, and/or central nervous system (CNS) processing. Despite the increasing identification of distinct pathophysiology, there is not a unifying putative mechanism, and patients are grouped clinically by symptoms, so that IBS is appropriately designated as a syndrome rather than a disease.

Rao SSC, Parkman HP, McCallum RW, eds.
Handbook of Gastrointestinal Motility and Functional Disorders (pp 221-239).
© 2015 Taylor & Francis Group.

PATHOPHYSIOLOGY

Factors That Increase Vulnerability of Developing Irritable Bowel Syndrome

Genetic Factors

IBS aggregates in families. In one case-control study of 477 IBS patients and 1492 of their first-degree relatives, compared to 297 controls and 936 of their first-degree relatives, 50% of IBS relatives had IBS compared to 27% of control relatives, which corresponded to an odds ratio of 2.75 (95% CI of 2.01 to 3.76).[3] While twin studies suggest heritability, there is also likely a strong influence of environment, such as the presence of IBS in the mother or father and the parental response to a child's abdominal pain.[4] At least 60 genes have been studied in IBS, but a consistent predisposition has not been identified.[5]

Prior Gastrointestinal Infection

Postinfectious IBS (PI-IBS) is the acute onset of IBS in an individual without a history of it, immediately following an acute illness characterized by 2 or more of the following: fever, vomiting, diarrhea, or a positive bacterial stool culture.[1] Gastroenteritis is an important risk factor for IBS, increasing the risk 2-fold. The risk is even greater in those with preexisting GI conditions such as gastroesophageal reflux disease (GERD) or dyspepsia, a history of more severe diarrheal illness, younger age, female gender, chronic stressful life events, or psychological comorbidities.[6] Postinfectious IBS is most often characterized by diarrhea or mixed bowel habit. The incidence varies from 3.7% to 36%.[6] Studies have demonstrated that PI-IBS can occur following bacterial infections such as *Campylobacter jejuni* or *Escherichia coli* O157:H7, viral gastroenteritis such as *Norovirus*, and parasitic infections such as *Giardiasis*.[6]

Stressful Life Events

There is an association between IBS symptoms and current life stress for many patients.[7] The development of PI-IBS is also associated with stressful life events at the time of the GI infection.[6] IBS patients have a higher prevalence of early adverse life events (EALs) or traumatic experiences during childhood, including but not limited to, maladjusted relationships with a parent or primary caregiver; severe illness or death of a parent; and physical, sexual, or emotional abuse.[8,9] Events during infancy such as perinatal gastric suctioning have also been associated with IBS.[8] Patients with IBS have a higher prevalence of general trauma, physical punishment, emotional abuse, and sexual abuse; emotional abuse was the strongest predictor of IBS in one study.[9] There is also evidence that IBS is a component of the "Gulf War Syndrome." In a study of Gulf War–era U.S. Navy Seabees, who have been considered to be among the most symptomatic Gulf War veterans, those who had been deployed to the Persian Gulf were more than three times more likely to have IBS when compared with Seabees deployed elsewhere or not deployed.[10]

Pathophysiologic Mechanisms

Although there is no consensus on the pathogenesis of IBS, one unifying theme of IBS pathophysiology is that the symptoms result from dysregulation of the "brain–gut axis," which manifests as enhanced visceral perception (Figure 18-1). Evidence suggests that IBS is multifactorial and that the symptom constellation may arise from several etiologies that can differ within subgroups of patients. There is currently no single biomarker that can encompass the different pathophysiologic mechanisms of IBS.

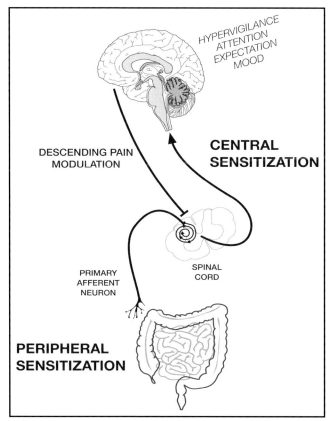

Figure 18-1. Factors that contribute to enhanced visceral perception include peripheral sensitization, central sensitization, descending pain modulation, and psychological and cognitive factors such as mood and attention.

Enhanced Visceral Perception

A unifying theory in the pathogenesis of IBS and other FGIDs is that there is a dysregulation in the complex interplay among the gut lumen, mucosa, enteric nervous system (ENS), and the CNS, as well as communication between these domains, that results in altered sensation and motility.[11] Enhanced perception of visceral stimuli (Figure 18-2) can occur in IBS patients, either as a result of greater sensitivity of visceral afferent pathways or as central amplification of visceral afferent input. This phenomenon may represent dysfunction in any, or even a combination of, the components involved in gut sensation, including signal transmission from the gut, signal transmission to the CNS, and modulation and processing of sensation by the CNS. Brain imaging studies found that in response to rectal distention, IBS patients showed increased activation of areas associated with emotional arousal (pregenual anterior cingulate cortex [ACC], amygdala), as well as a midbrain region associated with endogenous pain modulation, while controls showed more consistent activation of the medial and lateral prefrontal cortex (PFC), which are important in descending pain modulation.[11] Changes in brain structure have also been associated with IBS.[11]

Increased perception in terms of decreased pressure thresholds and/or increased sensory ratings and viscerosomatic referral areas to rectal and/or colonic balloon distention using a computerized distention device (barostat) has been found in IBS patients vs healthy controls.[12] However, visceral hypersensitivity is not present in all IBS patients, and perception does not change in

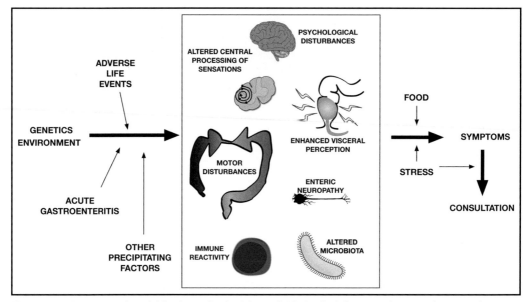

Figure 18-2. A conceptual model for the pathophysiology of IBS. On the left are predisposing factors and triggers. The middle panel illustrates disease mechanisms ranging from the brain to the gut. On the right are factors that can influence symptoms and illness behavior.

concert with symptom improvement; therefore, the use of visceral perception measured by the barostat has limited value as a biomarker.[12]

There is good evidence suggesting that experimental findings of increased sensitivity to rectal distention are influenced by stress and psychological factors, including hypervigilance and a tendency to report sensations as painful.[7,12]

Enhanced Stress Response

Evidence supports the association between chronic stress and IBS. Postinfectious IBS is predicted by psychological symptoms and stress.[6] Furthermore, experimental stress increases visceral sensitivity and gut permeability.[7] In addition, patients with IBS have an exaggerated increase in motility in response to stress.[7] The effect of stress on gut function and sensation likely results from alterations in the brain–gut axis. This is mediated by multiple factors, including the corticotropin-releasing factor (CRF)–hypothalamic pituitary adrenal (HPA) axis, the autonomic nervous system (ANS), and the immune system.

Autonomic Nervous System Dysregulation

Changes in autonomic tone are associated with bowel symptoms in IBS. Patients with IBS-D show evidence of enhanced adrenergic activation, and IBS-C patients show decreased vagal tone.[13] Both result in an imbalance favoring sympathetic over parasympathetic activity. The changes are predominantly seen in patients with more severe symptoms. A blunted ANS response has been associated with a greater duration of disease.[14]

Altered Gastrointestinal Transit and Motility

Altered colonic motility has long been recognized as a factor in IBS, and in early studies it was associated with psychological and physical stress.[7] Changes have included an increased number of rapid contractions in response to balloon distention and increased transit in IBS-D. Using a scintigraphic measurement of GI transit, colonic transit assessed at 24 and 48 hours was accelerated in 48% of IBS-D patients and delayed in 21% of IBS-C patients.[15] Prolonged transit was also correlated with visible abdominal distention but not with the symptom of bloating.[16]

Altered Immune Reactivity

Low-grade inflammation or immune activation is hypothesized to play a role in the pathophysiology of IBS through effects on visceral sensitivity and gut epithelial function. This is more apparent in patients with PI-IBS.[6] Studies in unselected IBS patients have demonstrated less consistent results.[17] Findings associated with IBS include increased lymphocytes in the blood or mucosa and increased mucosal mast cells, but these findings have not been reproduced in all studies. Studies have shown alteration in the cytokine profiles in IBS patients, but there has been more evidence for blood levels than colonic mucosal levels.[17]

Increased Gut Permeability

Gut permeability is frequently measured in the experimental setting by ingestion of molecular probes, which are excreted and can be measured in the urine.[18] Increased gut permeability may play a role in the interaction between stress, immune activation, dysbiosis, and hypersensitivity within the gut in IBS. Several studies have found increased permeability in the small intestine and colon in IBS patients.[18] Expression and cellular distribution of tight junction proteins are also altered in patients with IBS-D.[18] Permeability has been linked to abdominal pain and enhanced visceral perception in patients with IBS.[18] The association between increased permeability and IBS is strongest in PI-IBS[6] and IBS-D.[18]

Gut Microbiota

There is evidence that alterations in gut microbiota may play a role in IBS. The role of small intestinal bacterial overgrowth (SIBO) in IBS is controversial, due in part to the fact that methods available to diagnose SIBO have not been validated. Results of studies comparing fecal microbiota in IBS and controls have been inconsistent, but several have shown increased members of the phylum Firmicutes and reduced Bacteroidetes.[19] Some studies have shown fewer *Lactobacillus* and *Bifidobacterium* in IBS, but this may be related to the frequency of lactose intolerance in IBS patients, as these organisms thrive on dairy products. Diet can affect IBS symptoms, and this may be related to changes in the microbiota.[19]

Bile Acid Processing

The presence of bile acids in the colon and rectum is known to increase secretion, motility, and visceral sensitivity to rectal distention. A recent study using 23-seleno-25-homo-tauro-cholic acid (SeHCAT) scanning showed that bile acid malabsorption was present in 51% of patients with chronic diarrhea. About 20% of these patients had IBS-D, and 27% of this subgroup had evidence of bile acid malabsorption.[20] Thus, increased levels of colonic bile acids may be a relevant mechanism in some patients.

DIAGNOSIS

The key symptom of IBS is chronic or recurrent abdominal pain and/or discomfort associated with altered bowel habits. Patients with IBS also commonly report symptoms of gas, bloating, abdominal pain or fullness, and fullness in the rectum. In the absence of a biomarker, diagnosis is based on symptoms. The Rome III criteria for the diagnosis of IBS were published in 2006 and are listed in Table 18-1, along with other supporting symptoms that are suggestive, but not currently required, for the diagnosis of IBS.[1] It should be noted that diagnostic criteria, including the Rome III criteria, were developed to subgroup a more homogenous patient population for the purposes of clinical research and have limited diagnostic accuracy to distinguish IBS from organic disease.[21]

IBS is subgrouped by predominant bowel habit. Because stool form was found to be the best predictor of predominant bowel habit in IBS, stool form rather than frequency determines bowel

---

TABLE 18-1

ROME III CRITERIA AND SUPPORTIVE SYMPTOMS[1]

THE SYMPTOM-BASED ROME III CRITERIA FOR THE DIAGNOSIS OF IBS

These criteria should be met for the last 3 months, with symptom onset at least 6 months prior to diagnosis.

Recurrent abdominal pain or discomfort* at least 3 days per month in the last 3 months that is associated with 2 or more of the following:

- Improvement with defecation
- Onset associated with a change in frequency of stool
- Onset associated with a change in form (appearance) of stool

* Discomfort means an uncomfortable sensation not described as pain.

SUPPORTIVE SYMPTOMS (NONDIAGNOSTIC)

- Abnormal stool frequency (< 3 bowel movements per week or > 3 bowel movements per day)
- Abnormal stool form (lumpy/hard stool or loose/watery stool)
- Defecation straining, urgency, or a feeling of incomplete evacuation
- Passing mucus
- Bloating

---

habit subclassification according to the Rome III criteria.[1] These criteria are outlined in Table 18-2. Bowel symptoms fluctuate frequently over time for many patients with IBS.[22]

The differential diagnosis for the symptoms of IBS is shown in Table 18-3. Use of the symptom-based Rome III criteria[1] and evaluation for alarm signs or symptoms, as well as excluding celiac disease in some populations, are sufficient to make the diagnosis of IBS. While the presence of "red flags" or alarm signs and symptoms may indicate a need for further diagnostic workup, most patients with red-flag symptoms have not been found to have an organic disorder to explain their IBS symptoms.[23] According to the American College of Gastroenterology (ACG) Task Force on IBS, alarm features include rectal bleeding; weight loss; iron-deficiency anemia; nocturnal symptoms; and a family history of colon cancer, IBD, or celiac disease.[24]

The use of routine blood tests, such as a complete blood count, metabolic panel, thyroid function tests, and inflammatory markers such as erythrocyte sedimentation rate and C-reactive protein are use to exclude other diagnoses in IBS is not recommended by the ACG Task Force.[24] Although a meta-analysis found that biopsy-confirmed celiac disease was more common in individuals with suspected IBS than healthy controls (OR of 4.34 and 95% CI: 1.78 to 10.6), a more recent multicenter study in the United States found the prevalence of biopsy-confirmed celiac disease among nonconstipated IBS patients diagnosed by Rome II criteria to be similar to that in asymptomatic controls (2/492 [0.4%] with IBS vs. 2/458 [0.4%] controls, $p > 0.99$).[25] Nonetheless, cost-effectiveness studies have determined that testing for celiac disease in IBS-D and IBS-M patients is a cost-effective approach when the prevalence of celiac disease is at least 1%.[26] The ACG Task Force on IBS recommends that colonoscopy need not be performed in patients under the age of 50 with typical symptoms of IBS and without alarm features (Grade 1B).[24] This is based on the low pretest probability of Crohn disease, ulcerative colitis, and colonic neoplasia in this group.[27]

TABLE 18-2		
IRRITABLE BOWEL SYNDROME SUBTYPES BY BOWEL HABIT[1]		
	PERCENT OF STOOLS THAT MEET THE DESCRIPTION (OVER THE PRECEDING 3 MONTHS)	
*Subtype**	*Hard or Lumpy Stools (Bristol type 1-2)*	*Loose or Watery Stools (Bristol type 6-7)*
IBS with constipation (IBS-C)	≧ 25%	< 25%
IBS with diarrhea (IBS-D)	< 25%	≧ 25%
Mixed IBS (IBS-M)[†]	≧ 25%	≧ 25%
Unsubtyped IBS (IBS-U)	< 25%	< 25%

* The word *with* is preferred to *predominant* due to symptom instability.

† Patients with both diarrhea and constipation that may alternate within hours or days were previously classified as IBS-A according to the Rome II criteria, but should now be referred to as IBS-M. The category of alternating IBS (IBS-A) should be reserved for patients with bowel habits that have changed over time (eg, weeks to months).

EPIDEMIOLOGY

IBS has a very high prevalence, although it varies based on geographical region, diagnostic criteria, and population studied (eg, health care seeking vs community). A recent systematic review and meta-analysis of prevalence found values ranging from 1% to 45%,[28] and varies depending on the symptom-based criteria that is used. Up to 70% of patients with IBS symptoms do not seek health care. When studies were restricted to population-based studies using the Rome criteria (described in the section on diagnosis), the pooled prevalence (total N = 32,638) was 7% with a 95% confidence interval of 6% to 8%.[24]

The prevalence of IBS bowel habit subtypes can vary due to different subclassification criteria and populations. One systematic review found that the prevalence among IBS bowel habit subtypes were similar in population-based studies from the United States using the Manning criteria, while European studies showed a greater prevalence of IBS-C or IBS-A using the Rome I or II criteria compared to IBS-D.[28]

Gender and age can affect the prevalence of IBS. In a recent meta-analysis that pooled data from population-based studies (total N = 188,229), the odds of having IBS were higher among women with an OR of 1.7 and a 95% CI of 1.5 to 1.8.[29] The increased prevalence was stable across geographic regions. Women with IBS were more likely to have IBS-C and less likely to have IBS-D.[29] IBS is more commonly diagnosed in patients under the age of 50.

Studies demonstrate that patients with IBS have poor health-related quality of life (HRQOL). Impairment in HRQOL is comparable or even lower to other chronic disorders such as GERD, diabetes, hypertension, depression, and end-stage renal disease dependent on dialysis.[30] The severity of abdominal pain and psychological distress are strong predictors of poor HRQOL.[31]

IBS patients with comorbid somatic disorders report more severe IBS symptoms and lower HRQOL.[32] Many disorders common in the general population are more common in IBS. Common coexistent conditions include fibromyalgia, headaches, cystitis, pelvic pain, and psychiatric disorders.[33] It has been hypothesized that the comorbidity does not result from any specific

---

TABLE 18-3
DIFFERENTIAL DIAGNOSIS OF IRRITABLE BOWEL SYNDROME

IBS-C

- Hypothyroidism

IBS-D/M

- Carbohydrate maldigestion
- Bile acid malabsorption
- Chronic pancreatitis
- Gastrointestinal infection
- Inflammatory bowel disease
- Hyperthyroidism
- Carcinoid tumor

IBS-MULTIPLE SUBTYPES

- Celiac disease
- Food intolerance
- Small intestine bacterial overgrowth
- Enteric neuropathy or myopathy
- Malignancy
- Medication side effects
- Gynecologic conditions (eg, endometriosis)
- Psychological conditions (eg, depression, anxiety)
- Other functional gastrointestinal disorders (eg, functional abdominal pain syndrome, functional dyspepsia)

---

disease associations, but rather from "hypervigilance for noticing somatic sensations and a lower threshold for consulting a physician."[33] There is also a higher prevalence of psychiatric disorders in the IBS population than in controls. This is true in the community (prevalence of 18%),[34] in clinics (prevalence of 40% to 60%),[35] and in referral centers (prevalence for lifetime history of 94%).[34] Evidence suggests that psychiatric disorders influence health care seeking, rather than being the primary cause.

IBS is associated with significant cost and health care use. In 2004, there were 3.1 million ambulatory care visits with IBS noted as a diagnosis, and 52.5% listed IBS as the first diagnosis. The rate of visits for women was 4.4 times the rate for men.[36] The indirect and direct costs for IBS totaled $1.01 billion.[37] IBS accounts for 10% to 15% of primary care visits and 25% to 50% of gastroenterology visits. In addition to direct medical expenses, indirect costs to society include those that are due to work absenteeism and impaired work productivity.[38] IBS patients are also more likely to seek health care and incur costs for non-GI symptoms. Some of the costs may be accounted for by the increased number of non-GI physical complaints (eg, headaches, myalgias) in IBS patients. The tendency to seek care may relate to illness behaviors.

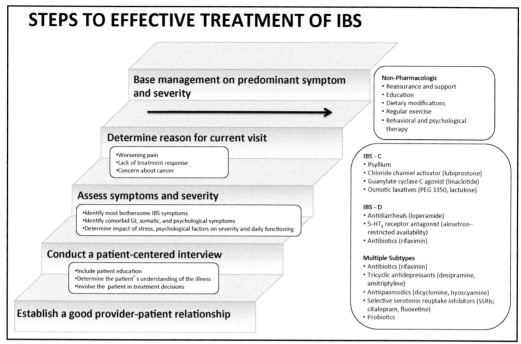

Figure 18-3. An approach to the treatment of IBS.

TREATMENT

An approach to the management of IBS is outlined in Figure 18-3. The reasons for a patient's visit can vary. Some patients seek care out of fear that they have a life-threatening illness such as colon cancer. These patients may find relief in receiving a positive diagnosis, reassurance, and education and may not require pharmacotherapy. However, patients with moderate to severe abdominal pain and bowel symptoms often require pharmacological and/or psychological therapies.

A good health care provider–patient relationship is the cornerstone of effective care of the patient with IBS. The quality of this relationship has been shown to improve patient outcomes. Elements of a good provider–patient relationship include a nonjudgmental patient-centered interview, a careful and cost-effective evaluation, inquiry into the patient's understanding of the illness, patient education, and involvement of the patient in treatment decisions. Addressing psychosocial factors is an important part of the interview and may improve health status and treatment response.[39]

Diet and Physical Activity

Many patients report an inconsistent symptom response to certain foods, and a 1- to 2-week food and symptom diary can help identify potential, consistent food triggers. While most patients cannot completely control symptoms through diet alterations alone, including elimination diets, diet-related exacerbations may be minimized. Common food triggers include high-fat foods, raw fruits and vegetables, and caffeinated beverages.

Studies suggest that a gluten-free diet can decrease IBS symptoms, although they have relatively small sample sizes. In one study, IBS patients who had symptomatically responded to a gluten-free diet were randomly assigned to a 3-day rechallenge of gluten-containing bread and a muffin versus gluten-free bread and muffin. Thirteen of 19 (68%) in the gluten group compared to 6 of 15 (40%) in the gluten-free group did not have adequate symptom control ($P=0.0001$).[40] Interestingly, the patients in the gluten group reported increased tiredness, while the gluten-free group did not. In another trial, a gluten-free diet improved stool frequency in IBS-D patients, particularly among patients who were positive for HLA-DQ2/8.[41]

Some patients may have symptoms related to excess fructose and short-chain fatty acids as well as sugar alcohols. These entities include fermentable oligosaccharides, disaccharides, monosaccharides, and polyols, which are collectively referred to by the acronym FODMAPs. A high-FODMAPs diet can result in increased small bowel water content due to the high osmotic load and gas production from bacterial fermentation, and can cause colonic dilation and a laxative effect.[42] Diets high in FODMAPs have been shown to result in increased hydrogen and methane gas production in both IBS patients and healthy controls, and among patients this was associated with GI symptoms.[43] A recent crossover study comparing a low-FODMAPs diet to an Australian diet with high-FODMAPs foods demonstrated a reduction in overall and individual IBS symptoms in patients.[44] A follow-up study by the same group found that gluten challenge did not have significant effects on GI symptoms in IBS patients with nonceliac gluten sensitivity who responded to a low-FODMAPs (including gluten avoidance) diet.[45] This study suggests that avoidance of gluten is not the predominant reason patients respond to a low-FODMAPs diet.

Increased physical activity has been studied in IBS. In one small (N = 102) randomized clinical trial (RCT) of physical activity and IBS, 20 to 60 minutes of moderate to vigorous activity 3 to 5 times weekly resulted in lower symptom severity after 12 weeks in comparison to usual activity.[46] Patients in the intervention group were also less likely to have experienced worsening of their IBS symptoms.

Pharmacologic Therapies

Pharmacologic therapies are outlined in Tables 18-4 to 18-6. The evidence-based recommendations from the most recent publication of the ACG Task Force are included in the tables.[47] It is important to note that the strength of recommendation is not based only on the quality of the evidence but takes into account benefits vs risk, patient-related factors, and cost. The reasons for the recommendations are discussed in the referenced monograph.[47]

Therapies for Irritable Bowel Syndrome With Constipation

Dietary Bulking Agents

Bulking agents include psyllium, methylcellulose, corn fiber, calcium polycarbophil, and ispaghula husk. A recent systematic review and meta-analysis published by the Cochrane Collaboration concluded that there was no benefit from the use of bulking agents for the treatment of IBS.[48] The review included 12 studies; 6 used soluble fiber (all used ispaghula or psyllium) and 6 used insoluble fiber (wheat bran, fruit fiber).[48] However, since that review, psyllium has been studied in an RCT in a primary care setting.[49] In this study, which is the largest study, patients receiving psyllium were more likely to report adequate relief of IBS symptoms in comparison to those receiving placebo. Of note, all studies were in IBS and not specifically IBS-C and no study reported results by predominant bowel habit. Anecdotal experience is that bulking agents are more effective in IBS-C than other subtypes of IBS.

Laxatives

There are limited data on the use of laxatives in IBS. Polyethylene glycol (PEG) was found to be effective in treating constipation symptoms in IBS-C but not abdominal pain.[50]

Chloride Channel Activator

The chloride channel (ClC-2) activator lubiprostone acts luminally to increase intestinal secretion. Two 12-week RCTs evaluated the efficacy of lubiprostone at a dose of 8 mcg twice daily

TABLE 18-4

EVIDENCE-BASED PHARMACOLOGICAL TREATMENT OF CONSTIPATION

AGENT (CLASS)	DOSE	NNT (95% CI)*	RECOMMENDATION (STRENGTH, QUALITY OF EVIDENCE)[47]	COMMENT
Psyllium/ispaghula (bulking agent)	20 to 25 g/day	7 (4 to 25)[47] 7 trials (N = 499)	Provides overall symptom relief (weak, moderate)	All studies recruited patients regardless of predominant symptom
Polyethylene glycol (osmotic laxative)	13.8 g PEG 3350 + E in 125 mL water, 1 to 3 times/day	2 trials (N = 166); Not effective for pain or overall symptoms; NNT for increased stool frequency: 5 (3 to 28)[50]	Is not effective for overall symptoms and pain (week, very low)	The larger trial of PEG[2] was published after the guidelines and was not included in the evidence grading.
Lubiprostone (chloride channel activator)	8 mcg twice daily	12 (8 to 25)[47] 3 trials (N = 1366)	Superior to placebo for IBS-C (strong, moderate)	Also available in 24 mcg twice daily for CIC
Linaclotide (guanylate cyclase C agonist)	290 mcg daily	6 (5 to 8) 3 trials (N = 2028)	Superior to placebo for IBS-C (strong, high)	Also approved for the treatment of CIC at a dose of 145 mcg daily

*To prevent one additional patient from having persistent symptoms.

IBS, irritable bowel syndrome; NNT, number needed to treat; CI, confidence interval; g, grams; mcg, micrograms; CIC, chronic idiopathic constipation.

			TABLE 18-5		
		EVIDENCE-BASED PHARMACOLOGICAL TREATMENT OF DIARRHEA			
AGENT (CLASS)	DOSE	NNT (95% CI)*	RECOMMENDATION (STRENGTH, QUALITY OF EVIDENCE)	COMMENT	
Loperamide (antidiarrheal)	Up to 4 mg 4 times daily	Studied in 2 poor-quality trials (N of 42)	Insufficient evidence to recommend (strong, very low)		
Rifaximin (antibiotic)	550 mg 3 times daily for 10 days	9 (6 to 12)[47] 5 trials (N = 1805)	Effective for symptoms and bloating in non-C IBS (weak, moderate)	Retreatment studies are ongoing	
Alosetron (5-HT3 agonist)	0.5 to 1 mg twice daily	8 (5 to 17)[47] 8 trials (N = 4987)	Effective in women with IBS-D (weak, moderate)	In the United States, only available under a risk management program for women with severe IBS-D	

*To prevent one additional patient from having persistent symptoms

IBS, irritable bowel syndrome; NNT, number needed to treat; CI, confidence interval; mg, milligrams

in patients with IBS-C.[51] The primary efficacy endpoint was assessed using a Likert scale with stringent responder definition. Responder rates were significantly higher in patients receiving lubiprostone compared to those on placebo (17.9% vs 10.1%). Lubiprostone also improved stool consistency, straining, abdominal pain/discomfort, HRQOL, and constipation severity. An open-label extension of the trial for up to 52 weeks showed a lasting benefit and that the drug was well tolerated; while nausea did occur in 11%, most who experienced nausea had only a single episode.

Guanylate Cyclase C Agonist

Linaclotide is a minimally absorbed, 14-amino acid peptide that binds to and activates guanylate cyclase C on the luminal surface of the intestinal epithelium, increasing levels of intra- and extracellular cyclic guanosine monophosphate (cGMP), which results in increased luminal secretion of chloride and bicarbonate via the cystic fibrosis transmembrane conductance regulator (CFTR). In clinical trials, linaclotide has shown efficacy in the treatment of bowel and abdominal symptoms in patients with chronic idiopathic constipation (CIC) and IBS-C.[52,53] Linaclotide was safe and well tolerated, with the most common adverse effect being diarrhea, which occurred on linaclotide compared to placebo with an RR of 4.7 (95% CI: 2.8 to 7.9). In post hoc analyses, the development of diarrhea was not associated with decreased treatment satisfaction in IBS-C or CIC patients.

TABLE 18-6

EVIDENCE-BASED PHARMACOLOGICAL TREATMENT OF VARIOUS IRRITABLE BOWEL SYNDROME SUBTYPES

AGENT (CLASS)	DOSE	NNT (95% CI)*	RECOMMENDATION (STRENGTH, QUALITY OF EVIDENCE)[47]	COMMENT
Probiotics	Various	7 (4 to 12)[47] 23 (N=2575)	Improve global symptoms, bloating and flatulence (weak, low)	Higher quality of evidence for *Bifidobacterium infantis* 35624[62] and *Bifidobacterium animalis*[64]
Antidepressants as a class		4 (3 to 6)[47] 17 trials (N=1084)	Effective in symptom relief (weak, high)	TCAs are more efficacious for pain relief and constipating side effects may be helpful in IBS-D
Selective serotonin reuptake inhibitors (SSRIs)	10 to 100 mg daily	Global symptoms: 3 (2 to 25)[48]		
Tricyclic antidepressants (TCAs)	10 to 200 mg daily	Global symptoms: 4 (2 to 7)[48] Abdominal pain: 4 (6 to 25)[48]		

(continued)

TABLE 18-6 (CONTINUED)
EVIDENCE-BASED PHARMACOLOGICAL TREATMENT OF VARIOUS IRRITABLE BOWEL SYNDROME SUBTYPES

AGENT (CLASS)	DOSE	NNT (95% CI)*	RECOMMENDATION (STRENGTH, QUALITY OF EVIDENCE)[47]	COMMENT
Antispasmodics as a class		5 (4 to 9)[47] 23 (N=2154)	Provide short-term symptomatic relief (weak, low)	
Hyoscine/scopolamine	10 mg 3 times daily	Global symptoms: 3 (2 to 25)[61]		
Alverine citrate 60mg + simethicone 300mg	3 times daily	Abdominal pain: 8 (4 to 33)[68]		
Otilonium bromide	40 mg 3 times daily	Pain: 7 (4 to 40)[69]		
Peppermint oil	~ 200 mg 3 times daily	3 (2 to 4)[47] 5 trials (N=482)	Superior to placebo for IBS symptoms (weak, moderate)	

* To prevent one additional patient from having persistent symptoms.

IBS, irritable bowel syndrome; NNT, number needed to treat; RCT, randomized controlled trial; CI, confidence interval; mg, milligrams

Therapies for Irritable Bowel Syndrome With Diarrhea

Antidiarrheals

Antidiarrheal agents are frequently used in IBS with diarrheal symptoms. The only agent that has been evaluated in RCTs is loperamide, which acts directly on intestinal smooth muscle via the opioid receptor to inhibit peristalsis and prolong transit time. It had no effect on global IBS symptoms or pain, but was effective in reducing stool frequency.[24] Although antidiarrheals can be used regularly with doses up to 4 mg four times daily, they are more commonly used on an as-needed basis, such as before leaving the house, a long car trip, meal, or a stressful event.

Antibiotics

Small intestinal bacterial overgrowth and dysbiosis have been theorized to play a role in IBS.[19] Rifaximin is an antibiotic that has very low systemic absorption and broad-spectrum activity against gram-positive and gram-negative aerobes and anaerobes. Two phase III RCTs showed significant improvement for the primary endpoint of the adequate relief of IBS symptoms in patients with non-IBS-C who were treated with 550 mg of rifaximin three times daily compared to placebo.[54] Rifaximin was also significantly more likely to improve bloating than placebo (OR = 1.55; 95% CI = 1.23 to 1.96; NNT = 10).[55] In a recent study, patients receiving rifaximin (n = 1103) and placebo (n = 829) had a similar incidence of drug-related adverse effects (12.1% vs 10.7%), serious adverse effects (1.5% vs 2.2%), GI-associated adverse effects (12.2% vs 12.2%), and infection-associated adverse effects (8.5% vs 9.5%). There were no cases of *Clostridium difficile* colitis or deaths.[56] Randomized placebo-controlled trials to evaluate the efficacy of retreatment with rifaximin in IBS-D patients who experienced symptom response with an initial course of rifaximin are currently ongoing.

5-HT3 Antagonists

5-HT3 receptor antagonists have both central and peripheral effects and slow gut transit and reduce visceral hypersensitivity. In high-quality RCTs, alosetron consistently improved abdominal pain and GI symptoms in IBS-D patients.[57,58] There is evidence for efficacy in women and in men, with one trial showing an increased rate of adequate relief of IBS symptoms in men.[58]

Alosetron is currently available under a risk evaluation and mitigation strategy (REMS) for women with severe IBS-D. It can be prescribed for women with severe IBS-D who have symptoms refractory to traditional treatments, starting at a lower dose (0.5 mg twice daily) but can be increased if needed to the original Food and Drug Administration (FDA)–approved dose of 1 mg twice daily. This restriction is due to the occurrence of GI-related serious adverse events, including ischemic colitis and serious complications of constipation. These events occurred at a rate of 1.1/1000 patient years for ischemic colitis and 0.66/1000 patient years for serious complications of constipation.[59] All of the alosetron-using patients with ischemic colitis had a reversible colopathy without long-term sequelae, and most cases occurred within the first month of treatment.[59] Recently, adjudication of reports of ischemic colitis and serious complications of constipation over the past 9 years of the REMS was performed.[60] The incidence rates of ischemic colitis (1.03 cases/1000 patient years) and serious complications of constipation (0.25 cases/1000 patient years) are low.

Ramosetron and ondansetron are other 5-HT3 receptor antagonists that have been shown to reduce IBS symptoms for IBS-D and have not been not associated with ischemic colitis or serious complications of constipation.

Therapies for Multiple Subtypes of Irritable Bowel Syndrome

Antispasmodics

Antispasmodics work by having a direct effect on intestinal smooth muscle or via their anti-cholinergic or antimuscarinic properties. A Cochrane Group systematic review and meta-analysis pooled results from 29 studies (2333 total patients) and found that there was a beneficial effect for antispasmodics over placebo for improvement of abdominal pain (RR = 1.32; 95% CI = 1.12 to 1.55; NNT = 7), global assessment (RR = 1.49; 95% CI = 1.25 to 1.77; NNT = 5), and symptom score (RR = 1.86; 95% CI = 1.26 to 2.76; NNT = 3).[48] Subgroup analyses for different types of antispasmodics found statistically significant benefits for cimetropium/dicyclomine, peppermint oil, pinaverium, and trimebutine.[48] Similar results were found with the systematic review and meta-analysis performed by the ACG.[61] Antispasmodics may be particularly beneficial in reducing postprandial IBS symptoms.

Probiotics

Probiotics are live organisms that, when administered in adequate quantities, confer a health benefit to the host. There is evidence that they have effects that may target some of the patho-physiologic mechanisms involved in IBS, such as visceral hypersensitivity, altered motility, gut permeability, and the composition of the microbiota. Probiotics have also been shown to have anti-inflammatory effects.[19]

While many species of probiotics subjectively reduced flatulence and bloating, the only one that showed good evidence for global improvement in IBS symptoms was *Bifidobacterium infantis*.[62] However, there is also evidence of improvement in symptoms, particularly gas, bloating, and flatulence, with other probiotics, such as VSL#3[63] and *Bifidobacterium animalis* DN-173 010.[64] It should be noted that there is considerable heterogeneity among trials. Many trials are small or of poor quality, and the question remains as to whether it is even appropriate to pool the results of trials of different probiotic species.

Antidepressants

The rationale for using antidepressants in IBS is that these agents may alter pain perception via a central modulation of visceral afferent input, alter GI transit, decrease firing of primary sensory afferent nerve fibers, and treat comorbid psychological symptoms. Antidepressants that have been studied in IBS include tricyclic antidepressants (TCAs), selective serotonin reuptake inhibitors (SSRIs), and to a lesser extent, serotonin-norepinephrine reuptake inhibitors (SNRIs).

Results of the systematic review and meta-analysis published by the Cochrane Group showed a beneficial effect for antidepressants over placebo for improvement of abdominal pain (RR = 1.49; 95% CI = 1.05 to 2.12; NNT = 5), global assessment (RR = 1.57; 95% CI = 1.23 to 2.00; NNT = 4), and symptom score (RR = 1.99; 95% CI = 1.32 to 2.99; NNT = 4).[48] Another meta-analysis by Ford et al[65] found similar results and significant benefit for both TCAs and SSRIs. The most common side effects associated with TCAs include dry mouth, constipation, and drowsiness. Selective serotonin reuptake inhibitors are generally better tolerated than TCAs, and they are commonly used in IBS, though most trials have been small.

Nonpharmacologic Therapies

Psychological Therapies

The rationale behind psychological treatments is based on the knowledge that symptom exacerbations are triggered by stressful life events in many patients, the high prevalence of comorbid psychiatric disorders, and the influence of the brain over perception of visceral pain.[66] Five treatment modalities that have been tested in RCTs are cognitive behavioral therapy (CBT), hypnosis, psychodynamic interpersonal therapy, relaxation training, and biofeedback.[66] The ACG Task

Force on IBS concluded that cognitive therapy, dynamic psychotherapy, and hypnotherapy, but not relaxation therapy, were more effective than usual care in relieving global symptoms of IBS.[24] Mindfulness is a technique that encourages regulation of attentional focus to thoughts, feelings, and bodily sensations. There is preliminary evidence to suggest that mindfulness therapy improved bowel symptoms and HRQOL in comparison to the control intervention, which was participation in a support group.[67]

REFERENCES

1. Longstreth GF, Thompson WG, Chey WD, Houghton LA, Mearin F, Spiller RC. Functional bowel disorders. *Gastroenterology.* 2006;130(5):1480-1491.
2. Camilleri M. Peripheral mechanisms in irritable bowel syndrome. *N Engl J Med.* 2012;367(17):1626-1635.
3. Saito YA, Petersen GM, Larson JJ, et al. Familial aggregation of irritable bowel syndrome: a family case-control study. *Am J Gastroenterol.* 2010;105(4):833-841.
4. Levy RL. Exploring the intergenerational transmission of illness behavior: from observations to experimental intervention. *Ann Behav Med.* 2011;41(2):174-182.
5. Saito YA. The role of genetics in IBS. *Gastroenterol Clin North Am.* 2011;40(1):45-67.
6. Grover M, Camilleri M, Smith K, Linden DR, Farrugia G. On the fiftieth anniversary. Postinfectious irritable bowel syndrome: mechanisms related to pathogens. *Neurogastroenterol Motil.* 2014;26(2):156-167.
7. Chang L. The role of stress on physiologic responses and clinical symptoms in irritable bowel syndrome. *Gastroenterology.* 2011;140(3):761-765.
8. Chitkara DK, van Tilburg MAL, Blois-Martin N, Whitehead WE. Early life risk factors that contribute to irritable bowel syndrome in adults: a systematic review. *Am J Gastroenterol.* 2008;103(3):765-774.
9. Bradford K, Shih W, Videlock EJ, et al. Association between early adverse life events and irritable bowel syndrome. *Clin Gastroenterol Hepatol.* 2012;10(4):385-390, e381-383.
10. Gray GC, Reed RJ, Kaiser KS, Smith TC, Gastanaga VM. Self-reported symptoms and medical conditions among 11,868 Gulf War-era veterans. *Am J Epidemiol.* 2002;155(11):1033-1044.
11. Mayer EA, Tillisch K. The brain-gut axis in abdominal pain syndromes. *Ann Rev Med.* 2011;62:381-396.
12. Keszthelyi D, Troost FJ, Masclee AA. Irritable bowel syndrome: methods, mechanisms, and pathophysiology. Methods to assess visceral hypersensitivity in irritable bowel syndrome. *Am J Physiol Gastrointest Liver Physiol.* 2012;303(2):G141-G154.
13. Aggarwal A, Cutts TF, Abell TL, et al. Predominant symptoms in irritable bowel syndrome correlate with specific autonomic nervous system abnormalities. *Gastroenterology.* 1994;106(4):945-950.
14. Cheng P, Shih W, Alberto M, et al. Autonomic response to a visceral stressor is dysregulated in irritable bowel syndrome and correlates with duration of disease. *Neurogastroenterol Motil.* 2013;25(10):e650-659.
15. Camilleri M, McKinzie S, Busciglio I, et al. Prospective study of motor, sensory, psychologic, and autonomic functions in patients with irritable bowel syndrome. *Clin Gastroenterol Hepatol.* 2008;6(7):772-781.
16. Agrawal A, Houghton LA, Reilly B, Morris J, Whorwell PJ. Bloating and distension in irritable bowel syndrome: the role of gastrointestinal transit. *Am J Gastroenterol.* 2009;104(8):1998-2004.
17. Hughes PA, Zola H, Penttila IA, Blackshaw LA, Andrews JM, Krumbiegel D. Immune activation in irritable bowel syndrome: can neuroimmune interactions explain symptoms? *Am J Gastroenterol.* 2013;108(7):1066-1074.
18. Camilleri M, Madsen K, Spiller R, Greenwood-Van Meerveld B, Verne GN. Intestinal barrier function in health and gastrointestinal disease. *Neurogastroenterol Motil.* 2012;24(6):503-512.
19. Mayer EA, Savidge T, Shulman RJ. Brain-gut microbiome interactions and functional bowel disorders. *Gastroenterology.* 2014;146(6):1500-1512.
20. Gracie DJ, Kane JS, Mumtaz S, Scarsbrook AF, Chowdhury FU, Ford AC. Prevalence of, and predictors of, bile acid malabsorption in outpatients with chronic diarrhea. *Neurogastroenterol Motil.* 2012;24(11):983-e538.
21. Ford AC, Bercik P, Morgan DG, Bolino C, Pintos-Sanchez MI, Moayyedi P. Validation of the Rome III criteria for the diagnosis of irritable bowel syndrome in secondary care. *Gastroenterology.* 2013;145(6):1262-1270, e1261.
22. Palsson OS, Baggish JS, Turner MJ, Whitehead WE. IBS patients show frequent fluctuations between loose/watery and hard/lumpy stools: implications for treatment. *Am J Gastroenterol.* 2012;107(2):286-295.
23. Whitehead WE, Palsson OS, Feld AD, et al. Utility of red flag symptom exclusions in the diagnosis of irritable bowel syndrome. *Aliment Pharmacol Ther.* 2006;24(1):137-146.
24. Brandt LJ, Chey WD, Foxx-Orenstein AE, et al. An evidence-based position statement on the management of irritable bowel syndrome. *Am J Gastroenterol.* 2009;104(Suppl 1):S1-S35.
25. Cash BD, Rubenstein JH, Young PE, et al. The prevalence of celiac disease among patients with nonconstipated irritable bowel syndrome is similar to controls. *Gastroenterology.* 2011;141(4):1187-1193.

26. Spiegel BMR, DeRosa VP, Gralnek IM, Wang V, Dulai GS. Testing for celiac sprue in irritable bowel syndrome with predominant diarrhea: a cost-effectiveness analysis. *Gastroenterology*. 2004;126(7):1721-1732.

27. Chey WD, Nojkov B, Rubenstein JH, Dobhan RR, Greenson JK, Cash BD. The yield of colonoscopy in patients with non-constipated irritable bowel syndrome: results from a prospective, controlled U.S. trial. *Am J Gastroenterol*. 2010;105(4):859-865.

28. Lovell RM, Ford AC. Global prevalence of and risk factors for irritable bowel syndrome: a meta-analysis. *Clin Gastroenterol Hepatol*. 2012;10(7):712-721.

29. Lovell RM, Ford AC. Effect of gender on prevalence of irritable bowel syndrome in the community: systematic review and meta-analysis. *Am J Gastroenterol*. 2012;107(7):991-1000.

30. El-Serag HB, Olden K, Bjorkman D. Health-related quality of life among persons with irritable bowel syndrome: a systematic review. *Aliment Pharmacol Ther*. 2002;16(6):1171-1185.

31. Naliboff BD, Kim SE, Bolus R, Bernstein CN, Mayer EA, Chang L. Gastrointestinal and psychological mediators of health-related quality of life in IBS and IBD: a structural equation modeling analysis. *Am J Gastroenterol*. 2012;107(3):451-459.

32. Lackner JM, Ma CX, Keefer L, et al. Type, rather than number, of mental and physical comorbidities increases the severity of symptoms in patients with irritable bowel syndrome. *Clin Gastroenterol Hepatol*. 2013;11(9):1147-1157.

33. Whitehead WE, Palsson OS, Levy RR, Feld AD, Turner M, Von Korff M. Comorbidity in irritable bowel syndrome. *Am J Gastroenterol*. 2007;102(12):2767-2776.

34. Walker EA, Katon WJ, Jemelka RP, Roy-Byrne PP. Comorbidity of gastrointestinal complaints, depression, and anxiety in the Epidemiologic Catchment Area (ECA) Study. *Am J Med*. 1992;92(1A):26S-30S.

35. Drossman DA, Camilleri M, Mayer EA, Whitehead WE. AGA technical review on irritable bowel syndrome. *Gastroenterology*. 2002;123(6):2108-2131.

36. Everhart JE, Ruhl CE. Burden of digestive diseases in the United States part II: lower gastrointestinal diseases. *Gastroenterology*. 2009;136(3):741-754.

37. Everhart JE. *Functional Intestinal Disorders*. Washington, DC: U.S. Government Printing Office: U.S. Department of Health and Human Services, Public Health Service, National Institutes of Health, National Institute of Diabetes and Digestive and Kidney Diseases;2008.

38. Spiegel B, Strickland A, Naliboff BD, Mayer EA, Chang L. Predictors of patient-assessed illness severity in irritable bowel syndrome. *Am J Gastroenterol*. 2008;103(10):2536-2543.

39. Chang L, Drossman D. Optimizing patient care: the psychological interview in irritable bowel syndrome. *Clin Perspect*. 2002;5(6):336-342.

40. Biesiekierski JR, Newnham ED, Irving PM, et al. Gluten causes gastrointestinal symptoms in subjects without celiac disease: a double-blind randomized placebo-controlled trial. *Am J Gastroenterol*. 2011;106(3):508-514; quiz 515.

41. Vazquez-Roque MI, Camilleri M, Smyrk T, et al. A controlled trial of gluten-free diet in patients with irritable bowel syndrome-diarrhea: effects on bowel frequency and intestinal function. *Gastroenterology*. 2013;144(5):903-911, e903.

42. Murray K, Wilkinson-Smith V, Hoad C, et al. Differential effects of FODMAPs (fermentable oligo-, di-, mono-saccharides and polyols) on small and large intestinal contents in healthy subjects shown by MRI. *Am J Gastroenterol*. 2014;109(1):110-119.

43. Ong DK, Mitchell SB, Barrett JS, et al. Manipulation of dietary short chain carbohydrates alters the pattern of gas production and genesis of symptoms in irritable bowel syndrome. *J Gastroenterol Hepatol*. 2010;25(8):1366-1373.

44. Halmos EP, Power VA, Shepherd SJ, Gibson PR, Muir JG. A diet low in FODMAPs reduces symptoms of irritable bowel syndrome. *Gastroenterology*. 2014;146(1):67-75, e65.

45. Biesiekierski JR, Peters SL, Newnham ED, Rosella O, Muir JG, Gibson PR. No effects of gluten in patients with self-reported non-celiac gluten sensitivity after dietary reduction of fermentable, poorly absorbed, short-chain carbohydrates. *Gastroenterology*. 2013;145(2):320-328, e321-323.

46. Johannesson E, Simren M, Strid H, Bajor A, Sadik R. Physical activity improves symptoms in irritable bowel syndrome: a randomized controlled trial. *Am J Gastroenterol*. 2011;106(5):915-922.

47. Ford AC, Moayyedi P, Lacy BE, et al. American College of Gastroenterology monograph on the management of irritable bowel syndrome and chronic idiopathic constipation. *Am J Gastroenterol*. 2014:109 Suppl 1: S2-S26.

48. Ruepert L, Quartero AO, de Wit NJ, van der Heijden GJ, Rubin G, Muris JW. Bulking agents, antispasmodics and antidepressants for the treatment of irritable bowel syndrome. *Cochrane Database Syst Rev*. 2011(8):CD003460.

49. Bijkerk CJ, de Wit NJ, Muris JW, Whorwell PJ, Knottnerus JA, Hoes AW. Soluble or insoluble fibre in irritable bowel syndrome in primary care? Randomised placebo controlled trial. *BMJ*. 2009;339:b3154.

50. Chapman RW, Stanghellini V, Geraint M, Halphen M. Randomized clinical trial: macrogol/PEG 3350 plus electrolytes for treatment of patients with constipation associated with irritable bowel syndrome. *Am J Gastroenterol*. 2013;108(9):1508-1515.

51. Drossman DA, Chey WD, Johanson JF, et al. Clinical trial: lubiprostone in patients with constipation-associated irritable bowel syndrome: results of two randomized, placebo-controlled studies. *Aliment Pharmacol Ther*. 2009;29(3):329-341.

52. Layer P, Stanghellini V. Review article: linaclotide for the management of irritable bowel syndrome with constipation. *Aliment Pharmacol Ther.* 2014;39(4):371-384.

53. Videlock EJ, Cheng V, Cremonini F. Effects of linaclotide in patients with irritable bowel syndrome with constipation or chronic constipation: a meta-analysis. *Clin Gastroenterol Hepatol.* 2013;11(9):1084-1092, e1083.

54. Pimentel M, Lembo A, Chey WD, et al. Rifaximin therapy for patients with irritable bowel syndrome without constipation. *N Engl J Med.* 2011;364(1):22-32.

55. Menees SB, Maneerattannaporn M, Kim HM, Chey WD. The efficacy and safety of rifaximin for the irritable bowel syndrome: a systematic review and meta-analysis. *Am J Gastroenterol.* 2012;107(1):28-35; quiz 36.

56. Schoenfeld P, Pimentel M, Chang L, et al. Safety and tolerability of rifaximin for the treatment of irritable bowel syndrome without constipation: a pooled analysis of randomised, double-blind, placebo-controlled trials. *Aliment Pharmacol Ther.* 2014;39(10):1161-1168.

57. Cremonini F, Nicandro JP, Atkinson V, Shringarpure R, Chuang E, Lembo A. Randomised clinical trial: alosetron improves quality of life and reduces restriction of daily activities in women with severe diarrhoea-predominant IBS. *Aliment Pharmacol Ther.* 2012;36(5):437-448.

58. Chang L, Ameen VZ, Dukes GE, McSorley DJ, Carter EG, Mayer EA. A dose-ranging, phase II study of the efficacy and safety of alosetron in men with diarrhea-predominant IBS. *Am J Gastroenterol.* 2005;100(1):115-123.

59. Chang L, Chey WD, Harris L, Olden K, Surawicz C, Schoenfeld P. Incidence of ischemic colitis and serious complications of constipation among patients using alosetron: systematic review of clinical trials and post-marketing surveillance data. *Am J Gastroenterol.* 2006;101(5):1069-1079.

60. Tong K, Nicandro JP, Shringarpure R, Chuang E, Chang L. A 9-year evaluation of temporal trends in alosetron postmarketing safety under the risk management program. *Therap Adv Gastroenterol.* 2013;6(5):344-357.

61. Ford AC, Talley NJ, Spiegel BM, et al. Effect of fibre, antispasmodics, and peppermint oil in the treatment of irritable bowel syndrome: systematic review and meta-analysis. *BMJ.* 2008;337:a2313.

62. Whorwell PJ, Altringer L, Morel J, et al. Efficacy of an encapsulated probiotic Bifidobacterium infantis 35624 in women with irritable bowel syndrome. *Am J Gastroenterol.* 2006;101(7):1581-1590.

63. Kim HJ, Vazquez Roque MI, Camilleri M, et al. A randomized controlled trial of a probiotic combination VSL# 3 and placebo in irritable bowel syndrome with bloating. *Neurogastroenterol Motil.* 2005;17(5):687-696.

64. Guyonnet D, Chassany O, Ducrotte P, et al. Effect of a fermented milk containing Bifidobacterium animalis DN-173 010 on the health-related quality of life and symptoms in irritable bowel syndrome in adults in primary care: a multicentre, randomized, double-blind, controlled trial. *Aliment Pharmacol Ther.* 2007;26(3):475-486.

65. Ford AC, Quigley EM, Lacy BE, et al. Effect of antidepressants and psychological therapies, including hypnotherapy, in irritable bowel syndrome: systematic review and meta-analysis. *Am J Gastroenterol.* 2014.

66. Palsson OS, Whitehead WE. Psychological treatments in functional gastrointestinal disorders: a primer for the gastroenterologist. *Clin Gastroenterol Hepatol.* 2013;11(3):208-216.

67. Gaylord SA, Palsson OS, Garland EL, et al. Mindfulness training reduces the severity of irritable bowel syndrome in women: results of a randomized controlled trial. *Am J Gastroenterol.* 2011;106(9):1678-1688.

68. Ford AC, Brandt LJ, Young C, Chey WD, Foxx-Orenstein AE, Moayyedi P. Efficacy of 5-HT3 antagonists and 5-HT4 agonists in irritable bowel syndrome: systematic review and meta-analysis. *Am J Gastroenterol.* 2009;104(7):1831-1843.

69. Wittmann T, Paradowski L, Ducrotte P, Bueno I, Andro Delestrain MC. Clinical trial: the efficacy of alverine citrate/simethicone combination on abdominal pain/discomfort in irritable bowel syndrome: a randomized, double-blind, placebo-controlled study. *Aliment Pharmacol Ther.* 2010;31(6):615-624.

70. Clave P, Acalovschi M, Triantafillidis JK, et al. Randomised clinical trial: otilonium bromide improves frequency of abdominal pain, severity of distention and time to relapse in patients with irritable bowel syndrome. *Aliment Pharmacol Ther.* 2011;34(4):432-442.

19

Slow Transit Constipation

Richard J. Saad, MD, MS

KEY POINTS

- Dyssynergic defecation must be excluded or identified and corrected before pursuing colonic transit testing.
- Objective testing of colonic transit is essential to make a diagnosis of slow transit constipation.
- Upper gastrointestinal dysmotility and coexisting psychiatric disorders must be excluded before pursuing elective subtotal colectomy for slow transit constipation.

DEFINITION

Slow transit constipation (STC) represents a well-recognized subtype of chronic constipation, and is characterized by delayed passage of fecal contents through the colon. Although severe cases of constipation marked by stasis of the bowels were first reported in 1909, the term *STC* was not introduced until 1986. Chronic constipation caused by intestinal stasis was initially termed *Arbuthnot Lane's disease* in deference to the British surgeon, Sir William Arbuthnot, who reported on a small case series of young women with severe refractory constipation symptoms responding favorably to subtotal colectomy in 1909.[1] It was not until 1968 that the concept of "constipation with slow intestinal transit rate" was introduced by Hinton et al[2] to describe constipation marked by a delayed elimination of orally ingested radiopaque pellets. Two decades later, the term *idiopathic slow transit constipation* was coined by Preston and Lennard-Jones[3] to define a series of 64 young women with severe constipation and delayed elimination of radiopaque markers in the absence of a structural disorder of the colon. The present term, *STC*, refers to individuals meeting the current clinical criteria for chronic constipation as defined by the Rome III working group, in the absence of secondary causes for the constipation symptoms and objectively demonstrating delayed passage of luminal contents of the colon (Table 19-1). Although the term *colonic inertia* is occasionally used

Rao SSC, Parkman HP, McCallum RW, eds.
Handbook of Gastrointestinal Motility and Functional Disorders (pp 241-252).

TABLE 19-1
CLINICAL CRITERIA FOR SLOW TRANSIT CONSTIPATION
1. Six or more months of 2 or more of the following symptoms occurring for more than 25% of defecations during the last 3 months:[34]
• Straining
• Passage of lumpy or hard stools
• Sensation of incomplete evacuation
• Sensation of anorectal obstruction or blockage
• Manual maneuvers to facilitate defecation
• Fewer than 3 defecations per week
2. The passage of loose stool is rarely present in the absence of laxative use
3. Failure to fulfill diagnostic criteria for irritable bowel syndrome
4. Exclusion of secondary causes of constipation, including structural, metabolic, and drug-induced causes
5. Objective evidence of delayed colonic transit on physiologic testing

interchangeably with STC, this term more accurately refers to a subtype of STC in which there is an absent or reduced colonic motility response to either a meal or a pharmacologic colonic stimulant such as bisacodyl or neostigmine.[4]

EPIDEMIOLOGY

The exact prevalence of STC in the general population is unknown. Epidemiologic studies collectively suggest a median constipation prevalence of 16% in the general adult population and 33% in those aged 60 years or older.[4] After excluding the secondary causes of chronic constipation, STC constipation is believed to represent one of the three major subtypes of chronic primary constipation. As is the case for constipation in general, it is presumed that mild cases of STC respond to lifestyle and/or dietary changes, as well as treatment with laxatives. There are no studies providing insight on the prevalence of STC in those seeking care in the primary care setting for chronic constipation. Limited epidemiologic studies in the tertiary care setting suggest an STC prevalence of 27% to 47% in those seeking specialty care for refractory chronic constipation.[5,6] It is important to understand that over one-half of cases of STC had coexistent pelvic floor dysfunction, suggesting that isolated STC only represents 15% to 20% of those with refractory chronic constipation.[7]

PATHOPHYSIOLOGY

Clinically, STC represents a constellation of refractory constipation syndromes characterized by a delay in stool transit through the colon, presumably as a result of disordered colonic motility. The constipation symptoms of STC can be lifelong, implying a congenital disorder, or they may arise later in life, either spontaneously or following a specific event. For example, STC has been reported in association with anorexia nervosa and those with excessive methane production by colonic flora.[7-9] The transit delay can vary widely in terms of its severity and response to therapy. The delayed transit may involve the entire colon or a segment of the colon, such as the right colon, left colon, or rectosigmoid. Furthermore, there may be a coexistent disorder of the pelvic floor and/or anorectal function that is discussed in a separate chapter. Pelvic floor dysfunction should be identified and ideally treated before pursuing tests for STC.

Similar to the heterogeneity in the presentation of STC, the purported pathophysiological mechanisms are equally diverse. Through colonic manometry, STC can be subtyped as a myopathic versus a neuropathic disorder of the colon. Indeed, several alterations in colonic function have been described using manometry, including impairment of phasic colonic motor activity, altered gastrocolonic meal response, and diminished waking response of the colon.[7] Reported alterations in motor activity have included decreased number, frequency, duration, and velocity of high-amplitude, propagated contractions; decreased overall colonic tone; and autonomic dysfunction.[7]

A variety of histologic abnormalities have been reported in STC, including decreased numbers of interstitial cells of Cajal (ICC), argyrophilic neurons, neurofilaments, and/or overall nerve fibers. Interstitial cells of Cajal are electrically active cells believed to act as the pacemaker for the intestines through their generation of slow waves in smooth muscle. The colon of those with STC has been shown to have a decreased density of ICC throughout, including the cecum, ascending colon, transverse colon, and sigmoid colon.[10]

Several abnormalities in neurotransmitter activity have also been described in STC, including reductions in excitatory neurotransmitters and increases in inhibitory neurotransmitters. For example, there have been reports of reductions in acetylcholine release and increased release of nitric oxide and adenosine triphosphate.[11] It should be realized that studies have been conflicting on many other neurotransmitters, including vasoactive intestinal polypeptide, neuropeptide Y, substance P, and serotonin.[11]

Diagnosis

As implied by its name, the diagnosis of STC requires specialized physiologic testing that provides objective evidence for a delay in transit of material through the colon. Physiologic studies for this purpose include the radiopaque marker transit test, scintigraphy, and the wireless motility capsule (Table 19-2).[7] Colonic manometry may provide additional information on colonic function in the evaluation of medically refractory STC.[7] Given the limited prevalence of STC in chronic constipation, high incidence of coexistent defecatory disorders, and limitation of testing, such physiologic testing should be reserved for those cases failing medical therapy in which all secondary causes of constipation and defecatory disorders have been excluded. Figure 19-1 provides a suggested algorithm for the role of physiologic testing in the assessment of suspected STC.

Radiopaque Marker Testing

Radiopaque marker testing (ROM) (Figure 19-2) provides the most widely available and inexpensive modality for the assessment of STC. However, it is important to understand that ROM provides an assessment of whole gut transit and not colon transit, as the markers are ingested orally and must pass through the stomach and the small bowel before traversing the colon. Consequently, it may be necessary to exclude delayed gastric and small bowel transit before concluding that an individual has STC. This is particularly important when considering surgical intervention for medically refractory STC. Radiopaque markers may consist of small plastic pieces, beads, or rings. The most commonly utilized markers are Sitzmarks (Konsyl Pharamaceuticals). Two ROM protocols are most commonly employed. The Hinton method is a 5-day ROM study providing a

TABLE 19-2
TESTS FOR COLON TRANSIT

	DEFINITION OF DELAYED TRANSIT	ADVANTAGES	DISADVANTAGES
5-day ROM test	Six or more retained markers on x-ray imaging 5 days (120 hours) after marker ingestion	Widely available Simple Inexpensive	Measures whole gut transit, not colonic transit Only provides qualitative data regarding transit Radiation exposure associated with x-ray Lack of standardization
7-day ROM test	Greater than 67 retained markers from the sum total of x-ray imaging on days 4 and 7	Widely available Inexpensive Provides quantitative data regarding colon transit Can provide estimation of segmental colonic transit	Measures whole gut transit, not colonic transit More complex than 5-day ROM study Radiation exposure associated with x-rays Lack of standardization
Scintigraphy	A numeric value of overall colon transit time based on the geometric center of radiolabeled marker This value varies by the center performing the study	Short testing time frame (24 to 72 hours) Provides colonic transit time	Limited availability Expensive Radiation exposure Lack of standardization
Wireless motility capsule	A colon transit time of greater than 59 hours (time from entrance into the terminal ileum to capsule exit from the body)	Office-based testing Standardized Provides simultaneous assessment of gastric, small bowel, and colonic transit time No radiation	Limited availability Expensive Potential for test failure and capsule retention

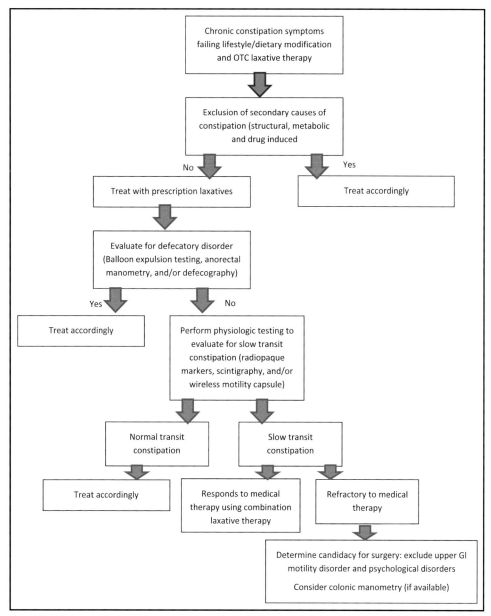

Figure 19-1. Diagnostic algorithm for STC.

qualitative assessment of colonic transit,[12] whereas the Metcalf method is a 7-day study providing a more quantitative assessment of colonic transit.[13] The Hinton method entails the ingestion of 24 markers followed by the performance of a standard abdominal x-ray 5 days later. The presence of more than 5 markers on the x-ray indicates delayed colonic transit. With the Metcalf method, 24 markers are ingested on days 1, 2, and 3 followed by the performance of abdominal x-rays on days 4 and 7. A total marker count from the 2 x-rays exceeding 67 indicates a delayed colonic transit. This methodology provides a more detailed assessment of transit time as well as an estimation of segmental colonic transit (right colon, left colon, rectosigmoid colon). Variations in ROM methodology have been reported with alterations in the marker ingestion scheme or x-ray imaging schedule. Regardless of the ROM methodology pursued, a bowel cleansing is not necessary prior to testing. Since many laxatives are likely to impact marker transit, it is strongly recommended that

Figure 19-2. Example of radiopaque marker study in slow transit constipation. Notice the large number of retained radiopaque markers scattered throughout the colon on this x-ray taken on day 4 of the 7-day ROM study. A wireless motility capsule study was performed simultaneously in this patient (the large cylindrical radiopaque shape in the left-lower quadrant is the wireless motility capsule, which did pass several days later).

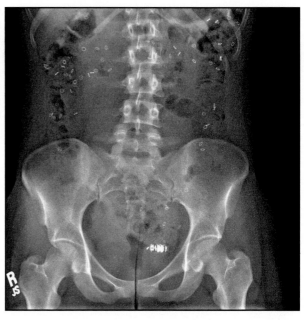

laxative use be suspended during ROM testing. It is also important to hold medications known to slow gastrointestinal transit during ROM testing, specifically all opioid analgesics and antispasmodics. Given the variability in testing methodology and lack of standardization, repeat testing should be considered if clinically indicated.

Scintigraphy

Radionuclide gamma scintigraphy represents an alternative to ROM. Although a shorter study than ROM, generally taking 24 to 72 hours depending on the protocol, scintigraphy is of limited availability, is more expensive, is associated with radiation exposure, and generally lacks standardization for test interpretation. Scintigraphic measurement of colonic transit has been described using one of two methods.[14] One approach entails the coingestion of 111-indium diethylenetriamine penta-acetic acid in water along with scrambled egg radiolabeled with 99-m technetium sulphur colloid as part of a liquid–solid gastric scintigraphic study. An alternative approach involves the ingestion of a pH-sensitive methacrylate-coated capsule containing 111-indium-labeled activated charcoal particles, which dissolves on entrance into the alkaline terminal ileum releasing the charcoal particles. Colonic transit time is then calculated through localization of the geometric center of the radiolabeled marker 24, 48, and/or 72 hours following ingestion of the meal. A variety of methods have been proposed for the assessment of the geometric center; however, no standardized or universally agreed-upon approach exists.[15] As is the case for ROM testing, laxatives and other medications known to alter gastrointestinal transit should be held or avoided during scintigraphy.

Wireless Motility Capsule

The wireless motility/pH capsule (WMC) is an orally ingested, nondigestible device (26.8 mm × 11.7 mm in size) that provides simultaneous assessment of regional and whole gut transit. The WMC study can be performed in the office setting with the patient presenting for transit testing following an overnight fast. The WMC is ingested following the consumption of a standardized 260 Kcal nutrient bar consisting of 17% protein, 66% carbohydrates, 2% fats, and 3% fiber (Smartbar) with 50 mL of water. The patient is then provided with a small external data recorder

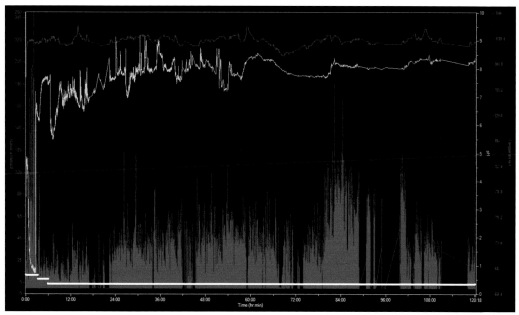

Figure 19-3. Wireless motility capsule recording in STC. Temperature is represented by the blue tracing, pH by the green tracing, and intraluminal pressure by the red tracing. The calculated gastric emptying time is 2 hours and 35 minutes (demonstrated by the abrupt rise in pH as the capsule leaves the acidic environment of the stomach) and represented by the first white hash mark at the bottom of the graph. The calculated small bowel transit time is 4 hours. The time of entrance into the small bowel and its delivery into the cecum (demonstrated by the abrupt drop in pH as the capsule enters the acid environment of the cecum) is represented by the second white hash mark at the bottom of the graph. The calculated colon transit time is 113 hours. The time of entrance into the cecum and its exit from the body (demonstrated by the abrupt drop in temperature as the capsule exits the body) is represented by the third white hash mark at the bottom of the graph.

to be worn on a specially designed belt that needs to be kept within 5 feet of the body for the 5-day testing period. Temperature, luminal pressure, and luminal pH are continuously recorded by the capsule and sent to the external recorder via a transmitter operating at a wavelength of 434 MHz. A combination of pH and temperature profiles is used to calculate the gastric, small bowel, colonic, and whole gut transit time (Figure 19-3). The WMC has been validated in the measurement of colonic transit time in chronic constipation.[16] A colonic transit time of >59 hours has been defined as one of delayed colon transit.[16] Limitations of this testing modality include cost, availability, test failure, and the rare risk of capsule retention, which may require endoscopic or surgical extraction.[16] Once again, laxatives and other medications known to alter gastrointestinal transit should be held during WMC testing.

Colonic Manometry

Colonic manometry provides a sensorimotor evaluation of the colon that is reserved for the assessment of medically refractory STC. It consists of either a water-perfused or solid-state manometric probe, which may also include a 10-cm polyethylene balloon at the proximal end serving as a barostat. The device is placed through the anus and advanced to the mid-descending colon or ascending colon[17] using a colonoscope, with or without fluoroscopic assistance. Colonic manometry can be performed in the laboratory setting using a stationary manometric-barostat device in which data are collected over a period of 6 hours. Alternatively, the solid-state manometric probe with portable recorder can be used in the ambulatory setting in which data are collected over a period of 24 hours. Manometric parameters, including the gastrocolonic response following a meal

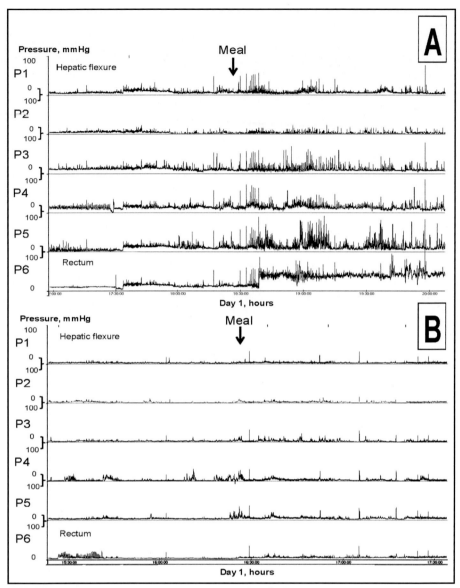

Figure 19-4. Colonic manometry tracing in STC. Samples of colonic manometry: Report A represents a normal manometry. Report B represents the manometry pattern in an individual with a neuropathic slow transit constipation.

(Figure 19-4), waking response, and pattern of high-amplitude propagated contractions, allow for subtyping of STC as one of colonic neuropathy, colonic myopathy, or normal manometry.[17] Use of the optional colonic barostat allows for the assessment of colonic sensation. This manometric assessment may help direct treatment, as STC with myopathy or normal manometry is more likely to respond to medical therapy as opposed to those cases of neuropathy (see Figure 19-4), which are more responsive to surgical intervention.[17] For a variety of reasons, including very limited availability (only performed at a few highly specialized centers), expense, need for specialized training, and discomfort, as well as inconvenience to the patient, colonic manometry is considered an adjunct to colonic transit testing in STC and not an absolute necessity.

TREATMENT

The treatment of STC can be challenging. Patients may present with a variety of chronic and bothersome symptoms, including infrequent bowel movements, the passage of hard stool, straining, sensation of incomplete evacuation, sensation of blockage in the anus, bloating, nausea, abdominal pain, abdominal distention, and diminished appetite. These long-standing and often refractory symptoms may also be associated with considerable anxiety, frustration, and depressed mood. The initial approach to treatment should include obtaining a careful history, establishing a secure diagnosis, and setting realistic goals with the patient. When taking the history, particular attention should be given to prior therapies and their reasons for failure. A careful review of all medications, both prescription and over-the-counter agents, is important at the outset, as these can have a significant impact on bowel motility and measured transit time. Not only must delayed colon transit be objectively demonstrated, but other secondary causes of constipation and altered colon transit also must be excluded, particularly that of a drug-induced constipation. It is essential to assess for functional outlet obstruction, not only from structural sources including rectocele or enterocele, but also as a result of dyssynergic defecation. There could also be a coexistent condition of small bowel bacterial overgrowth, which should be treated if identified. Coexistent psychological disorders are common in this population and can negatively impact symptoms and response to treatment. If identified, they need to be considered and properly addressed. Most importantly, define realistic goals with the patient both in terms of anticipated treatment response as well as potential side effects of therapy. This is particularly important if surgical intervention is being entertained.

Medical Therapy

Although STC is frequently refractory to initial trials of laxative therapy, a combination of laxatives with complementary mechanisms of action may be effective and well tolerated. The patient should be encouraged to maintain dietary fiber and/or fiber supplementation as tolerated; however, increasing fiber intake is unlikely to provide additional benefit. Increased dietary fiber has minimal effect in STC,[18] and it has been this author's experience that symptoms of abdominal distention and bloating typically worsen with increased dietary fiber intake. Furthermore, water-soluble fiber supplements such as psyllium may improve stool consistency and increase stool frequency; however, there is no effect on colon transit.[19] Osmotic laxatives such as polyethylene glycol (PEG) and lactulose have consistently demonstrated efficacy in the treatment of chronic constipation. Both PEG and lactulose have demonstrated acceleration in colon transit in small studies.[20,21] There are no published clinical trials assessing the saline laxative magnesium; however, anecdotally speaking, magnesium is a relatively safe and effective alternative osmotic agent used in the treatment of constipation. The stimulant laxative bisacodyl has demonstrated promotility effects in some cases of STC.[22] If an osmotic agent has been used in the past and not found to be effective, its use in combination with a stimulant laxative may be effective and well tolerated. Although osmotic and stimulant laxatives are likely to improve stool form and frequency, there is little effect on abdominal pain and bloating.[23] The effect of the chloride channel activator lubiprostone in STC remains largely unknown. There is some emerging evidence that it may accelerate colonic transit in those with constipation and delayed colon transit.[24] The effect of the guanylate cyclase C activator linaclotide in STC also remains unknown. However, linaclotide has demonstrated acceleration of colonic transit in irritable bowel syndrome with constipation.[25] Although not available in the United States, the serotonin receptor agonist prucalopride has accelerated colonic transit, as well as addressed constipation symptoms in STC.[26]

Other agents to consider in the treatment of STC include the synthetic prostaglandin analog misoprostol and the alkaloid antigout agent colchicine.[27] Two months of colchicine 1 mg/day was

TABLE 19-3
SUGGESTED PHARMACOLOGIC TREATMENT STRATEGIES FOR SLOW TRANSIT CONSTIPATION

	SUGGESTED DOSING SCHEME	PRACTICAL POINTS
Osmotic + stimulant laxative	Polyethylene glycol (PEG) 3350 17 to 34 grams once daily + Bisacodyl 5 to 10 mg every evening	Lactulose likely to promote more bloating than PEG Generally well tolerated Consider senna as alternative to bisacodyl for cramping with use
Secretagogue + stimulant	Lubiprostone 24 mcg twice daily + Bisacodyl 5 to 10 mg every evening Linaclotide 145 to 290 mcg once daily + Bisacodyl 5 to 10 mg every evening	Lubiprostone should be dosed with food Linaclotide should be taken in the fasting state to reduce occurrence of diarrhea Start with secretagogue alone and add stimulant if needed Consider senna as alternative to bisacodyl for cramping with use
Osmotic + stimulant laxative + misoprostol Secretagogue + stimulant + misoprostol	Polyethylene glycol (PEG) 3350 17 to 34 grams once daily + Bisacodyl 5 to 10 mg every evening + Misoprostol Lubiprostone 24 mcg twice daily + Bisacodyl 5 to 10 mg every evening + Misoprostol Linaclotide 145 to 290 mcg once daily + Bisacodyl 5 to 10 mg every evening + Misoprostol	Start with a low dose of misoprostol at 200 mcg once daily and increase slowly as needed every 1 to 2 weeks to maximum of 400 mcg tid Maximum dose studied in constipation was 400 mcg tid, although this dose is not well tolerated Misoprostol contraindicated in pregnancy; use carefully in women of child-bearing age Long-term safety of misoprostol unknown
Osmotic + stimulant laxative + colchicine Secretagogue + stimulant + colchicine	Polyethylene glycol (PEG) 3350 17 to 34 grams once daily + Bisacodyl 5 to 10 mg every evening + Colchicine Lubiprostone 24 mcg twice daily + Bisacodyl 5 to 10 mg every evening + Colchicine Linaclotide 145 to 290 mcg once daily + Bisacodyl 5 to 10 mg every evening + Colchicine	Starting dose of colchicine should be 0.6 to 1 mg once daily Maximum dose of colchicine should be 0.6 mg tid Long-term safety of colchicine unknown Remain vigilant for rare side effects with colchicine to include myopathy, neuropathy, bone marrow suppression, severe pancytopenia

superior to placebo in the treatment of constipation symptoms associated with STC.[27] Misoprostol was tested on 18 adults with refractory constipation in an open-labeled study at total daily doses ranging from 600 to 2400 mcg.[28] One-third of the patients dropped out during the 4-week trial due to side effects (symptoms were largely dose dependent). In those completing the trial, mean bowel frequency increased from once every 11.25 to 4.8 days. A dose of 400 mcg/day increased colonic motility in 5 patients. The long-term safety in the treatment of constipation is unknown for both agents; furthermore, misoprostol has a pregnancy Category X designation.

The author has found a variety of combination laxative regimens effective in the treatment of STC. See Table 19-3 for suggested combination dosing regimens for STC. For episodic symptomatic fecal loading associated with STC, it may be necessary to pursue a bowel purge using one of the approved bowel purgatives for colonoscopy.

Surgical Therapy

Subtotal colectomy with ileorectal anastomosis should be considered for STC that is refractory to medical therapy.[4] The overall rate of satisfaction with surgical therapy is reported to be 86% (range: 39% to 100%).[29] Proper patient selection, as well as a candid and thorough discussion regarding the anticipated outcomes and potential side effects of therapy, is essential for success. Pelvic floor dysfunction and a generalized gastrointestinal motility disorder should be excluded in surgical candidates.[4] Caution should be exercised in patients with a psychological disorder or history of sexual abuse, given the potential negative impact on surgical outcomes for STC.[29] It has been suggested that colonic manometry can be used to predict better surgical outcomes, as STC due to colonic neuropathy responds better to surgical intervention than myopathic STC.[17] Patients considering surgical therapy should be informed that symptoms of abdominal pain and bloating are unlikely to respond, and that the constipation symptoms are frequently replaced with diarrheal symptoms. It is also important to make patients aware of the potential complications associated with surgery. Overall postoperative mortality in 25 case series is 2.6% (range 0% to 15%).[29] Other complications include postoperative ileus, small bowel obstruction, wound infection, anastomotic leaks, anastomotic stricture, diarrhea, and fecal incontinence. In general, the outcomes with subtotal colectomy are superior to that of hemicolectomy or other forms of segmental colectomy.[4] Another surgical intervention that has not gained wide acceptance in the adult population is the performance of antegrade colonic enema via an appendiceal conduit or indwelling cecostomy catheter.

Emerging Therapies

Several emerging therapies for STC are under further investigation. Neuromodulation through implanted sacral nerve stimulation or transcutaneous electrical stimulation may play a future role in medically refractory STC.[30] Other surgical interventions reported to be effective in small case series of STC include colonic bypass with cecorectal anastomosis,[31] colonic pacing via surgical placement of a colonic electrical stimulator,[32] and percutaneous tibial nerve stimulation.[33]

REFERENCES

1. Lane WA. An address on chronic intestinal stasis. *Br Med J.* 1909;1(2528):1408-1411.
2. Hinton JM, Lennard-Jones JE. Constipation: definition and classification. *Postgrad Med J.* 1968;44(515):720-723.
3. Preston DM, Lennard-Jones JE. Severe chronic constipation of young women: "idiopathic slow transit constipation." *Gut.* 1986;27(1):41-48.
4. Bharucha AE, Pemberton JH, Locke GR, 3rd. American Gastroenterological Association technical review on constipation. *Gastroenterology.* 2013;144(1):218-238.
5. Mertz H, Naliboff B, Mayer E. Physiology of refractory chronic constipation. *Am J Gastroenterol.* 1999;94(3): 609-615.

6.   Surrenti E, Rath DM, Pemberton JH, Camilleri M. Audit of constipation in a tertiary referral gastroenterology practice. *Am J Gastroenterol.* 1995;90(9):1471-1475.

7.   Rao SS. Constipation: evaluation and treatment of colonic and anorectal motility disorders. *Gastrointest Endosc Clin N Am.* 2009;19(1):117-139, vii.

8.   Ghoshal UC, Srivastava D, Verma A, Misra A. Slow transit constipation associated with excess methane production and its improvement following rifaximin therapy: a case report. *J Neurogastroenterol Motil.* 2011;17(2): 185-188.

9.   Hadley SJ, Walsh BT. Gastrointestinal disturbances in anorexia nervosa and bulimia nervosa. *Curr Drug Targets CNS Neurol Disord.* 2003;2(1):1-9.

10. Lyford GL, He CL, Soffer E, et al. Pan-colonic decrease in interstitial cells of Cajal in patients with slow transit constipation. *Gut.* 2002;51(4):496-501.

11. Knowles CH, Martin JE. Slow transit constipation: a model of human gut dysmotility. Review of possible aetiologies. *Neurogastroenterol Motil.* 2000;12(2):181-196.

12. Hinton JM, Lennard-Jones JE, Young AC. A new method for studying gut transit times using radioopaque markers. *Gut.* 1969;10(10):842-847.

13. Metcalf AM, Phillips SF, Zinsmeister AR, MacCarty RL, Beart RW, Wolff BG. Simplified assessment of segmental colonic transit. *Gastroenterology.* 1987;92(1):40-47.

14. Rao SS, Camilleri M, Hasler WL, et al. Evaluation of gastrointestinal transit in clinical practice: position paper of the American and European Neurogastroenterology and Motility Societies. *Neurogastroenterol Motil.* 2011;23(1):8-23.

15. Madsen JL. Scintigraphic assessment of gastrointestinal motility: a brief review of techniques and data interpretation. *Clin Physiol Funct Imaging.* 2013.

16. Saad RJ, Hasler WL. A technical review and clinical assessment of the wireless motility capsule. *Gastroenterol Hepatol.* 2011;7(12):795-804.

17. Singh S, Heady S, Coss-Adame E, Rao SS. Clinical utility of colonic manometry in slow transit constipation. *Neurogastroenterol Motil.* 2013;25(6):487-495.

18. Voderholzer WA, Schatke W, Muhldorfer BE, Klauser AG, Birkner B, Muller-Lissner SA. Clinical response to dietary fiber treatment of chronic constipation. *Am J Gastroenterol.* 1997;92(1):95-98.

19. Ashraf W, Park F, Lof J, Quigley EM. Effects of psyllium therapy on stool characteristics, colon transit and anorectal function in chronic idiopathic constipation. *Aliment Pharmacol Ther.* 1995;9(6):639-647.

20. Bassotti G, Fiorella S, Roselli P, Modesto R. Use of polyethylene glycol solution in slow transit constipation. *Ital J Gastroenterol Hepatol.* 1999;31(Suppl 3):S255-256.

21. Pontes FA, Silva AT, Cruz AC. Colonic transit times and the effect of lactulose or lactitol in hospitalized patients. *Eur J Gastroenterol Hepatol.* 1995;7(5):441-446.

22. Herve S, Savoye G, Behbahani A, Leroi AM, Denis P, Ducrotte P. Results of 24-h manometric recording of colonic motor activity with endoluminal instillation of bisacodyl in patients with severe chronic slow transit constipation. *Neurogastroenterol Motil.* 2004;16(4):397-402.

23. Dinning PG, Hunt L, Lubowski DZ, Kalantar JS, Cook IJ, Jones MP. The impact of laxative use upon symptoms in patients with proven slow transit constipation. *BMC Gastroenterol.* 2011;11:121.

24. Saad R, Nahlawi L, Chey WD. Effect of the chloride channel activator, lubiprostone, on gastrointestinal and colonic transit, motility and pH in patients with the irritable bowel syndrome and constipation (IBS-C) (Abstract). *Am J Gastroenterol.* 2013;108(S1):S565.

25. Andresen V, Camilleri M, Busciglio IA, et al. Effect of 5 days of linaclotide on transit and bowel function in females with constipation-predominant irritable bowel syndrome. *Gastroenterology.* 2007;133(3):761-768.

26. Emmanuel AV, Roy AJ, Nicholls TJ, Kamm MA. Prucalopride, a systemic enterokinetic, for the treatment of constipation. *Aliment Pharmacol Ther.* 2002;16(7):1347-1356.

27. Taghavi SA, Shabani S, Mehramiri A, et al. Colchicine is effective for short-term treatment of slow transit constipation: a double-blind placebo-controlled clinical trial. *Int J Colorectal Dis.* 2010;25(3):389-394.

28. Roarty TP, Weber F, Soykan I, McCallum RW. Misoprostol in the treatment of chronic refractory constipation: results of a long-term open label trial. *Aliment Pharmacol Ther.* 1997;11(6):1059-1066.

29. Bove A, Bellini M, Battaglia E, et al. Consensus statement AIGO/SICCR diagnosis and treatment of chronic constipation and obstructed defecation (part II: treatment). *World J Gastroenterol.* 2012;18(36):4994-5013.

30. van Wunnik BP, Baeten CG, Southwell BR. Neuromodulation for constipation: sacral and transcutaneous stimulation. *Best Pract Res Clin Gastroenterol.* 2011;25(1):181-191.

31. Zhao S, Kong B, Chen Q, Zhao F. Colonic bypass: an alternative approach to slow transit constipation in elderly patients. *Int J Colorectal Dis.* 2011;26(9):1215-1216.

32. Martellucci J, Valeri A. Colonic electrical stimulation for the treatment of slow-transit constipation: a preliminary pilot study. *Surg Endosc.* 2013.

33. Collins B, Norton C, Maeda Y. Percutaneous tibial nerve stimulation for slow transit constipation: a pilot study. *Colorectal Dis.* 2012;14(4):e165-170.

34. Longstreth GF, Thompson WG, Chey WD, Houghton LA, Mearin F, Spiller RC. Functional bowel disorders. *Gastroenterology.* 2006;130(5):1480-1491.

Dyssynergic Defecation and Constipation

Gina Sam, MD, MPH and Satish S.C. Rao, MD, PhD, FRCP

KEY POINTS

- Dyssynergic defecation is a common clinical problem, affecting over one-third of patients with chronic constipation, with an approximate prevalence of 7% in the general population.

- It is characterized by incoordination of the muscles involved in achieving normal defecation.

- Chief symptoms include prolonged and excessive straining, feeling of incomplete evacuation, hard stools, and use of digital maneuvers to evacuate, with or without infrequent defecation.

- Digital rectal examination can detect dyssynergia with >80% accuracy, but it requires confirmation with physiological tests.

- Anorectal manometry, together with balloon expulsion test, is the gold standard for an objective diagnosis of dyssynergic defecation, together with modified Rome III criteria.

- Biofeedback therapy has been demonstrated to be an effective treatment modality, both in the short-term and the long-term management of this condition and is the mainstay of current treatment approaches, along with laxatives and supportive therapy.

Constipation is a common problem in Western countries, with an average prevalence of 15% in the population.[1] It negatively impacts the quality of life and is one of the leading reasons for a medical consultation. Most patients who experience constipation will respond to changing their diet, adding fiber, or taking laxatives. Patients who do not respond to these measures fall into the group of patients often referred to as idiopathic chronic constipation, many of whom have an evacuation disorder.[1] Approximately 33% of patients with chronic constipation have an evacuation disorder, and most will be classified as dyssynergic defecation.[2] The term dyssynergic defecation is also known as anismus, pelvic floor dyssynergia, obstructive defecation, paradoxical puborectalis contraction, pelvic outlet obstruction, or spastic pelvic floor syndrome.[2]

Rao SSC, Parkman HP, McCallum RW, eds.
Handbook of Gastrointestinal Motility and Functional Disorders (pp 253-264).
© 2015 Taylor & Francis Group.

DEFINITION

Dyssynergic defecation occurs when there is incoordination of the push effort generated by the abdominal, rectal, and pelvic floor muscles and the relaxation induced by the puborectalis and anal sphincter muscle. This leads to an inability to have a complete bowel movement.[2]

EPIDEMIOLOGY

Constipation is a common complaint. In a telephone interview of 10,018 individuals at least 18 years old, the prevalence was estimated at 14.7%.[1] Functional constipation was reported by 3.6% of responders and difficult defecation was reported by 13.8% in a questionnaire survey of 5430 households in the United States.[1] The exact prevalence is underestimated because most patients do not seek out medical care.

Constipation affects women more than men, with a female to male ratio of 2.2:1.1,[2] advanced age has been associated with an increase in prevalence, with patients over the age of 65 reporting more hard stools and straining. The prevalence of constipation was found to be 2-fold higher in African Americans, in nursing home residents, and in patients with lower socioeconomic status (income < $20,000 per year).[1]

Economic Burden

Constipation is a disease associated with a huge economic burden. It was estimated in one study that in 2001, the cost of treating constipation with over-the-counter (OTC) laxatives in the United States was $835 million.[2,3] Another study in 2007 estimated that of 76,854 patients enrolled in a medical program, it cost $18,891,008 over a 15-month period in expenditures for patients with constipation. This was an average cost of $246 per patient.[3] On the other hand, the indirect costs from constipation are high as well, including 2.4 days/month due to missing work or school. One study reported 13.7 million days of restricted activity every year due to constipation.[4]

Psychological Distress and Abuse

It has been reported in several studies that there is an increase in anxiety, depression, obsessive compulsiveness, psychoticism, and somatization among patients experiencing constipation. One study compared patients with dyssynergic defecation to slow transit constipation, and it was found that paranoid ideation and hostility subscores were higher in patients with dyssynergia compared to the slow transit constipation group or healthy controls.[5]

ETIOLOGY

The cause of dyssynergic defecation is unclear. A prospective study by Rao et al[6] of 100 patients with dyssynergic defecation reported that the problem began in childhood in 31% of patients; after a pregnancy, trauma, or back injury in 29% of patients; and in 40% of patients, there was no identifiable cause. The majority of cases of dyssynergic defecation occur during adulthood. In these patients, approximately 17% had a history of sexual abuse, 43% reported hard stools often, and 16% reported hard stool intermittently.[6] It is possible that dyssynergic defecation occurs due to excessive straining to expel hard stools over a prolonged period of time.[6]

PATHOPHYSIOLOGY

Based on early studies, it has been proposed that dyssynergic defecation is due to the paradoxical contraction or involuntary anal spasm during defecation. Past attempts of Botox (botulinum toxin) injection of the anal sphincter and anal myomectomy had minimal improvement in defecation.[2] One prospective study of patients with dyssnergic defecation showed that there was an inability to coordinate the abdominal, rectoanal, and pelvic floor muscles during defecation. This inability includes impaired rectal contraction (61%), paradoxical anal contraction (78%), or inadequate anal relaxation.[7] Therefore, the incoordination or the muscles working against each other is the primary dysfunction in dyssynergic defecation.[7]

Clinical Features

The key features that patients with dyssynergic defecation report include excessive straining (84%), a feeling of incomplete evacuation (76%), the passage of hard stools (65%), abdominal bloating (74%), a stool frequency of fewer than 3 bowel movements per week (62%), and digital maneuvers (35%), but is usually not reported by the patient.[6] It is important to ask patients about various digital maneuvers that help evacuate stool such as digital disimpaction or splinting the vagina or buttock muscles to have a bowel movement. Many patients do not feel comfortable sharing this information unless they are specifically asked.

One study of 134 patients reported that having 2 or fewer stools/week, laxative dependence, and constipation since childhood was associated with slow transit constipation, but backache, heartburn, anorectal surgery, and a lower prevalence of normal stool frequency were associated with dyssynergic defecation. This study concluded that symptoms can be utilized as good predictors of transit time, but are not good predictors of dyssynergic defecation.[8]

It has been reported that patients who have defecation disorders do exhibit psychological abnormalities. One disorder that has been associated with defecation disorder is obsessive compulsive disorder. Here the patient believes that a bowel movement should occur daily, and if it does not occur, the patient has to use laxatives, enemas, or suppositories to have a bowel movement. Some patients may also experience a phobia of stool impaction. This has been shown to occur in children who use a minor disturbance in defecation to gain attention. Various psychosocial issues, including interparental or parental/child conflicts or sibling rivalry may contribute to the problem. One study showed that if there is parental detachment during childhood, this can lead to problems with bowel problems in adulthood.[2,6]

DIAGNOSIS

The diagnostic criteria for dyssynergic defecation include the fulfillment of the Rome III criteria for functional constipation and manometric evidence of a dyssnergic pattern, with one other quantifiable measure of dyssynergic defecation, including balloon expulsion test, delay of colonic transit time, or defecography showing incomplete evacuation (Table 20-1).[9,10]

Performing a complete digital rectal exam (DRE) is an important part of the clinical evaluation.[2,10,11] The first step is to inspect the anorectum to look for any skin excoriations, skin tags, anal fissures, hemorrhoids, or anal fistula.[2,10,11] The perineal sensation and the anocutaneous reflex can be assessed by gently stroking the perianal skin with a cotton bud or a blunt needle in all four quadrants. A normal response will cause the external anal sphincter to contract.[2,10,11] If there is no contraction of the external anal sphincter, this may suggest a neuropathy.[2,10,11]

Table 20-1
Diagnostic Criteria for Dyssynergic Defecation*

A) Rome III criteria for functional constipation

Two or more of the following with at least 25% defecation:

Straining

Lumpy or hard stools

Sensation of incomplete evacuation

Fewer than 3 bowel movements per week

Sensation of anorectal obstruction or blockage

Manual maneuvers to facilitate defecation (digital evacuation, support of pelvic floor)

B) During repeated attempts to defecate, must demonstrate dyssynergic pattern of defecation by anorectal manometry or electromyography

C) Patient must demonstrate one other abnormal test:

   1) Abnormal balloon expulsion test (> 1 minute)

   2) Prolonged colonic transit time (Sitzmarks/scintigraphy)

   3) Abnormal defecography (> 50% barium retention)

*Must include A, B, and C

On digital examination, a mass, stricture, internal hemorrhoid, spasm, blood, or stool may be present.[2] If there is stool in the rectal vault and the patient is unaware, this may be due to rectal hyposensitivity.[2,10] The resting tone of the anal sphincter is evaluated, and then the patient is asked to squeeze to evaluate the anal sphincter and the puborectalis muscle. Then the patient is asked to bear down to mimic defecation, and the examiner can evaluate the relaxation of the external anal sphincter and/or the puborectalis muscle, along with perineal descent.[10,11] If the patient paradoxically contracts during this maneuver, it is highly suspicious for dyssynergic defecation.[10,11] The DRE has a high sensitivity for identifying dyssynergic defecation.[11] The DRE is an extremely useful tool in the workup of dyssynergic defecation, but there is a lack of knowledge on performing a proper exam.[10,11] A survey of 256 students in their final year of medical school found that 17% had never performed a DRE and 48% were unsure of their findings.[11] The sensitivity and specificity of DRE in evaluation of dyssynergic defecation is 75% and 87%, respectively.[11]

Anorectal Manometry

Anorectal manometry measures the rectal and anal pressure at rest and during attempted defecation and is also able to assess rectal sensation, rectoanal reflexes, and rectal compliance.[2,10,12] It is essential for the diagnosis of dyssynergic defecation. Anorectal manometry rules out Hirschsprung disease.[2,10,12] During the test, a balloon is distended in the rectum and there is a reflex that causes the internal anal sphincter to relax. This is mediated by the myenteric plexus. In Hirschsprung disease, this reflex is absent. Anorectal manometry is key for detecting abnormalities during attempted defecation.[2,10,12] During the maneuver when a patient mimics defecation or bearing down, there should be a rise in the rectal pressure along with relaxation of the external anal sphincter.[2,10,12] This is a voluntary response and is primarily learned. If the patient is unable

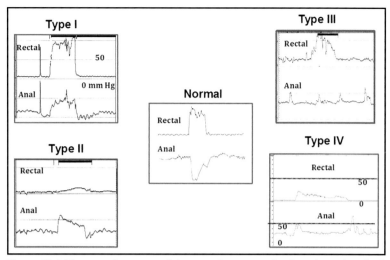

Figure 20-1. There are four types of dyssynergic patterns that have been described. Type I: The patient can generate adequate push effort but has a paradoxical increase in the anal sphincter pressure. Type II: The patient is unable to generate an adequate push effort and has paradoxical anal sphincter contraction. Type III: The patient can generate an adequate push force but has an absent or incomplete anal sphincter relaxation (< 20%). Type IV: The patient is unable to generate an adequate push effort and has an absent or incomplete anal sphincter relaxation.

to relax the external anal sphincter and/or the puborectalis, it indicates dyssynergic defecation (Figure 20-1).[2,10,12] There are 4 subtypes described by Rao et al.[9]

Anorectal manometry is also able to detect sensory dysfunction.[2,10,12] In patients who have dyssynergic defecation, the first sensation and the threshold for the desire to defecate were found to be higher in 60% of patients.[12] This also can be due to increased rectal compliance. Some patients may have difficulty relaxing the external anal sphincter due to performing the test in a laboratory setting.

There is a new high-resolution anorectal manometry system that performs manometric recordings using 12 circumferential pressure sensors and provides a detailed topographical plot. It provides high-resolution intraluminal pressure changes and increased anatomical detail, providing a better assessment of the defecatory disorders (Figure 20-2).[13,14]

Balloon Expulsion Test

A 50-mL balloon filled with warm water or a silicone-filled stool-like device such as a fecom is placed into the rectum; the patient is given a stopwatch and is left alone on a commode or toilet and stops the watch when the balloon is expelled.[2,10,12] Patients with normal defecation are able to expel the balloon in 1 minute. If the patient has difficulty expelling the balloon in this period, dyssynergic defecation should be suspected. The balloon expulsion test has a specificity of 80% to 90% and a negative predictive value of 97% for diagnosing dyssynergic defecation.[2,10,12] It has a sensitivity of 50%, but is useful to identify constipated patients who do not have dyssynergia.[2,10,12]

Colonic Transit Study

Dyssynergic defecation can coexist with two-thirds of patients with slow transit constipation, and it is important to differentiate between patients with isolated dyssynergic defecation or dyssynergic defecation with slow transit constipation.[2,10] A Sitzmarks (Konsyl) study can measure the colonic transit time by administering 24 radiopaque markers and doing a plain abdominal x-ray on

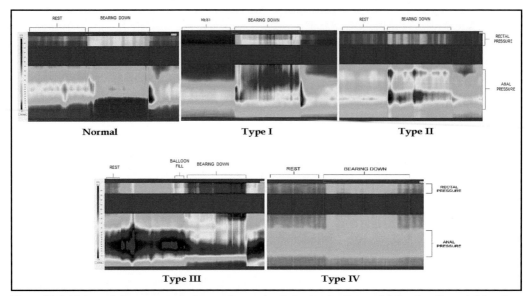

Figure 20-2. High-resolution manometry image of normal and abnormal patterns of defecation. Normal defecation: High-resolution image of a healthy patient showing manometric and topographic features during an attempted defecation. The upper part of the panel shows pressure changes from the rectum indicating that the patient generated a good push effort. The lower part of the panel shows topographic images from the entire anal canal and puborectalis showing that both anal sphincter and puborectalis relaxed normally with a drop in the pressure indicated by the colors getting lighter. Type I: High-resolution manometry image of a patient with constipation showing manometric and topographic features during attempted defecation maneuver. The upper part of the panel shows pressure changes from the rectum indicating that the patient generated a good push effort. The lower part of the panel shows topographic images from the entire canal and puborectalis, showing that both anal sphincter and puborectalis increased pressure consistent with dyssynergic defecation. Type II: High-resolution manometry image of a patient with constipation showing manometric and topographic features during attempted defecation maneuver. The upper part of the panel shows pressure changes from the rectum, indicating that the patient was unable to generate a good push effort. The lower part of the panel shows topographic images from the entire canal and puborectalis, showing that both anal sphincter and puborectalis increased pressures consistent with dyssynergic defecation. Type III: High-resolution manometry image of a patient with constipation showing manometric and topographic features during attempted defecation maneuver. The upper part of the panel shows pressure changes from the rectum indicating that the patient was able to generate a good push effort. The lower part of the panel shows topographic images from the entire canal and puborectalis, showing that both the anal sphincter and puborectalis have an absent or incomplete anal sphincter relaxation (< 20%) consistent with dyssynergic defecation. Type IV: High-resolution manometry image of a patient with constipation showing manometric and topographic features during attempted defecation maneuver. The upper part of the panel shows pressure changes from the rectum indicating that the patient was unable to generate a good push effort. The lower part of the panel shows topographic images from the entire canal and puborectalis, showing that both anal sphincter and puborectalis have an absent or incomplete anal sphincter relaxation.

day 5. An abnormal colonic transit time is when there are more than 20% of the markers or more than 5 markers on day 5.[10]

Colonic Transit Scintigraphy

Colonic transit scintigraphy can be used in patients who have suspected colonic dysmotility or diffuse motility disorders affecting the entire gastrointestinal tract. This test will determine whether a constipated patient has slow transit time and can influence the management of this disorder.

There are two methods for performing colonic transit scintigraphy.[15] The first method involves colon transit of 111-In diethylene triamine pentaacetic acid (DTPA)–labeled water consumed in a standard solid-liquid meal for gastric scintigraphy. The second method involves a capsule that contains 111-In absorbed on activated charcoal and coated with a pH-sensitive polymer, methacrylate, that dissolves in the terminal ileum's alkaline environment, thus releasing the radioisotope into the lumen.[15] The colonic transit scintigraphy can be used to measure colonic transit in patients with constipation or diarrhea and is available at certain dedicated centers.[15]

Wireless Motility Capsule Test

The wireless motility capsule (SmartPill, Covidien) is a wireless capsule that measures the pH, temperature, and pressure of the whole gastrointestinal tract.[16] It measures the gastric, small bowel, and colonic transit time and the whole gut transit time without any radiation. It has been recommended by the American Neurogastroenterology and Motility Society as a standardized method to measure normal colonic transit and slow transit.[15] It has been approved by the Food and Drug Administration (FDA) for evaluating colonic transit time in patients suspected to have chronic constipation and in those with suspected gastroparesis.[15,16] It has good device agreement with Sitzmarks studies and picks up upper gut dysmotility in 20% to 25% of patients.[15,16]

Three-Dimensional Endoanal Ultrasonography

The anal sphincter can be assessed using three-dimensional endoanal ultrasonography and is useful in assessing the sphincter integrity and volume, and can also determine whether there are any fistulous tracks or abscesses.[17]

Defecography/Magnetic Resonance Defecography

Defecography and magnetic resonance imaging (MRI) defecography are two imaging methods that may identify dyssynergic defecation. During a defecography, barium paste is inserted into the patient's rectum and videofluoroscopy records anatomic and functional changes as the patient attempts to expel the barium paste.[18] A patient who has dyssynergic defecation may have poor activation of the levator muscles, prolonged time to expel the barium or retained barium in the rectal vault, or absence of a stripping wave in the rectum.

MRI defecography allows visualization of the pelvic soft tissue structures and does not subject the patient to radiation.[18] Dynamic pelvic MRI defecography allows imaging of the pelvic anatomy in dynamic motion. In one controlled trial MRI defecography identified difficulty with evacuation and/or squeeze in 94% of patients with suspected dyssynergic defecation.[18]

MANAGEMENT OF DYSSYNERGIC DEFECATION

Standard Treatment and Other Medical Options

The medical treatment of this disorder is to avoid medications that can cause constipation such as narcotics, increasing the intake of fiber, increasing fluid intake, physical activity, and timed toilet training. It is recommended to have 20 to 25 grams of fiber daily.[2,10,19] There is currently insufficient data to support supplementation with a synthetic fiber supplement. On the other hand, the American College of Gastroenterology (ACG) Task Force and a systematic review determined that psyllium, a natural fiber supplement, was given a grade B recommendation.[19] Medications that promote bowel movements such as stool softeners, stimulant laxatives (senna or bisacodyl or castor oil), or osmotic laxatives (magnesium sulfate, lactulose, sorbitol, or mannitol) can be

Table 20-2

Summary of the Randomized Controlled Trials of Biofeedback Therapy for Dyssynergic Defecation

	CHIARIONI ET AL[21]	RAO ET AL[22]	RAO ET AL[23]	HEYMEN ET AL[24]	CHIARIONI ET AL[25]
Trial design	Biofeedback vs PEG 14.6 g	Biofeedback vs standard vs sham biofeedback	Biofeedback vs standard therapy	Biofeedback vs diazepam 5 mg vs placebo	Biofeedback for slow transit vs dyssynergia
Subjects and randomization	104 women 54 biofeedback 55 polyethylene glycol	77 (69 women) 1:1:1 distribution	52; short-term therapy 26=long-term study 12=biofeedback 13=standard therapy	84 (71 women) 30 biofeedback 30 diazepam 24 placebo	52 (49 women) 34 dyssynergia 12 slow transit 6 mixed
Duration and number of biofeedback sessions	3 months and 1 year 5 weekly, 30-minute training sessions performed by physician investigator	3 months, biweekly, 1 hour, maximum of 6 sessions over 3 months, performed by biofeedback nurse therapist	1 year; 6 active therapy sessions and 3 reinforcement sessions at 3-month intervals	6 biweekly, 1-hour sessions	5 weekly 30-minute training sessions, performed by physician investigator
Outcome measures	Global improvement of symptoms Worse=0 No improvement=1 Mild=2 Fair=3 Major improvement=4	1. Presence of dyssynergia 2. Balloon expulsion time 3. No. of CSBM 4. Global satisfaction	No. of CSBM; secondary outcome; presence of dyssynergia; balloon expulsion time; global satisfaction	Global symptom relief	Symptom improvement None=1 Mild=2 Fair=3 Major=4

(continued)

TABLE 20-2 (CONTINUED)

SUMMARY OF THE RANDOMIZED CONTROLLED TRIALS OF BIOFEEDBACK THERAPY FOR DYSSYNERGIC DEFECATION

	CHIARIONI ET AL[21]	RAO ET AL[22]	RAO ET AL[23]	HEYMEN ET AL[24]	CHIARIONI ET AL[25]
Dyssynergia corrected or symptoms improved	79.6% reported major improvement at 6 and 12 months; 81.5% reported major improvement at 24 months	Dyssynergia corrected at 3 months in 79% with biofeedback vs 4% sham and 6% in standard group; CSBM=biofeedback group vs. sham or standard, p<0.05	No. of CSBM/week increased significantly in biofeedback ($p<0.001$); dyssynergia pattern normalized ($p<0.0010$); balloon expulsion improved ($p<0.001$); colonic transit normalized ($p<0.01$)	70% improved with biofeedback compared to 38% with placebo and 30% with diazepam	71% with dyssynergia and 8% with slow transit alone reported fair improvement in symptoms
Conclusions	Biofeedback was superior to laxatives	Biofeedback was superior to sham feedback and standard therapy	Biofeedback is superior to standard therapy	Biofeedback is superior to placebo and diazepam	Biofeedback benefits dyssynergia and not slow transit constipation

	RAO ET AL[26]	GO ET AL[27]
Trial design	Home biofeedback therapy vs office biofeedback therapy	Biofeedback on quality of life and cost effectiveness. Compared whether biofeedback at home has improvement in quality of life compared to office biofeedback
Subjects and randomization	100 subjects (96 women); 83 completed; 45=office biofeedback; 38=home biofeedback	50 subjects; Office 42.4 years vs home 27.1 years; Similar baseline demographics, gender, and constipation

(continued)

Table 20-2 (continued)
Summary of the Randomized Controlled Trials of Biofeedback Therapy for Dyssynergic Defecation

	RAO ET AL[26]	GO ET AL[27]
Duration and number of biofeedback sessions	Office biofeedback: 6 biweekly sessions of pelvic floor and simulated defecation along with laxatives and home exercises Home therapy biofeedback: Given LCD to practice 20 minutes 2 to 3 times a day	6 sessions of home biofeedback 6 sessions of office biofeedback SF-36 QOL questionnaire at week 0 and 3 months after home therapy of office therapy
Primary outcomes	Change in the number of CSBM/week Dyssynergia pattern Balloon expulsion time Bowel satisfaction score	1. Examine effects of biofeedback on quality of life 2. To compare changes of QOL in dyssynergic patients after home or office biofeedback therapy 3. Evaluate whether QOL with each treatment is equivalent
Dyssynergia corrected or symptoms improved	No. of CSBM/week: similar in both groups $P<0.0001$ Bowel satisfaction: p similar in both groups $p<0.0012$ Balloon expulsion time improved in both groups $p<0.0301$ Dyssynergic pattern: No improvement	Physical conditioning: improvement in both groups $p=0.0003$ Role Physical: improved $p=0.0004$ Bodily pain improvement $p=0.0090$ General health improvement $p=0.0002$ Vitality improvement $p=0.0108$ Social functioning improvement $p=0.0383$ Role emotional improvement $p=0.0001$ Mental health improvement $p=0.0100$
Conclusions	Home biofeedback is safe and effective for dyssynergic defecation	Biofeedback, irrespective of home or office, improved quality of life in patients with dyssynergic defecation When compared to standard office, home biofeedback had equivalent QOL gains compared to the office biofeedback

helpful; however, the ACG Task Force stated that there is insufficient evidence for these treatment options. The ACG did give polyethylene glycol a grade A recommendation.[19] One study done over a 6-month period reported adequate relief of constipation in 52% of patients treated with polyethylene glycol compared to 11% treated with placebo.[19]

Lubiprostone is a chloride channel-2 activator used for patients with chronic constipation.[20] Lubiprostone 24 mcg twice daily was found to be more effective than placebo in improving stool frequency and symptoms in chronic constipation.[20] Linaclotide, a guanylate cyclase-C agonist at a dose of 145 mcg/day was found to provide rapid and sustained improvement of bowel symptoms, global relief, and improved quality of life and is currently FDA-approved for irritable bowel syndrome with constipation and chronic constipation.[20] Prucalopride, a 5-hydroxytrypatmine-4 receptor agonist at a dose of 2 to 4 mg daily has been shown to be effective in the treatment of chronic constipation, but is not approved yet in the United States.[20] Medications used for chronic constipation have not been validated in patients with dyssynergic defecation.

Biofeedback Therapy

This treatment has been shown to be effective in patients with dyssynergic defecation. The primary goal of biofeedback is to restore normal defecation using "operant conditioning" techniques.[2,10] More specifically, the goals of biofeedback are to correct the dyssynergia in coordination of the abdominal, rectal, and anal sphincter muscles and also improve rectal sensory perception in patients who have difficulty with sensation in the rectum.[2,10] The process of biofeedback involves placing a manometry catheter into the rectal vault and showing the patient visual images of what occurs during various maneuvers such as squeezing the anal sphincter and bearing down.[2,10] This provides instant visual imagery to teach patients how to retrain the brain to relax the anal sphincter. A biofeedback session is usually 1 hour long, and the patient performs various exercises using visual and verbal feedback provided by a biofeedback therapist, who can be a trained nurse, physician, or a physical therapist.[2,10]

Randomized controlled trials have demonstrated that biofeedback is superior to sham, standard therapy, or laxatives in the treatment of dyssynergic defecation (Table 20-2).[21-24] It was not shown to be effective for patients with isolated slow transit constipation.[25] One randomized controlled trial showed that there was sustained improvement of bowel symptoms and anorectal function up to 1 year after when compared to standard treatment with laxatives.[23] Home biofeedback has been shown to be as effective[26] and more cost effective than office biofeedback.[26,27] Home biofeedback involves using a probe in the rectum, which is attached to a liquid crystal display box, and this will give the patient the ability to visualize the exercises and their performance. The study found that when home biofeedback was compared to office biofeedback, there was no difference between the two treatments. There was significant improvement in the number of complete spontaneous bowel movements per week, dyssynergic pattern, balloon expulsion time, and bowel satisfaction score. Recent studies suggest that biofeedback therapy alters gut-brain-gut communication and thereby leads to improvement of bowel symptoms.

Dyssynergic defecation is a common problem that affects 33% of patients with chronic constipation. Timely recognition with a careful evaluation of symptoms, DRE, and diagnostic tests such as anorectal manometry and balloon expulsion test should provide definitive diagnosis. Biofeedback therapy along with supportive therapy including laxatives can be effective in its management.

References

1. Higgins PD, Johanson JF. Epidemiology of constipation in North America: a systematic review. *Am J Gastroenterol.* 2004;99(4):750-759.
2. Rao SSC. Dyssynergic defecation and biofeedback therapy. *Gastroentol Clin North Am.* 2008;37:569-586.
3. Singh G, Lingala V, Wang H, et al. Use of health care resources and cost of care for adults with constipation. *Clin Gastroenterol Hepatol.* 2007;5(9):1053-1058.

4. Dennison C, Prasad M, Lloyd A, Bhattacharyya SK, Dhawan R, Coyne K. The health-related quality of life and economic burden of constipation. *Pharmacoeconomics.* 2005;23(5):461-476.

5. Rao SS, Seaton K, Miller MJ, et al. Psychological profiles and quality of life differ between patients with dyssynergia and those with slow transit constipation. *J Psychosom Res.* 2007;63(4):441-449.

6. Rao SS, Tuteja AK, Vellema T, Kempf J, Stessman M. Dyssynergic defecation: demographics, symptoms, stool patterns, and quality of life. *J Clin Gastroenterol.* 2004;38(8):680-685.

7. Rao SSC, Welcher K, Leistikow J. Obstructive defecation: a failure of recto-anal coordination. *Am J Gastroenterol.* 1998;93:1042-1050.

8. Glia A, Lindberg G, Nilsson LH, Mihocsa L, Akerlund JE. Clinical value of symptom assessment in patients with constipation. *Dis Colon Rectum.* 1999;42(11):1401-1408.

9. Rao SSC, Mudipalli RS, Stessman M, et al. Investigation of the utility of colorectal function test and Rome II criteria in dyssynergic defecation (anismus). *Neurogastroenterol Motil.* 2004;16:589-596.

10. Rao SS. Approach to the patient with constipation. In: Yamada T et al, eds. *Principles of Clinical Gastroenterology* (5th ed); 2008:373-398.

11. Tantiphlachiva K, Rao P, Attaluri A, Rao SS. Digital rectal examination is a useful tool for identifying patients with dyssynergia. *Clin Gastroenterol Hepatol.* 2010;8(11):955-960.

12. Rao SSC, Patel RS. How useful are manometric tests of anorectal function in the management of defecation disorders. *Am J Gastroenterol.* 1997;92:469-475.

13. Noelting J, Ratuapli SK, Bharucha AE, Harvey DM, Ravi K, Zinsmeister AR. Normal values for high-resolution anorectal manometry in healthy women: effects of age and significance of rectoanal gradient. *Am J Gastroenterol.* 2012;107(10):1530-1536.

14. Bharucha AE, Wald AM. Anorectal disorders. *Am J Gastroenterol.* 2010;105(4):786-794.

15. Rao, SS, Camilleri M, Hasler WL, et al. Evaluation of gastrointestinal transit in clinical practice: position paper of the American and European Neurogastroenterology and Motility Societies. *Neurogastroenterol Motil.* 23;1:8-23.

16. Rao SS, Juo B, McCallum RW, et al. Investigation of colonic and whole-gut transit with wireless motility capsule and radiopaque markers in constipation. *Clin Gastroenterol Hepatol.* 2009;7:537-544.

17. Coss-Adame E, Rao SS, Valestin J, et al. high definition anorectal manometry (3-D) and pressure topography in healthy subjects. *Clin Gastroenterol Hepatol.* In press.

18. Bharucha AE, Fletcher JG, Seide B, Riederer SJ, Zinsmeister AR. Phenotypic variation in functional disorders of defecation. *Gastroenterology.* 2005;128(5):1199-1210.

19. American College of Gastroenterology Chronic Constipation Task Force. An evidence- based approach to the management of chronic constipation in North America. *Am J Gastroenterol.* 2005;100 (Suppl 1):S1-4.

20. Singh S, Rao SS. Pharmacologic management of chronic constipation. *Gastroenterol Clin North Am.* 2010;39(3):509-527.

21. Chiarioni G, Whitehead WE, Pezza V, Morelli A, Bassotti G. Biofeedback is superior to laxatives for normal transit constipation due to pelvic floor dyssynergia. *Gastroenterology.* 2006;130(3):657-664.

22. Rao SS, Seaton K, Miller M, et al. Randomized controlled trial of biofeedback, sham feedback, and standard therapy for dyssynergic defecation. *Clin Gastroenterol Hepatol.* 2007;5:331-338.

23. Rao SS, Valentin J, Brown CK, et al. Long-term efficacy of biofeedback therapy with dyssynergic defecation: randomized control trial. *Am J Gastroenterol.* 2010;105:890-896.

24. Heymen S, Scarlett Y, Jones K, et al. Randomized controlled trial shows biofeedback to be superior to alternative treatments for patients with pelvic floor dyssynergia-type constipation. *Dis Colon Rectum.* 2007. A randomized clinical trial. *Gastroenterology.* 2011;140:S52.

25. Chiarioni G, Salandini L, Whitehead WE. Biofeedback benefits only patients with outlet dysfunction, not patients with isolated slow transit constipation. *Gastroenterology.* 2005;129:86-97.

26. Rao SSC, Valestin J, Brown C, et al. Home or office biofeedback therapy for dyssynergic defecation: randomized controlled trial. *Gastroenterology.* 2011;140:S160.

27. Go J, Valestin J, Brown CK, et al. Is biofeedback therapy effective in improving quality of life in dyssynergic defecation? A randomized clinical trial. *Gastroenterology.* 2011;140:S52.

21

Fecal Incontinence

William E. Whitehead, PhD; Steve Heymen, PhD;
and Giuseppe Chiarioni, MD

KEY POINTS

- Fecal incontinence (FI) is highly prevalent (8.4% of adults) but underdiagnosed and undertreated.

- Continence is maintained by multiple mechanisms with built-in compensatory mechanisms, so no single physiological deficit is sufficient to cause FI, and most patients have multiple deficits.

- Medical history and physical examination are sufficient to identify most risk factors and initiate treatment; referral for specialized tests provides objective information regarding underlying mechanisms.

- Conservative treatment—patient education, diet and medications to normalize stool consistency, and pelvic floor exercises—yields clinically meaningful improvement in 50% to 75% of patients but rarely leads to complete continence.

- Treatments available by specialist referral—biofeedback, sacral nerve stimulation, injectable bulking agents—in appropriately selected patients yield continence in 20% to 44% and reports of adequate relief in up to 76%.

- Patients with known risk factors—diarrhea, urgency, diabetes mellitus, irritable bowel syndrome, neurological disorders—should be screened even if they do not mention fecal incontinence.

DEFINITION AND TERMINOLOGY

FI refers to recurring uncontrolled passage of solid or liquid stool for a period of at least 3 months in an individual with a developmental age of at least 4 years.[1] Soiling of underwear or pads with mucus or stains is included in this definition even if no significant amount of solid or

Rao SSC, Parkman HP, McCallum RW, eds.
Handbook of Gastrointestinal Motility and Functional Disorders (pp 265-278).
© 2015 Taylor & Francis Group.

liquid stool is passed. Mucus (ie, clear or yellow slime with no brown streaks) has been treated inconsistently in published studies, but should be included in the definition because soiling is difficult to reliably distinguish from solid and liquid stool loss, and it has a negative impact on quality of life. Unintended passage of gas (flatus) is not included in the definition of FI because it occurs frequently in most people.[2] However, readers should be aware that the term *anal incontinence*, used mostly by surgeons, includes accidental loss of flatus.

Validated questionnaires that measure the severity of FI can be used to compare patients to each other and to compare published studies. The Fecal Incontinence Severity Index (FISI)[3] inquires about the frequency of four types of incontinence—solid, liquid, mucus, and gas—and weights each response based on the overall severity judgments of a group of patients; these weighted responses are summed together to compute the severity index. The Fecal Incontinence and Constipation Assessment (FICA)[4] is an alternative questionnaire that has the advantage of including the volume of stool lost in the calculation of the severity index. The Fecal Incontinence Quality of Life Scale (FIQL)[5] is a validated disease-specific questionnaire for measuring quality-of-life impact.

Daily symptom diaries are often used as an alternative to these retrospective questionnaires and have the advantage of providing more information on the triggers for FI events; for this reason, symptom diaries are frequently used to guide adjustments to the treatment regimen. However, paper diaries will be inaccurate if patients forget to complete the diary on some days and attempt to enter the missing data just prior to clinic visits. In clinical trials, this limitation may be overcome by requiring patients to report on symptoms by telephone or Internet on a daily basis and sending them reminders if they fail to report on time.

The term *fecal incontinence* is used by physicians and researchers to communicate with each other, but this term is not understood by some patients and is avoided by other patients because of embarrassment. Many patients prefer the term *accidental bowel leakage* (ABL).[6]

Pathophysiology

Continence depends on multiple mechanisms (Figure 21-1) and because of this redundancy a deficit in any one of these mechanism may not result in FI. Consequently, FI usually has multiple causes (eg, diarrhea plus external anal sphincter [EAS] weakness).

Rectum

The rectum is a specialized segment of the large intestine whose functions are (1) to store stool prior to defecation and (2) to signal the brain through afferent pathways that stool has entered the rectum. The walls of the rectum are composed primarily of longitudinally oriented smooth muscle fibers, which normally offer little resistance to being slowly stretched; consequently, when new stool enters the rectum, these smooth muscle fibers relax to accommodate the increased volume with little or no increase in intrarectal pressure. However, when distended beyond a critical threshold or when distended very rapidly, the rectal smooth muscles contract reflexively. These phasic reflex contractions last 20 to 30 seconds and may empty the rectum unless opposed by a strong voluntary contraction of the striated pelvic floor muscles.

In addition to these relatively brief phasic contractions, the rectal smooth muscle exhibits tonic contractions—prolonged waves of contraction and relaxation lasting many minutes—that are referred to as smooth muscle tone. Smooth muscle tone increases immediately after meal ingestion and in response to anxiety; conversely, muscle tone decreases during relaxation. Smooth muscle tone influences the threshold for conscious perception of rectal filling and the threshold for reflex phasic contractions. Consequently, people become aware of more rectal sensations after meals, and rectal evacuation of stool or gas is more likely soon after a meal and when the individual is anxious. There is a greater risk of FI at these times.

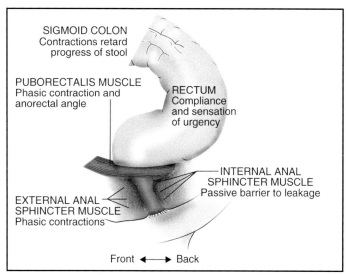

Figure 21-1. Sagittal view of the anatomy of the anal canal and rectum with text labels to identify anatomical components and mechanisms for continence.

Afferent nerve endings that give rise to conscious sensations are presumed to lie in the walls of the rectum. They are activated both by passive distention of the rectum and by the contraction of the rectal smooth muscle. The subjective quality of these sensations ranges from a sensation of gas or movement in the rectum through a normal urge to defecate ("call to stool"), and it can reach an almost intolerable sensation of strong urgency. The sensation of gas or movement in the rectum is triggered by passive distention of the rectum with small amounts of gas or stool, whereas normal urge is elicited by larger volumes or by increased smooth muscle tone. The sensation of intolerable urge occurs when the rectal smooth muscle contracts reflexively. The ability to consciously perceive rectal distention is a critical warning cue that tells the central nervous system (CNS) when to voluntarily contract the pelvic floor muscles to prevent FI. When these sensations are absent or attenuated (rectal hyposensitivity), as they are in patients with spinal cord transection or peripheral nerve injury, the risk of *passive* FI is greatly increased. Conversely, when the rectum is hypersensitive to rectal distention due to increased smooth muscle tone, the risk of *urge*-related FI is greatly increased.

Internal Anal Sphincter

The anal canal is surrounded by both the internal anal sphincter (IAS), which is composed of smooth muscle that is not under voluntary control, and the EAS, which is composed of striated muscles that are subject to voluntary control. The IAS normally remains contracted (submaximal contraction) and causes the pressure in the anal canal to be approximately 40 to 70 mm Hg at rest—well above the pressure normally found in the rectum, which is usually below 10 mm Hg. This anorectal pressure gradient functions as a passive barrier to leakage of gas and liquid from the rectum.

To allow defecation to occur, the tonic contraction of the IAS is reflexively inhibited in response to increased distention of the rectum; this is called the rectoanal inhibitory reflex (RAIR). During defecation, the RAIR is normally triggered by voluntarily contracting abdominal wall muscles and simultaneously lowering the diaphragm. However, prolonged inhibition of the IAS can also be produced by the accumulation of a large mass of stool in the rectum. Decreased resting pressure in the anal canal can also be caused by surgical division or traumatic tears in the IAS. Decreased IAS pressure from either fecal impaction or sphincter injury is a risk factor for passive FI.

The RAIR is also called the *"sampling reflex"*—a term used to identify one of the functions of this reflex, which is to expose the rectal contents to the more sensitive nerve endings in the anal canal. This helps the individual discriminate whether the rectal contents are solid, liquid, or gas. Gas may be passed unintentionally during the RAIR, but the individual can voluntarily contract the striated EAS during this RAIR to prevent the passage of solids, liquids, and even gas.

External Anal Sphincter

The EAS is a striated muscle that is innervated by the pudendal nerve and is under voluntary control. The voluntary contraction of this muscle in response to the perception of rectal distention is one of the most important continence mechanisms. This response is learned during early childhood and may occur without conscious effort or attention because it is so well rehearsed; however, unless the individual is able to consciously perceive rectal distention, they are at high risk for passive FI.

The puborectalis is another striated muscle that shares innervation from the pudendal nerve and normally contracts at the same time. It loops behind the rectum at the junction between the anal canal and rectum; it supports the rectum and helps to maintain an angle of approximately 90 degrees between the rectum and the anal canal to prevent the passage of solid stool into the anal canal. When voluntarily contracted, it further elevates the rectum and sharpens the anorectal angle. During defecation, the puborectalis is voluntarily relaxed to allow the rectum to funnel formed stool into the anal canal. The puborectalis is one of the muscles that are collectively referred to as the levator ani muscles, with the others being the ileorectalis and the coccygeus muscles.

DIAGNOSIS

The diagnosis of FI is based on the patient's report of symptoms; no diagnostic tests are required. However, identification of the pathophysiological mechanisms contributing to FI is important to guide the choice of treatment. Table 21-1 lists the most common medical conditions associated with FI and the types of pathophysiological mechanisms associated with them.

History

Diarrhea is consistently found in surveys to be a risk factor for FI. Therefore, if the medical history suggests FI is caused or exacerbated by diarrhea, it is appropriate to take immediate steps to identify the cause of diarrhea and treat it, or, if it is chronic, to prescribe dietary fiber or antidiarrheal medications to normalize stool consistency.

Other risk factors that are identified by the medical history are cognitive and mobility impairment. Dementia is a frequent contributor to FI and presents unique challenges for management because the patient may not be able to comply with treatment recommendations without assistance from a caregiver. Mobility impairment is also a frequent risk factor and may benefit from having a home health care nurse or physical therapist visit the patient's home to assess barriers to self-toileting and make recommendations for assistive devices and improved access to the toilet.

TABLE 21-1
PHYSIOLOGICAL MECHANISMS RESPONSIBLE FOR FECAL INCONTINENCE

CATEGORY	PHYSIOLOGICAL MECHANISM	CLINICAL SETTING
Functional causes	Fecal impaction leads to reflex dilation of IAS with overflow	Disordered defecation; spinal cord injury
	Diarrhea with rapid transit and loose/watery stools	IBS; infectious or chronic diarrhea
	Social indifference	Dementia, retardation, psychosis
Sphincter weakness	IAS or EAS tears	Obstetric injury, MVA, foreign body trauma
	Pudendal nerve injury	Obstetric injury, diabetes mellitus, multiple sclerosis
	CNS injury	Spina bifida, traumatic spinal injury, stroke, multiple sclerosis
Hyposensitive rectum	Afferent nerve injury leads to inability to detect rectal filling	Diabetic neuropathy, spinal cord injury, multiple sclerosis
Hypersensitive rectum	Noncompliant rectum leads to irresistible urgency	Ulcerative proctitis, radiation injury, rectal resection
Obstructed sphincter closure	Mucus secretion from exposed rectal mucosa or leakage of liquid stool	Rectal prolapse, prolapsed hemorrhoids

IBS, irritable bowel syndrome; IAS, internal anal sphincter; EAS, external anal sphincter; CNS, central nervous system; MVA, motor vehicle accident.

Digital Rectal Exam: Test for Fecal Impaction

Fecal impaction is a common cause of FI in children and in sedentary elderly patients. It can be detected by digital rectal examination (DRE) revealing a mass of solid stool in the rectum, and if found, the patient should be treated for constipation (see treatment section). However, if the patient has persistent fecal impaction, evaluate for an evacuation disorder by anorectal manometry and balloon evacuation testing according to the guidelines of the American College of Gastroenterology.[7] If the digital rectal exam identifies a rectal mass other than stool or identifies blood in the stool, a colonoscopy may be indicated to rule out rectal cancer.

Digital Rectal Examination: Squeeze Pressures in the Anal Canal

The examiner should place a gloved finger tip in the anal canal with one hand and place the other hand on the patient's abdomen as shown in Figure 21-2 and Figure 21-3A. Then instruct

Figure 21-2. Examiner with right index finger in patient's anus and left hand on patient's abdomen.

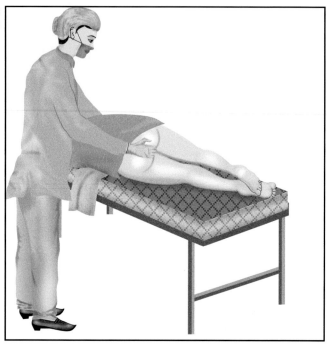

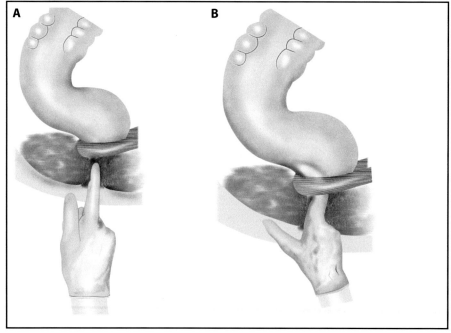

Figure 21-3. Technique of digital rectal exam. In panel A, the examiner evaluates the external anal sphincter by putting a finger tip into the anus and instructing the patient to squeeze as if holding back stool. In panel B, the examiner evaluates the strength of the puborectalis muscle by hooking a finger tip over the posterior rim of the rectum and instructing the patient to pull up or squeeze.

the patient to squeeze as if holding in a bowel movement. The pressure on the finger in the anal canal will indicate the strength of the EAS, while the hand on the patient's abdomen will allow the examiner to judge whether the patient inappropriately contracts their abdominal wall when squeezing to hold in stool. To assess the strength of the puborectalis muscle, the examiner inserts a finger deeper into the anal canal and hooks it over the posterior rim of the rectum, as shown in Figure 21-3B. When the patient squeezes, the puborectalis will be appreciated as a pulling up against the fingertip.

Digital Rectal Examination: Resting Anal Canal Pressure

The integrity of the IAS is assessed by noting how much pressure is felt around a finger in the anal canal (Figure 21-3A) when the patient is instructed to relax. If resting pressure is low, the examiner should check for fecal impaction by DRE because distention of the rectum by a large fecal impaction may reflexively dilate the internal sphincter. If no fecal impaction is detected, the patient is presumed to have a disruption of the IAS, but this should be confirmed by endoanal ultrasound or magnetic resonance imaging (MRI).

Physical Examination for Obstructed Defecation

An often neglected part of the physical examination is the test for prolapsed rectal mucosa or hemorrhoids. When the history indicates that FI consists exclusively of soiling or staining of underwear by mucus or streaks on underwear or pads, or when the patient reports a bulge from their rectum, the examiner should have the patient push to defecate while sitting on a commode chair and observe whether pushing causes prolapse of mucosa or hemorrhoids and whether the prolapsed tissue spontaneously retracts into the anal canal when the patient stops pushing. To minimize patient embarrassment, have them urinate to empty their bladder prior to this test and place a receptacle below the commode chair.

Anorectal Manometry

This test is performed with a tube that contains pressure sensors along its circumference to measure anal canal pressures and a balloon attached to the tip to measure sensory thresholds (first detectable volume of balloon distention in the rectum, threshold volume and pressure for urgency to defecate, and maximum tolerable volume) and compliance (resistance to distention) when the balloon is progressively inflated with air. Resting and squeeze pressures can be inferred from the digital rectal exam, although the anorectal manometry (ARM) provides more quantitative measures that can be compared to published normal ranges; see Figure 21-4 for an example of ARM performed using a high-resolution, solid-state ARM catheter. Sensory thresholds and rectal compliance require ARM. A high threshold for detecting the distention of the rectum (rectal hyposensitivity) is a risk factor for FI. Conversely, when progressive distention of the rectal balloon causes abnormally high balloon pressures (indicative of decreased smooth muscle compliance) and a report of a strong urge sensation, this hypersensitivity is an independent risk factor for FI.

Electromyographic Activity Recorded From the Anal Canal

By placing a probe in the anal canal that has stainless steel electrodes on its surface, it is possible to measure the averaged electromyographic (EMG) activity of the striated muscles surrounding the anal canal. The averaged EMG tracing provides a more direct indication of the innervation of the pelvic floor muscles than does ARM. However, the EMG does not replace the ARM because it does not measure sensory thresholds and compliance. The EMG is complementary to ARM

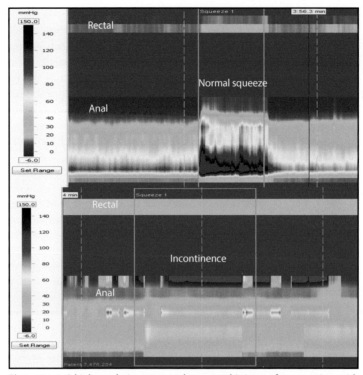

Figure 21-4. A high-resolution anorectal topographic image from a patient with fecal incontinence showing weak resting and squeeze sphincter pressures (lower panel) and an image from a normal subject showing normal sphincter responses (upper panel). (Reprinted with permission from Satish SC Rao, MD, PhD, FRCP.)

because it distinguishes neurological from morphological causes of low squeeze pressure, and it is also useful in the identification of patients with dyssynergic defecation (difficulty evacuating the rectum, which is a risk factor for fecal impaction and overflow FI).

Endoanal Ultrasonography and Magnetic Resonance Imaging

The gold standard for identifying and characterizing the severity of morphological abnormalities in the internal and external anal sphincters is endoanal ultrasound; see Figure 21-5 for an example. The reliability is somewhat greater for IAS defects than for EAS defects. Magnetic resonance imaging is emerging as a better test than EUS because it provides more easily interpreted images of the EAS and the puborectalis, but pelvic MRI is presently limited to a few tertiary medical centers.

In summary, most of the pathophysiological mechanisms that contribute to FI can be evaluated in the primary care physician's office based on a careful history, a digital rectal exam, and a physical examination (Figure 21-6). Only abnormalities in rectal sensation and compliance require referral to a specialist for further testing.

EPIDEMIOLOGY

The prevalence of FI in noninstitutionalized U.S. adults is estimated to be 8.4% with no significant difference between women (9.4%) and men (7.3%).[8] These prevalence rates are underestimates because the prevalence of FI in nursing homes is approximately 48%.[9] Prevalence increases

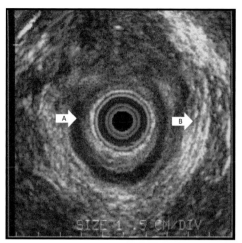

Figure 21-5. Ultrasound image showing disruption of the internal and external anal sphincter in a patient with a history of obstetric injury. The dark ring surrounding the anal canal at A is the internal anal sphincter, and the light-colored, hyperechoic fibers surrounding the internal anal sphincter at B are part of the external anal sphincter. In this image both the internal and external anal sphincter are interrupted in the anterior quadrant (top).

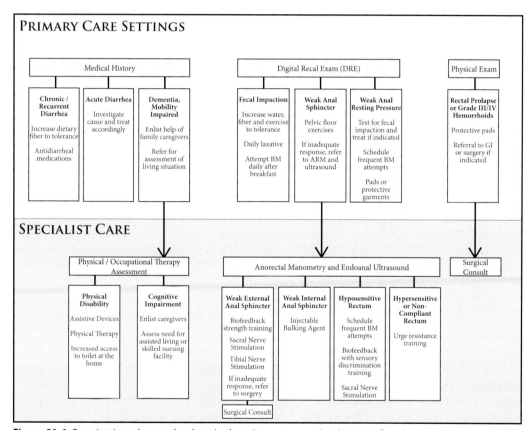

Figure 21-6. Examinations that can be done in the primary care setting (top panel) and examinations reserved for the specialist care setting (bottom panel). Treatment recommendations for the most common diagnostic findings are given in the vertical boxes.

with age from 2.9% in 20-year-olds to 16.2% in those aged 70 or older. There is no significant difference in FI rates between Whites, Blacks, and Hispanic Americans in the United States.[8]

The significant independent risk factors for FI in the largest population-based study done to date[8] were diarrhea (OR = 2.5), having ≥ 3 chronic illnesses (OR = 1.7), urinary incontinence (OR = 1.6), and diabetes mellitus (OR = 1.5). Factors sometimes described as risk factors but not found to be statistically significant in population-based studies after multivariate adjustment are female sex, parity, obesity, constipation, and socioeconomic status.

Most neurological disorders that affect the innervation of the pelvic floor are risk factors for FI. In addition, the gastrointestinal symptom of strong urge sensations prior to bowel movements is a significant predictor of FI even after adjustment for diarrhea.[10] Gastrointestinal disorders associated with FI include irritable bowel syndrome, inflammatory bowel disease, grade 3 or 4 hemorrhoids that obstruct closure of the anal sphincters, and rectal prolapse. For rectal prolapse and hemorrhoids, FI usually consists of soiling only. Patients with any of these risk factors should be screened for FI even if they do not volunteer this symptom.

TREATMENT

A large number of treatments have been proposed for FI, but published treatment trials offer only limited guidance for the following reasons: (1) randomized controlled trials have been limited to a few treatments that are, for the most part, only available at academic medical centers, while conservative treatments that could be employed in primary care are only supported by descriptive and anecdotal studies; (2) few comparative effectiveness studies have been reported; and (3) published randomized controlled trials have rarely structured enrollment criteria in a way that would permit evaluation of which treatments work for which patients. Therefore, the treatment algorithm shown in Figure 21-6 is heavily influenced by practical considerations and the experience of the authors.

Fiber and Drug Treatment of Diarrhea

Fiber is recommended as the first-line treatment for diarrhea-associated FI, although there is limited clinical trial data to support this recommendation.[11] Fiber is usually prescribed in doses of 3 to 4 grams, and can be titrated up to 16 grams daily if tolerated. If fiber supplementation fails to control diarrhea-associated FI, an antidiarrheal medication can be added. The published literature suggests that the preferred drug is loperamide 2 to 4 mg.[12] The Food and Drug Administration (FDA)–licensed indications for loperamide do not include the treatment of FI, but loperamide is commonly used for this purpose in clinical practice. See Omar and Alexander[12] for a systematic review of drug treatment for FI.

Treating "Overflow" Fecal Incontinence Secondary to Fecal Impaction

When fecal impaction is discovered by digital rectal exam, aggressive treatment is recommended to clear the impaction first, followed by a regimen to prevent recurrence. The maintenance regimen begins with increasing water, fiber, and exercise to tolerance. If this is insufficient, a daily laxative is recommended. Polyethylene glycol at a dose of 17 to 34 g/day (1 to 2 "caps full") is recommended, although other laxatives, suppositories, or enemas may also be effective. If this approach does not prevent recurring fecal impaction and overflow incontinence, referral to a specialist who can test for dyssynergic defecation is recommended,[7] and if this evaluation leads to a diagnosis of disordered defecation, biofeedback to teach relaxation of the pelvic floor is more effective than laxatives.[13]

Pelvic Floor Exercises

Patients with FI are routinely encouraged to perform pelvic floor exercises to strengthen the EAS and the puborectalis, but patients are rarely given specific training on how to do these exercises. The Mayo Clinic Health Letter on pelvic floor exercises provides good instructions, which can be downloaded from the Internet, printed, and distributed to patients (www.health-letter.mayoclinic.com/Editorial/Editorial.cfm/i/454/t/Pelvic_floor_exercises). However, indirect evidence indicates that pelvic floor exercises are more effective if taught during a digital rectal exam: the examiner can palpate the appropriate muscles to direct the patient's attention to which muscles to contract and can provide feedback to the patient on whether they are appropriately contracting the pelvic floor muscles and whether they are inappropriately contracting abdominal wall muscles when they try to squeeze. Two studies reported that pelvic floor exercises taught during digital rectal exam were as effective as biofeedback training using electronic devices,[14,15] but this requires confirmation.

When conservative management, including pelvic floor exercises, fails to provide adequate relief of FI, referral to a gastroenterologist for further testing is recommended. This examination may identify rectal hyposensitivity or noncompliance of the rectum as additional factors that have to be addressed to achieve an optimal outcome. The gastroenterologist will also be able to provide or refer the patient for specialized treatments such as biofeedback, sacral nerve stimulation, or tibial nerve stimulation (described later).

Medical Management of Weak Internal Anal Sphincter Resting Pressure

Low resting anal canal pressure is sometimes due to tonic reflex inhibition of the IAS secondary to fecal impaction. If suspected, clean out the rectum and reassess resting anal pressure after 1 hour. If this normalizes resting anal canal pressure, no further treatment of the IAS is needed. Teaching the patient with an IAS defect to keep the rectum relatively empty by attempting a bowel movement 3 times a day, even if no urge to defecate is felt, may also reduce the frequency and severity of FI. If this is ineffective, consider an injectable bulking agent. No drugs are available that reliably improve IAS resting pressure.

Injectable Bulking Agents

A recently published randomized clinical trial[16] shows that injecting dextranomer into the submucosal space surrounding the anal canal significantly improves FI, and follow-up publications show that the improvements are maintained for at least 24 months in most patients. Based on this evidence, the FDA has approved this treatment, which can be performed in an outpatient setting.

Biofeedback for Strength Training

Biofeedback has been used to treat FI since 1972. Many uncontrolled studies support its effectiveness, but randomized controlled trials have yielded inconsistent results, suggesting that outcomes depend on the training and experience of the therapist. The positive outcomes from the methodologically soundest study,[17] combined with long-term maintenance of benefits from biofeedback, have led the American College of Gastroenterology[7] and the American

Gastroenterological Association[18] to endorse biofeedback as the preferred treatment for patients who have not responded to conservative treatment.

As originally described, biofeedback is primarily a technique for improving the strength of the pelvic floor muscles: pressures or EMG activity recorded from sensors in the anal canal are amplified and displayed to the patient and the therapist to help both of them recognize when the patient is able to make small improvements in the strength of their pelvic floor contractions. Some biofeedback devices also display pressures in the rectum to help the patient recognize inappropriate contractions of the abdominal wall muscles during attempts to prevent incontinence.

Recent studies suggest that combining biofeedback with electrical stimulation of the anal canal may augment its effectiveness.[19] However, electrical stimulation to the anal canal without concomitant biofeedback is not effective.

Biofeedback for Sensory Training

When it was shown that neurological injuries resulting in loss of rectal sensation make an independent contribution to the development of FI, new biofeedback procedures were developed to explicitly focus on improving the ability of patients to recognize weak distention of the rectum. This sensory discrimination training is done by first identifying the smallest volume of rectal balloon distention the patient can detect (sensory threshold) and then presenting sample distentions above and below this threshold to teach the patient to recognize weaker rectal distentions. Sensory training was shown to improve clinical outcomes in patients with FI.[20]

Biofeedback for Urge Resistance Training

Another innovation in biofeedback training procedures was triggered by the recognition that some patients have a so-called *hypersensitive rectum*—they feel an excessively strong urge to defecate when the rectum is distended with small volumes of stool and they are unable to inhibit defecation. Urge resistance training was developed to treat this type of urge FI.[21] The first step is to slowly inflate a balloon in the rectum until the threshold for a strong urge is identified. Then some of the air is withdrawn from the balloon, and the patient is encouraged to relax using deep breathing. Subsequently, the balloon is slowly inflated again while challenging the patient to use relaxation to tolerate higher volumes of rectal balloon filling. Further research is needed to validate and refine this procedure.

Sacral Nerve Stimulation (Neuromodulation)

This surgical treatment involves continuously pulsed electrical stimulation of the sacral nerves near their exit from the spinal cord. It begins with a trial period in which fine wire electrodes are inserted percutaneously into the region of the sacral nerves and positioned so that electrical stimulation elicits a sphincter contraction. The leads are connected to a temporary electrical stimulator, which is worn outside the body for a period of 2 weeks. If this results in a 50% reduction in the frequency of FI, the electrical stimulator is permanently implanted subcutaneously, whereas if there is less than a 50% reduction in FI, the electrodes are withdrawn. A randomized controlled trial has shown that sacral nerve stimulation produces long-term benefits in more than two-thirds of FI patients undergoing permanent implantation. However, the mechanism is unknown, and when treatment outcomes were analyzed by intention-to-treat analysis, the median responder rate dropped to 59%.[22] The stimulator has to be explanted for battery replacement about every 7 years.

Tibial Nerve Stimulation

Intermittent electrical stimulation of the tibial nerve through percutaneous needle electrodes has also been shown to reduce the severity of FI.[23] However, this remains an investigational treatment because relatively few studies have been reported and the physiological rationale for the procedure is unclear.

SUMMARY

Several effective treatments are available for FI, and one can expect significant improvement in 65% to 75% and cure in 30% to 50%. Significant improvements can be achieved with conservative treatments consisting of patient education, diet, drug treatment of diarrhea and constipation, and pelvic floor exercises—all of which can be implemented in community-based practices. For patients who fail conservative management, specialized treatments such as injection of bulking agents, biofeedback with or without electrical stimulation, and electrical stimulation of the sacral nerve or tibial nerve are available by referral.

REFERENCES

1. Wald A, Bharucha AE, Enck P, Rao SSC. Functional anorectal disorders. In: Drossman DA, Corazziari E, Delvaux M, et al, eds. *Rome III: The Functional Gastrointestinal Disorders.* McLean, VA: Degnon Associates; 2006:639-685.
2. Whitehead WE, Borrud L, Goode PS, et al. Fecal incontinence in US adults: epidemiology and risk factors. *Gastroenterology.* 2009;137:512-517.
3. Rockwood TH, Church JM, Fleshman JW, et al. Patient and surgeon ranking of the severity of symptoms associated with fecal incontinence: the Fecal Incontinence Severity Index. *Dis Colon Rectum.* 1999;42:1525-1532.
4. Bharucha AE, Locke GR, III, Seide BM, Zinsmeister AR. A new questionnaire for constipation and faecal incontinence. *Aliment Pharmacol Ther.* 2004;20:355-364.
5. Rockwood TH, Church JM, Fleshman JW, et al. Fecal Incontinence Quality of Life Scale: quality of life instrument for patients with fecal incontinence. *Dis Colon Rectum.* 2000;43:9-16.
6. Brown HW, Wexner SD, Segall MM, Brezoczky KL, Lukacz ES. Accidental bowel leakage in the mature women's health study: prevalence and predictors. *Int J Clin Pract.* 2012;66:1101-1108.
7. Wald AB, Bharucha AE, Cosman BC, Whitehead WE. ACG Clinical Guidelines: Management of benign anorectal disorders. *Am J Gastroenterol.* 2014;109:1141-1157.
8. Ditah I, Devaki P, Luma HN, et al. Prevalence, trends, and risk factors for fecal incontinence in United States adults, 2005-2010. *Clin Gastroenterol Hepatol.* 2013.
9. Jones AL, Dwyer LL, Bercovitz AR, Strahan GW. The National Nursing Home Survey: 2004 overview. National Center for Health Statistics. Vital Health Stat 13(167). 2009.
10. Bharucha AE, Zinsmeister AR, Locke GR, et al. Risk factors for fecal incontinence: a population-based study in women. *Am J Gastroenterol.* 2006;101:1305-1312.
11. Coggrave M, Norton C, Cody JD. Management of faecal incontinence and constipation in adults with central neurological diseases. *Cochrane Database Syst Rev.* 2014;1:CD002115.
12. Omar MI, Alexander CE. Drug treatment for faecal incontinence in adults. *Cochrane Database Syst Rev.* 2013;6:CD002116.
13. Chiarioni G, Whitehead WE, Pezza V, Morelli A, Bassotti G. Biofeedback is superior to laxatives for normal transit constipation due to pelvic floor dyssynergia. *Gastroenterology.* 2006;130:657-664.
14. Norton C, Chelvanayagam S, Wilson-Barnett J, Redfern S, Kamm MA. Randomized controlled trial of biofeedback for fecal incontinence. *Gastroenterology.* 2003;125:1320-1329.
15. Solomon MJ, Pager CK, Rex J, Roberts R, Manning J. Randomized, controlled trial of biofeedback with anal manometry, transanal ultrasound, or pelvic floor retraining with digital guidance alone in the treatment of mild to moderate fecal incontinence. *Dis Colon Rectum.* 2003;46:703-710.
16. Maeda Y, Laurberg S, Norton C. Perianal injectable bulking agents as treatment for faecal incontinence in adults. *Cochrane Database Syst Rev.* 2013;2:CD007959.
17. Heymen S, Scarlett YV, Jones KR, Ringel Y, Drossman DA, Whitehead WE. Randomized controlled trial shows biofeedback to be superior to pelvic floor exercises for fecal incontinence. *Dis Colon Rectum.* 2009;52:1730-1737.
18. Whitehead WE, Bharucha AE. Diagnosis and treatment of pelvic floor disorders: what's new and what to do. *Gastroenterology.* 2010;138:1231-1235, e1-4.
19. Vonthein R, Heimerl T, Schwandner T, Ziegler A. Electrical stimulation and biofeedback for the treatment of fecal incontinence: a systematic review. *Int J Colorectal Dis.* 2013;28:1567-1577.

20. Chiarioni G, Bassotti G, Stegagnini S, Vantini I, Whitehead WE. Sensory retraining is key to biofeedback therapy for formed stool fecal incontinence. *Am J Gastroenterol.* 2002;97:109-117.
21. Whitehead WEP. Behavioral treatment of fecal incontinence. In: Mostofsky DI, ed. *Handbook of Behavioral Medicine.* 1st ed. New York: John Wiley & Sons; 2014:787.
22. Chiarioni G, Palsson OS, Asteria CR, Whitehead WE. Neuromodulation for fecal incontinence: an effective surgical intervention. *World J Gastroenterol.* 2013;19:7048-7054.
23. Thomas GP, Dudding TC, Rahbour G, Nicholls RJ, Vaizey CJ. A review of posterior tibial nerve stimulation for faecal incontinence. *Colorectal Dis.* 2013;15:519-526.

Anorectal Disorders
Fecal Impaction, Descending Perineum Syndrome, Rectocele, and Levator Ani Syndrome

Satish S.C. Rao, MD, PhD, FRCP and Kulthep Rattanakovit, MD

KEY POINTS

- Patients with anorectal disorders present to many specialists; it is important to recognize these problems, as strategies for treatment differ.

- Fecal impaction is the abnormal accumulation of large amounts of hard stool in the rectum and distal colon with near-total inability of the individual to evacuate these stools; disimpaction, often under sedation, and prevention of recurrence are keys for successful management.

- Descending perineum syndrome (DPS) is the excessive descent of the perineum several centimeters below the bony outlet of the pelvis during a straining effort, and can present with pain, straining, and/or difficulty with defecation and is often associated with dyssynergic defecation.

- Rectocele is a saccular protrusion of the rectal wall, usually toward the vagina, through the separations or tears of the fascia, typically in the rectovaginal septum. Patients with a rectocele may report incomplete evacuation, prolonged straining, vaginal splinting, and/or rectal pain, and are ideally managed conservatively, and rarely with surgery.

- Levator ani syndrome (LAS) is characterized by recurrent, chronic anorectal pain in the absence of infectious or inflammatory conditions of the anorectum. Its treatment remains unsatisfactory, but biofeedback therapy may be useful.

Rao SSC, Parkman HP, McCallum RW, eds.
Handbook of Gastrointestinal Motility and Functional Disorders (pp 279-289).
© 2015 Taylor & Francis Group.

Anorectal disorders are common and encompass many conditions that affect both defecation and continence. This chapter discusses several common entities that include fecal impaction, descending perineum syndrome (DPS), rectocele, and levator ani syndrome. Although there is some overlap among these conditions and more than one problem may coexist or confound or cause a pelvic floor disorder, with regard to symptoms and presentation, each of these conditions is discussed separately. An algorithm for a clinical approach and management is presented in Figures 22-1 and 22-2.

Fecal Impaction

Fecal impaction represents the abnormal accumulation of hard and compacted stool in the rectum, typically over several days to weeks, together with a near-total failure to evacuate these stools. It is commonly seen in older patients, with a prevalence of 40% in hospitalized older patients, but can occur in younger individuals.

Pathophysiology

Chronic constipation with pelvic floor dysfunction is the chief underlying mechanism.[1] Rectal hyposensitivity—either a primary problem or as a result of certain psychosocial and behavioral factors like decreased mobility, drugs that are constipating, and other conditions—may also lead to stool impaction; increased rectal compliance has also been described.[1] The factors contributing to fecal impaction are listed in Table 22-1.

Diagnosis and Evaluation

Fecal impaction usually presents with lower abdominal pain, distention, nausea, and vomiting. Occassionally with overflow incontinence; in severe cases, with colonic obstruction, stercoral ulceration; and rarely, with bowel perforation. Abdominal examination reveals stool that is palpable in a distended abdomen. Rectal examination may reveal impacted stool, but rarely the stool may be located more proximally; if so, a plain abdominal x-ray is required.

Digital Rectal Exam

Digital rectal examination (DRE) is an important diagnostic tool that can be performed at bedside. DRE may show the presence of stricture, spasm, tenderness, mass, blood, or stool. If stool is present in the rectum, patients should be asked about their awareness of it. Failure of awareness may suggest rectal hyposensitivity, and this is often seen in fecal impaction. Resting anal sphincter tone is assessed as the next step, followed by an assessment of squeeze tone. Next, the patient is asked to push and bear down as if to defecate. Normally, the examiner should feel relaxation of the external anal sphincter and/or the puborectalis muscle, together with perineal descent. Failure of this normal finding should raise a suspicion of dyssynergic defecation or an evacuation disorder. The examiner must also place his or her hand on the patient's abdomen to assess the push effort. DRE has a sensitivity of 75% and specificity of 87% for detecting dyssynergia.[2] Unfortunately, this examination is not performed by most physicians and trainees and merits emphasis during medical training.[3]

Evaluation

A plain abdominal x-ray often reveals fecal impaction. Sometimes, a computerized abdominal tomography scan may be required to evaluate extraintestinal structures that may be obstructing the colon to cause fecal impaction. Routine complete blood count, metabolic profile, calcium levels, and thyroid function test should be performed, along with a flexible sigmoidoscopy or

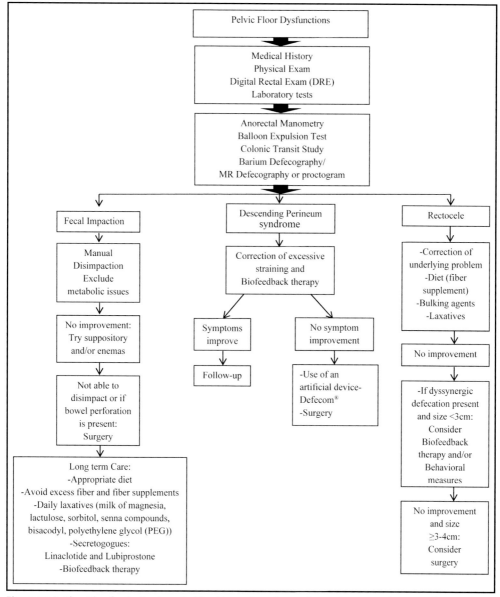

Figure 22-1. Algorithm for the treatment of fecal impaction, descending perineum syndrome, and rectocele.

colonoscopy to identify a secondary cause; if none are identified, colonic transit study, anorectal manometry, and balloon expulsion test should be performed to identify an underlying defecation disorder.

Anorectal Manometry

Anorectal manometry is essential for a diagnosis of dyssynergic defecation. It is the most reliable way of detecting dyssynergic defecation, especially when the patient is asked to attempt defecation on a commode.[4] During a bearing-down maneuver or defecation attempt, intrarectal pressure increases (≥ 40 mm Hg), accompanied by adequate decrease ($> 20\%$) in external anal sphincter pressure coinciding with the relaxation of the external anal sphincter. In dyssynergic defecation, this voluntary and learned response is impaired or uncoordinated; there is inadequate

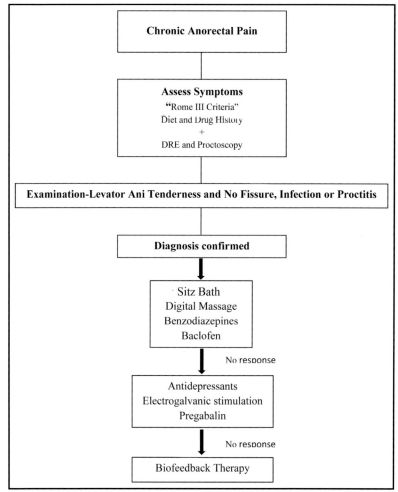

Figure 22-2. Algorithm for evaluation and management of levator ani syndrome.

increase in rectal pressure or impaired anal relaxation, or paradoxical anal sphincter contraction, or a combination of these mechanisms. At least four types of dyssynergia patterns have been recognized by Rao et al.[4]

Balloon Expulsion Test

This is a useful screening test to identify patients with dyssynergic defecation. Although its specificity is high (80% to 90%), it has low sensitivity (50%). The test is performed by placing a 4-cm-long rectal balloon filled with 50 cc of warm water.[4] After placement, the patient is given privacy and asked to expel the balloon. A stopwatch is provided to assess the time required for expulsion. Normal healthy subjects can usually expel a balloon in <1 minute.[4]

Management

An algorithmic approach for evaluation and management of fecal impaction is shown in Figure 22-1. Impacted stool should be removed manually, often under sedation. Milk and molasses or gastrografin enemas and bisacodyl suppositories may be needed to initiate disimpaction,

	TABLE 22-1	
	CAUSES OR CONDITIONS THAT PREDISPOSE TO FECAL IMPACTION	
CONSTIPATING MEDICATIONS	**NEUROLOGICAL DISEASES**	**OTHER REASONS**
Opioids	Cerebrovascular disease and stroke	Dehydration
Iron	Parkinson's disease	Immobility
Calcium channel blockers	Multiple sclerosis	Bed restraints
Antidepressants	Autonomic neuropathy	Mechanical obstruction
Anticholinergics	Spinal cord lesions	General weakness
Antacids	Dementia	
Diuretics	Endocrine and metabolic diseases	
Antihistamines	Diabetes mellitus	
Antiparkinsonian drugs	Hypothyroidism	
	Hyperparathyroidism	
	Chronic renal disease	
	Myopathic diseases	
	Amyloidosis	
	Scleroderma	

especially if the impaction is located more proximally; however, stool softeners have limited efficacy.[1] Surgery may be needed if disimpaction cannot be managed manually or if bowel perforation is present.[1]

Once impaction is managed, patients should be placed on an appropriate dietary regimen. Excess fiber and fiber supplements should be avoided. Patients must receive aggressive daily treatment with a laxative such as milk of magnesia, lactulose, sorbitol, senna compounds, bisacodyl, or polyethylene glycol (PEG). Similarly, lubiprostone and linaclotide may be beneficial. However, there are no studies of laxatives in patients with fecal impaction. In patients with dyssynergic defecation, biofeedback therapy is the treatment of choice. Biofeedback therapy was shown to be effective in dyssynergic defecation in randomized controlled trials (RCTs).[4] However, the efficacy of biofeedback has not been established in elderly patients or in fecal impaction. Further, multicenter cooperative studies are needed to assess the epidemiology and pathophysiology of fecal impaction—in particular, its etiology. There is also a lack of information regarding the outcomes of interventions and the best clinical approach.

DESCENDING PERINEUM SYNDROME

Definition

DPS is the excessive descent of the perineum several centimeters below the bony outlet of the pelvis during a straining effort. Its prevalence is unknown. DPS is associated with pelvic floor

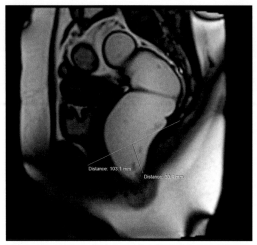 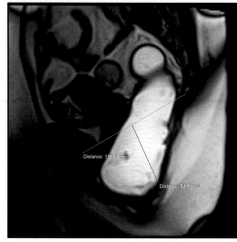

Figure 22-3. (A) Typical example of MR defecography images showing the anorectal morphology at rest. (B) MR defecography with bearing-down maneuver. When bearing down, it can be seen that there is excessive descent (> 3 cm) of the perineum and anorectal junction.

weakness[5] and other anorectal disorders, such as rectocele, solitary rectal ulcer syndrome (SRUS), or rectal prolapse.

Diagnosis and Evaluation

The patient may present with rectal and perineal pain, prolonged and excessive straining, feelings of incomplete evacuation and blockage during defecation, and/or fecal incontinence.[6] Passage of mucus and tenesmus are also common. A history of long-standing constipation and/or use of laxatives is usually present. This condition can be diagnosed with physical examination, particularly a detailed rectal examination. More recently, 3-D high-definition anorectal manometry and/or barium or magnetic resonance (MR) defecography has been shown to be useful in the diagnosis of DPS.

Magnetic Resonance Defecography

Magnetic resonance defecography is performed without radiation and with an open or closed system. This technique gives excellent details of all pelvic floor compartments, muscles, soft tissue, and supporting structures. In the open system, the images are acquired when the patient is in a physiologic sitting position, thereby simulating true defecation, whereas in a closed system, the patient is lying or in a supine position.[7,8] Recently, dynamic MR defecography with an open-configuration and low-field tilting MR system was shown to detect pelvic floor disorders more accurately in the orthostatic position than in the supine position.[8] Although this technique gives useful information, it is not widely available. A ≥ 3 cm descent of the perineum during straining or > 4 cm descent at rest is diagnostic of DPS. On defecography, the anorectal angle is more than 130 degrees at rest and increases to more than 155 degrees during straining (Figure 22-3). A perineometer may also be useful for diagnosis, because it can measure the length of perineal descent. An algorithmic approach for evaluation and management of descending perineum syndrome is shown in Figure 22-1.

Management

Treatment is mostly behavioral and consists of correcting the excessive straining behavior and dyssynergia. Pelvic floor retraining may be useful, and the extent of perineal descent may be a good predictor of its efficacy.[5] In a retrospective study of 9 patients who underwent retroanal levator plate myorrhaphy (RLPM),[9] there was a mean reduction of perineal descent of 1.08 cm and improvement of stress urinary incontinence, urgency, dysuria, fecal incontinence, dyschezia, dyspareunia, perineodynia, cystocele, and rectocele. However, RCTs are needed. Stapled transanal rectal resection (STARR) and stapled transanal prolapsectomy associated with perineal levatorplasty (STAPL) were found to be safe and effective; however, STARR caused less postoperative pain and better clinical outcomes compared to STAPL.[10] Another study showed that STARR is safe and effective.[11] An artificial device, Defecom—a polycarbonate plate with two separate holes for passing urine and stool, as well as a built-in hump that supports the perineum when sitting on a commode—may also be a good supportive approach. The Defecom together with biofeedback therapy may improve symptoms in about 50%. At present, there is no standard or approved medical, behavioral, or surgical therapy for DPS. Future efforts should be directed toward a better understanding of the pathophysiology; a better characterization of the phenotype, prevalence, and coexisting problems; and performing well-designed RCTs.

RECTOCELE

Epidemiology

Rectocele is usually asymptomatic, and hence its true prevalence is unknown.[9] In a cross-sectional analysis among women participating in the National Health and Nutrition Examination Survey between 2005 and 2006, the prevalence in the US female population was reported to be 23.7%. In a cohort study on young nulliparous women, the prevalence was 12% and its size ranged from 10 to 25 mm.[12] Postmenopausal women show higher prevalence of rectoceles, and it occurs in both multiparous and nulliparous women.[9]

Definition

Rectocele is the saccular protrusion of the rectal wall, usually towards the vagina, through the separations or tears of the fascia in the rectovaginal septum (anterior wall) and rarely towards the sacrum (posterior wall). Rectocele can be classified according to their anatomical position and size.[13] High rectoceles are associated with loss of support from the uterine body, midrectoceles lack support of the pelvic floor, and low rectoceles result from weakness of the perineal body.[9] Rectoceles can also be classified according to their size. Rectoceles >2 cm are regarded as a cutoff value for a clinically significant problem.[9]

Pathophysiology

Defects or weakness of the rectovaginal septum is believed to be the main cause.[9] Excessive straining and vaginal delivery with instrument use (ie, forceps) may cause weakness or defects in the rectovaginal fascia, weakness of the pelvic floor muscles, and damage to the pudendal nerve. As a result of the weakened pelvic floor, the vaginal outlet becomes bigger. Since the vagina cannot close during straining, the pressure gradient between the rectum (high pelvic pressure) and vagina (low atmospheric pressure) increases. The pressure gradient pushes the anterior rectal wall towards the vagina, eventually causing rectocele.[9] Pelvic floor disorders were found to be more common in women and associated with aging, pregnancy, parity, and instrumental delivery.[14] A higher body mass index and a history of constipation were associated with rectocele; a more recent study showed that paradoxical anal sphincter contraction was found to be higher (60%) in patients with rectocele than in patients without rectocele (24%), suggesting a correlation between rectocele and dyssynergic defecation.[15] Also, hysterectomy and intussusception have been found to be associated with rectoceles.[9]

Figure 22-4. Typical example of defecography images showing an anterior rectocele during a bearing-down maneuver.

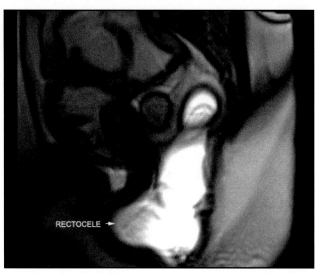

Clinical Presentation

Rectoceles that are <2 cm are clinically inconsequential and usually asymptomatic. Large rectoceles may be associated with symptoms of incomplete evacuation, prolonged straining, vaginal splinting, and rectal pain.[13] Dyspareunia, anorectal/vaginal pain, fecal soiling, and urologic symptoms are also reported by patients with rectocele.[9,15]

Diagnosis and Evaluation

A DRE performed during a straining maneuver may reveal outward bulging of the anterior rectal wall. A combined vaginal and DRE may also be helpful in the diagnosis of rectocele. Posterior rectocele is usually difficult to detect, but can be identified radiologically.

Defecography is considered the gold standard for the diagnosis of rectocele (Figure 22-4). It also reveals other pathologic findings, such as excessive perineal descent and rectal mucosal intussusception. Because rectocele is commonly reported on a defecogram even in healthy women, a clinical diagnosis should be based both on symptoms and defecography.[16] However, defecography findings cannot predict the clinical outcome of surgery.[9] Magnetic resonance not only detects rectocele, but can also provide dynamic multicompartment evaluation of the pelvis when both the dynamic and static sequences are used together.[17] A real-time continuous imaging with a dynamic true fast imaging with steady-state precession (FISP) sequence is suggested to be included in MR studies to evaluate pelvic floor dysfunction.[18] A recent study comparing dynamic anal endosonography and MR defecography in pelvic floor disorders revealed that the two techniques were similar with regard to the sensitivity, specificity, or positive and negative predictive values for detecting these disorders.[19] However, more internal anal sphincter defects were detected by dynamic anal endosonography, and this technique was reported to be better tolerated by patients when compared to dynamic MR or conventional defecography. In one study, rectocele <2.5 cm was found in 55% of patients with dyssynergic defecation diagnosed by anorectal manometry.[9] An algorithmic approach for evaluation and management of rectocele is shown in Figure 22-1.

Management

The first approach is the correction of any underlying problem. Diet with fiber supplements, bulking agents, laxatives, behavioral therapy, and timed-toilet training may be helpful. If

TABLE 22-2

ROME III DIAGNOSTIC CRITERIA FOR LEVATOR ANI SYNDROME

Chronic or recurrent rectal pain or aching

Episodes last 20 minutes or longer

Other causes of rectal pain such as ischemia, inflammatory bowel diseases, cryptitis, intramuscular abscess, anal fissure, hemorrhoids, prostatitis, and coccygodynia have been excluded

Tenderness during posterior traction on the puborectalis

*Criteria fulfilled for the last 3 months, with symptom onset at least 6 months prior to diagnosis

Adapted from Wald A, Bharucha AE, Enck P, Rao SSC. Functional anorectal disorders. *Rome III: The Functional Gastrointestinal Disorders*;2006: 639-685.

dyssynergic defecation is an underlying problem, biofeedback therapy is indicated before surgery. The underlying occult disorders like psychological distress, anismus, and rectal hyposensitivity should be corrected before considering surgery, since this can affect the outcome of surgery.[9] Patients who are symptomatic and who do not respond to conservative treatment and have a large rectocele (>3 or 4 cm) or have coexisting vaginal prolapse may be suitable candidates for surgery.[9] Posterior colporrhaphy is the standard surgical procedure, which can provide cure rates of up to 95%.[20] Both transanal and transvaginal techniques have been found to be effective in rectocele repair and may avoid postoperative dyspareunia; however, the transanal technique was associated with greater recurrence of rectocele.[21] The use of native tissue or a mesh seems to have similar outcomes when repairing a rectocele, but native tissue is generally regarded as the gold standard.[9] A recent study showed that transperineal repair of rectocele is superior to transanal repair.[9] Transperineal repair was also found to improve the functional outcomes and sensory thresholds such as urge to defecate. When a levatorplasty was added to the transperineal approach, the overall bowel function score increased significantly, but there were unwanted side effects such as dyspareunia.

LEVATOR ANI SYNDROME

Definition

LAS is characterized by chronic, recurrent anorectal pain, often described as a dull ache or pressure in the anorectal area or a feeling of "sitting on a ball."[22] The pain can be aggravated by riding or prolonged sitting or defecation. Unlike proctalgia fugax, the duration of pain in LAS usually lasts more than 30 minutes, often several hours.

As listed in Table 22-2, the following criteria have been proposed for the diagnosis of LAS. On physical examination, tenderness of the levator muscles (ileococcygeus, pubococcygeous, and puborectalis) is usually present.

Pathophysiology

Whether the LAS and proctalgia fugax are different entities or part of the same spectrum of anal hyperkinetic spastic disorders remains unsettled. Despite the absence of definite psychological traits, there is a correlation between presence of anorectal symptoms and stressful situations.[22,23]

Diagnosis

The diagnosis of LAS, in large part, rests on clinical findings. The classical history, together with tenderness of the levator muscles during physical exam, is often diagnostic. However, a detailed neurological and pelvic exam, as well as examination of the anorectal, prostate, and genital areas, should be performed to exclude other causes for pain. Anoscopy or flexible sigmoidoscopy may also help to exclude mucosal diseases such as anal fissure or inflammatory or neoplastic conditions that cause rectal pain.

Treatment

Different therapeutic modalities have been proposed for relieving LAS, as summarized in Figure 22-2.

Rectal Massage

This treatment consists of repeated massage of the puborectalis sling. It is performed by firmly moving the finger in the rectum in an anterior-posterior direction. If tolerated, it is recommended that the affected area should be massaged up to 50 times.[22] Grant et al reported the resolution of symptoms in 65% of 316 patients with LAS after 2 or 3 massages that were given 2 to 3 weeks apart in conjunction with hot sitz bath and diazepam.[22] Whether the massage, the warmth, or the smooth muscle relaxation with benzodiazepine offered the most relief is unclear. This study typifies the confounding literature on this topic. Also, botulinum toxin injection into the anal sphincter was shown to be ineffective in an RCT of LAS patients.[24]

Sitz Bath

Hot sitz bath is performed by immersion of the buttocks in warm water (40°C) for at least 20 minutes daily.[22] At this temperature, the anal canal pressure decreases in normals and in patients with proctalgia.[23]

Electrogalvanic Stimulation

The rationale with this technique is that a low-frequency (80 cycles per second) oscillating current, when applied to a muscle, induces fasciculation and fatigue, which may break the cycle of pain → spasm → pain.[25] An anal probe is inserted and connected to an electrogalvanic stimulator, which is set at a pulse frequency of 80 cycles per second and voltage 150 or 400 volts, depending on the patient's tolerance.[25-27] Each treatment lasts between 15 and 60 minutes and is delivered every other day. The treatment is well tolerated and without side effects.[25] Since the initial study by Sohn et al,[25] five other series have reported symptom improvement with electrogalvanic stimulation in 43% to 91% of patients with LAS.[25-29]

Biofeedback Therapy

Biofeedback training has been used in LAS with variable results. The objective is to train individuals to relax the external anal sphincter and thereby decrease the intra-anal resting pressure. In a large prospective RCT, a majority of patients with LAS were found to have dyssynergia defecation, and 87% responded to biofeedback therapy when compared to 45% and 22% who received electrogalvanic stimulation and massage for treatment.[30] Interestingly, only patients who had levator ani tenderness responded to treatment with biofeedback therapy.

Anorectal disorders are common. Their diagnosis and management options are continuing to evolve. Much more needs to be learned about the underlying mechanisms for these disorders, which in turn could pave the way for improved treatment strategies.

References

1. Rao SS, Go JT. Update on the management of constipation in the elderly: new treatment options. *Clin Interv Aging.* 2010;5:163-171.
2. Tantiphlachiva K, Rao P, Attaluri A, Rao SS. Digital rectal examination is a useful tool for identifying patients with dyssynergia. *Clin Gastroenterol Hepatol.* 2010;8:955-960.
3. Wong RK, Drossman DA, Bharucha AE, et al. The digital rectal examination: a multicenter survey of physicians' and students' perceptions and practice patterns. *Am J Gastroenterol.* 2012;107:1157-1163.
4. Rao SS. Dyssynergic defecation and biofeedback therapy. *Gastroenterol Clin North Am.* 2008;37:569-586.
5. Harewood GC, Coulie B, Camilleri M, Rath-Harvey D, Pemberton JH. Descending perineum syndrome: audit of clinical and laboratory features and outcome of pelvic floor retraining. *Am J Gastroenterol.* 1999;94:126-130.
6. Zhang B, Ding JH, Yin SH, Zhang M, Zhao K. Stapled transanal rectal resection for obstructed defecation syndrome associated with rectocele and rectal intussusception. *World J Gastroenterol.* 2010;16:2542-2548.
7. Flusberg M, Sahni VA, Erturk SM, Mortele KJ. Dynamic MR defecography: assessment of the usefulness of the defecation phase. *Am J Roentgenol.* 2011;196:W394-W399.
8. Fiaschetti V, Squillaci E, Pastorelli D, et al. Dynamic MR defecography with an open-configuration, low-field, tilting MR system in patients with pelvic floor disorders. *Radiol Med.* 2011;116:620-633.
9. Schey R, Cromwell J, Rao SS. Medical and surgical management of pelvic floor disorders affecting defecation. *Am J Gastroenterol.* 2012;107:1624-1634.
10. Boccasanta P, Venturi M, Salamina G, Cesana BM, Bernasconi F, Roviaro G. New trends in the surgical treatment of outlet obstruction: clinical and functional results of two novel transanal stapled techniques from a randomised controlled trial. *Int J Colorectal Dis.* 2004;19:359-369.
11. Pechlivanides G, Tsiaoussis J, Athanasakis E, et al. Stapled transanal rectal resection (STARR) to reverse the anatomic disorders of pelvic floor dyssynergia. *World J Surg.* 2007;31:1329-1335.
12. Dietz HP, Clarke B. Prevalence of rectocele in young nulliparous women. *Aust N Z J Obstet Gynaecol.* 2005;45:391-394.
13. Zbar AP, Lienemann A, Fritsch H, Beer-Gabel M, Pescatori M. Rectocele: pathogenesis and surgical management. *Int J Colorectal Dis.* 2003;18:369-384.
14. MacLennan AH, Taylor AW, Wilson DH, Wilson D. The prevalence of pelvic floor disorders and their relationship to gender, age, parity and mode of delivery. *BJOG.* 2000;107:1460-1470.
15. Mellgren A, López A, Schultz I, Anzén B. Rectocele is associated with paradoxical anal sphincter reaction. *Int J Colorectal Dis.* 1998;13:13-16.
16. Shorvon PJ, McHugh S, Diamant NE, Somers S, Stevenson GW. Defecography in normal volunteers: results and implications. *Gut.* 1989;30:1737-1749.
17. Foti PV, Farina R, Riva G, et al. Pelvic floor imaging: comparison between magnetic resonance imaging and conventional defecography in studying outlet obstruction syndrome. *Radiol Med.* 2012. [Epub ahead of print].
18. Hecht EM, Lee VS, Tanpitukpongse TP, et al. MRI of pelvic floor dysfunction: dynamic true fast imaging with steady-state precession versus HASTE. *Am J Roentgenol.* 2008;191:352-358.
19. Vitton V, Vignally P, Barthet M, et al. Dynamic anal endosonography and MRI defecography in diagnosis of pelvic floor disorders: comparison with conventional defecography. *Dis Colon Rectum.* 201;54:1398-1404.
20. Kudish BI, Iglesia CB. Posterior wall prolapse and repair. *Clin Obstet Gynecol.* 2010;53:59-71.
21. Nieminen K, Hiltunen KM, Laitinen J, Oksala J, Heinonen PK. Transanal or vaginal approach to rectocele repair: a prospective, randomized pilot study. *Dis Colon Rectum.* 2004;47:1636-1642.
22. Salvati E. The levator syndrome and its variant. *Gastroenterol Clin North Am.* 1987;16:71-78.
23. Dodi G, Bogoni F, et al. Hot or cold in anal pain? A study of the changes in internal sphincter pressure profiles. *Dis Colon Rectum.* 1986;29:248-251.
24. Rao SS, Paulson J, Mata M, et al. Effect of botulinum toxin on levator ani syndrome: a double-blind placebo-controlled study. *Aliment Pharmacol Ther.* 2009;29:985-991.
25. Sohn N, Weinstein MA, et al. The levator syndrome and its treatment with high-voltage electrogalvanic stimulation. *Am J Surg.* 1982;144:580-582.
26. Oliver GC, Rubin RJ, et al. Electrogalvanic stimulation in the treatment of levator syndrome. *Dis Colon Rectum.* 1985;28:662-663.
27. Billingham RP, Isler JT, et al. Treatment of levator syndrome using high-voltage electrogalvanic stimulation. *Dis Colon Rectum.* 1987;30:584-587.
28. Nicosia JF, Abcarian H. Levator syndrome: a treatment that works. *Dis Colon Rectum.* 1985;28:406-408.
29. Hull TL, Milson JW, et al. Electrogalvanic stimulation for levator syndrome: how effective is it in the long term? *Dis Colon Rectum.* 1993;36:731-733.
30. Chiarioni G, Nardo A, Vantini I, et al. Biofeedback is superior to electrogalvanic stimulation and massage for treatment of levator ani syndrome. *Gastroenterology.* 2010;138:1321-1329.
31. Wald A, Bharucha AE, Enck P, Rao SSC. Functional anorectal disorders. *Rome III: The Functional Gastrointestinal Disorders.* 2006:639-685.

23

Diabetes and the Gut

Christopher K. Rayner, MBBS, PhD, FRACP;
Karen L. Jones, Dip App Sci (Nuc Med), PhD; and
Michael Horowitz, MBBS, PhD, FRACP

KEY POINTS

- Type 1 and type 2 diabetes are associated with a variety of symptoms at all levels of the gastrointestinal tract.
- The relationship of gastrointestinal symptoms to motor dysfunction is relatively weak.
- Gastrointestinal motility and symptoms in diabetes may be exacerbated acutely by poor glycemic control.
- Recent studies indicate that the underlying pathophysiology of gut dysfunction in diabetes is heterogeneous.
- Gastrointestinal motor function, particularly the rate of gastric emptying, is a major determinant of postprandial glycemic control.

Diabetes mellitus can affect the motor, sensory, and secretory function of any segment of the gastrointestinal tract. Patients with type 1 diabetes may be at higher risk of gastrointestinal dysfunction due to a longer duration of disease, but the overall burden of disease is likely to be greater in patients with type 2 diabetes, rather than type 1, due its substantially higher prevalence in modern society.

Gut dysfunction typically presents with symptoms, and clinicians should specifically ask patients with diabetes about these, since they may not be spontaneously volunteered. Community-based patients with diabetes have an increased prevalence of symptoms related to both the upper and lower gastrointestinal tract, including reflux symptoms, dyspepsia, diarrhea, and constipation, and these appear to be worse in patients with poor glycemic control.[1] Women and patients with psychological comorbidity appear at greater risk, and not infrequently, there is a substantial adverse impact on quality of life.

Rao SSC, Parkman HP, McCallum RW, eds.
Handbook of Gastrointestinal Motility and Functional Disorders (pp 291-302).

Aside from symptoms, disordered gastrointestinal motility in patients with diabetes can manifest as disturbed glycemic control and impaired nutrition and absorption of oral medications. Given the rapid increase in the prevalence of type 2 diabetes worldwide, there are major implications for utilization of health care resources.

Gut dysfunction related to diabetes has long been attributed to the presence of autonomic neuropathy, although the relationship between disordered motility and the presence of demonstrable cardiac autonomic neuropathy (a surrogate for gastrointestinal autonomic dysfunction) is relatively weak.[2] Recent studies have revealed a heterogeneous mix of pathophysiology in patients with severe gastroparesis that offers potential for more specific treatment in the future.[3]

The purpose of this chapter is to document the spectrum of disordered gut function associated with diabetes, presented in an organ-based approach. The discussion will focus on the aspects of individual motility disorders that are specific to diabetes, since a more general approach to the diagnosis and treatment of these disorders is covered in the preceding chapters of this handbook.

ESOPHAGUS

Presentation

Disorders of esophageal motility in patients with diabetes can present with dysphagia or symptoms of gastroesophageal reflux; however, other specific causes of dysphagia must always be excluded. Gastroesophageal reflux can frequently be asymptomatic, particularly in the presence of established autonomic neuropathy,[4] and erosive disease has been associated particularly with the presence of peripheral neuropathy.[5] Patients with diabetes are at increased risk of esophageal candidiasis, which may present with odynophagia.

Pathophysiology

The first report of esophageal motor dysfunction in diabetes, dating from 1967, indicated that 12 of 14 patients with long-standing, predominantly insulin-treated diabetes had barium swallow abnormalities, including diminution of the primary peristaltic wave, the presence of tertiary contractions, and a marked delay in esophageal emptying.[6] The majority of these patients had evidence of autonomic and/or peripheral neuropathy, and many had gastrointestinal symptoms, although in only a minority were these clearly related to the esophagus.

Subsequent scintigraphic and manometric studies have indicated that esophageal motility and transit are abnormal in up to 50% of patients with long-standing diabetes, with a decrease in the number, amplitude, and velocity of peristaltic waves and an increase in simultaneous contractions in patients with both type 1 and 2 diabetes, although these correlate poorly with the presence of esophageal symptoms.

Delayed transit affects solids more than liquids and is related to peristaltic failure.[7] However, disordered esophageal motility appears to correlate poorly with the presence of delayed gastric emptying.[2]

Altered biomechanical properties have been observed in both animal models and humans with long-standing diabetes, with increased stiffness and diminished compliance of the esophageal body associated with reduced sensitivity to distension.[8] Electrophysiological studies indicate that peripheral conduction of sensory impulses in response to esophageal electrical stimulation is delayed, together with altered central processing within the insula, which may contribute to symptom generation.[9]

As in other regions of the gut, esophageal motility is affected by acute variations in the blood glucose concentration, with a substantial reduction in lower esophageal sphincter pressure and the velocity of peristalsis during marked hyperglycemia.[10]

Diagnosis

The investigation of esophageal symptoms in patients with diabetes follows a similar algorithm to nondiabetic patients. Endoscopy detects mucosal disease, while esophageal motor function is evaluated with manometry, and contrast video swallow radiology highlights both structural and functional disorders. Esophageal pH and impedance studies may be helpful in the assessment of gastroesophageal reflux; a high index of suspicion should be maintained, given the possibility of atypical or minimally symptomatic presentations.

Epidemiology

The prevalence of esophageal symptoms varies depending on whether study populations are derived from tertiary referral centers or from the community; reflux symptoms may affect around 40% in the former and 15% in the latter, but in each population, the prevalence remains greater than in controls. Meanwhile, dysphagia affects perhaps 25% of outpatients attending tertiary centers and 5% of patients in the community.[1]

Whether the risk of Barrett's esophagus is increased in diabetes has been controversial, but the presence of type 2 diabetes was recently identified as an independent risk factor in a large epidemiological study, even allowing for the association of type 2 diabetes with obesity.[11]

Treatment

Dysphagia and gastroesophageal reflux disease are treated similarly in patients with diabetes as in the general population. The limited studies available are inconsistent as to the benefit of prokinetic drugs for treating either esophageal dysmotility or acid reflux. Patients with delayed transit should be advised to drink a glass of water after taking oral medications to reduce the risk of "pill esophagitis."

STOMACH

Disordered gastric emptying is the most widely recognized motility disorder associated with diabetes, and has profound implications for overall management. The term *diabetic gastroparesis* was first proposed by Kassander in 1958,[12] and in most tertiary referral centers, diabetes is implicated in at least one-third of all patients presenting with gastroparesis.[13] The definition of diabetic gastroparesis requires careful documentation, since many patients have delayed emptying with few symptoms, while a few with "typical" symptoms are found to have abnormally rapid emptying.

Patients with diabetic gastropathy typically present with upper gastrointestinal symptoms. Early satiety and fullness relate most closely to the presence of delayed emptying[14]; fatigue is also commonly reported. When compared to patients with idiopathic gastroparesis, vomiting is more prominent and abdominal pain less so.[15] Despite a high prevalence of overweight and obesity, malnutrition remains a concern in these patients, though vitamin and mineral deficiencies are less common than in the idiopathic group.[16] Gastroparesis can interfere with the absorption of oral medications; this is mainly relevant for drugs with a short half-life or where rapid onset of action is needed, and applies to some oral hypoglycemic agents.[13]

Given the central role of the upper gut in determining postprandial blood glucose excursions, as discussed later in the section on treatment, it is not surprising that disordered glycemic control is a frequent complication of diabetic gastroparesis; indeed, in insulin-treated patients, otherwise unexplained hypoglycemic episodes may be the sole presenting feature of disordered gastric function.[17]

Patients with diabetes also have high rates of postprandial hypotension, which is at least as common as orthostatic hypotension in this group, putting them at increased risk of syncope and vascular events. In a group of recently diagnosed patients with type 2 diabetes, over 40% manifested a sustained fall in blood pressure of ≥ 20 mm Hg after an oral glucose drink.[18] In the broadest sense, this phenomenon represents a "gastrointestinal" disorder, since the fall in blood pressure was related to the rate of gastric emptying of glucose, such that those with more rapid emptying were at greater risk. This is consistent with the concept of "dumping syndrome" being related to falls in blood pressure, as well as a drop in blood glucose concentrations after an initial early peak in individuals who have rapid gastric emptying.

Pathophysiology

The motor abnormalities associated with disordered gastric emptying in diabetes include low fasting tone and impaired postprandial accommodation of the proximal stomach, antral hypo-motility, an increase in pyloric pressures, impaired antroduodenal coordination,[13] and disruption of the migrating motor complex. Disturbances of the gastric electrical rhythm are frequently observed, while there also appears to be hypersensitivity to proximal gastric distension.[19]

It has long been held that gastroparesis is a manifestation of irreversible autonomic neuropathy affecting the vagus nerve, which is supported by the finding of impaired pancreatic polypeptide secretion in response to sham feeding in patients with gastric dysfunction.[3] In the past 5 to 10 years, much more information has become available—facilitated by the establishment of the National Institutes of Health (NIH)–funded Gastroparesis Research Consortium—from analysis of full-thickness gastric biopsies taken from patients with severe gastroparesis, showing that over 80% have histologic changes, but that the pathogenesis is clearly heterogeneous. The most prominent abnormalities include loss or damage to the interstitial cells of Cajal (ICC), which fulfill a pacemaker function in the stomach, together with immune infiltration involving the myenteric plexus and loss of intrinsic nerves.[20] The patients in these studies represent the most severe end of the gastroparesis spectrum, and it remains to be seen whether the changes observed are representative of most patients with abnormal gastric emptying in the context of diabetes. A hallmark of diabetic gastroparesis is the presence of a thickened basal lamina around smooth muscle cells and nerves,[21] and inclusion bodies in the smooth muscle have also been reported.

The number of ICC has been shown to be inversely related to the proportion of a test meal retained in the stomach at 4 hours in diabetic, but not idiopathic, gastroparesis.[22] Loss and/or dysfunction of ICC may be related to reduced insulin or insulin-like growth factor-1 (IGF-1) signaling, with atrophy of smooth muscle and reduced production of stem cell factor—the latter is required for normal function and survival of the ICC.[3] Increased oxidative stress may be critical to the loss of ICC in diabetic gastroparesis. In a nonobese diabetic (NOD) mouse model, the loss of ICC could be reversed by antioxidant therapy with hemin or carbon monoxide.[23] Recent evidence indicates that altered expression of the Ano-1 gene, which is expressed in ICC and encodes a calcium-activated chloride channel, may contribute to the etiology of diabetic gastroparesis.[24]

Animal models of gastroparesis also demonstrate a preferential loss of inhibitory neurons expressing neuronal nitric oxide synthase (nNOS); accumulation of advanced glycation end products (AGEs), formed by glyco-oxidation during sustained hyperglycemia, may contribute. However, the decline in nNOS neurons is relatively modest in severe diabetic gastroparesis (20% vs. 40%), when compared to idiopathic, and the phosphodiesterase type 5 inhibitor sildenafil, which facilitates NO-mediated pathways, does not accelerate gastric emptying in diabetic gastroparesis.[19] Advanced glycation end products may also contribute to the structural remodeling observed in the esophagus, stomach, and small intestine in diabetes, which potentially affects both motility and mechanosensitivity.[8]

Acute changes in glycemia can reversibly affect the function of each segment of the gastrointestinal tract, although the magnitude and consistency of these effects remain contentious.[10] In the stomach, marked hyperglycemia (blood glucose about 15 mmol/L [270 mg/dL]) slows gastric emptying and impairs both fundic and antral motility while stimulating pyloric pressures, and even modest increases in the blood glucose concentration within the physiological postprandial range (about 8 mmol/L [140 mg/dL]) retard gastric emptying. Conversely, insulin-induced hypoglycemia accelerates gastric emptying, even in patients with long-standing type 1 diabetes—a phenomenon that may serve as a counter-regulatory mechanism to hasten the absorption of carbohydrates. The impact of chronic changes in glycemia on gastric motor function is less well established. Normalization of glycemia after combined pancreas–kidney transplantation has been variously reported either to reverse gastroparesis or have no impact. A recent report suggests normalization of delayed emptying can occur in type 2 patients once glycemia is controlled[25] and the acid–base balance stabilized.

Diagnosis

Methods used to measure the rate of gastric emptying in clinical practice are discussed in detail in the chapter on gastroparesis. In patients with diabetes, the blood glucose concentration should be monitored and ideally optimized (blood glucose 4 to 10 mmol/L [70 to 180 mg/dL]) during the evaluation, and medications that may affect gastric emptying should be temporarily withheld, if possible.

Scintigraphy remains the gold standard to measure gastric emptying, and recent attempts have been made towards international standardization of this investigation.[26] Stable isotope breath tests are relatively well validated for the measurement of gastric emptying and have the advantage of being able to be performed at the point of care, with subsequent centralized analysis of stored breath samples.[19] Evaluation of gastric emptying with the wireless motility capsule SmartPill (Given Imaging) is complicated by the fact that large indigestible solids tend to empty with the return of phase III of the migrating motor complex in the stomach after a meal, the timing of which differs from the emptying of nutrient liquids and digestible solids.

Techniques that provide information about gastric volume (magnetic resonance imaging, single photon emission computed tomography, ultrasound), tone and regional pressure events (barostat, manometry), or the gastric electrical rhythm (electrogastrography) remain essentially research tools.[19]

In the past decade, new questionnaires have been validated for the evaluation of gastrointestinal symptoms in diabetes, particularly for use in clinical trials. These include the Diabetes Bowel Symptom Questionnaire[27] and the Gastroparesis Cardinal Symptom Index (GCSI).[28] The latter originated as a diary that scored 9 symptoms in the domains of nausea/vomiting, fullness/early satiety, and bloating on a 0 (none) to 5 (very severe) scale over the preceding 2 weeks. A new daily diary format (GCSI-DD) may prove more responsive to changes in symptoms over the short term.

Epidemiology

Estimates of the prevalence of gastroparesis among patients with diabetes vary depending on how gastroparesis is defined and the nature of the population in question. A recent epidemiological study from Minnesota indicated that over a 10-year period, around 5% of patients with type 1 diabetes, but only 1% of patients with type 2 diabetes, develop gastroparesis (as determined by scintigraphy or the presence of "typical" symptoms).[29] This compares to a prevalence of gastroparesis in the general population of about 10/100,000 persons for men and about

---

TABLE 23-1
TREATMENT GOALS IN DIABETIC GASTROPARESIS

Optimize glycemia

- Attempt to match the timing of delivery of exogenous insulin to nutrient absorption (consider insulin pump)

Ensure adequate nutrition

- Consider jejunal feeding

Trial of prokinetic therapy

Consider symptom-specific therapy for nausea and abdominal pain

Address psychological comorbidities

40/100,000 persons for women.[30] However, the issue is complicated by the fact that the relationship between symptoms and the presence of delayed gastric emptying is weak in most cases, and many patients with abnormally slow emptying will be relatively or totally asymptomatic, yet potentially at risk of other complications such as poor glycemic control. Data from unselected patients with type 1 and type 2 diabetes attending a tertiary referral center indicate that up to 50% have delayed emptying for solids and/or nutrient liquids,[2] with an increased prevalence in females. There are considerable implications for health care utilization given the rising prevalence of type 2 diabetes, and U.S. data indicate escalating hospital admission rates for a diagnosis of gastroparesis in recent years.[31]

The prognosis of diabetic gastroparesis remains controversial. Recent retrospective data indicate that for patients with type 1 or type 2 diabetes, there is a 3-fold increase in the prevalence of cardiovascular disease among those with gastroparesis[32]; conversely, a cohort that was followed prospectively over 25 years displayed no increased risk of mortality among those with delayed gastric emptying[33]; moreover, the rate of gastric emptying tended to remain fairly stable over time.[34]

Treatment

The goals of treatment in diabetic gastroparesis need to be individualized for particular patients[19] and do not necessarily relate directly to acceleration of gastric emptying (Table 23-1). Not infrequently, the outcome of treatment is less than satisfactory, perhaps because the pathogenesis of symptoms remains poorly characterized. The primary aims may include relief of symptoms, improvement in nutrition, or optimization of glycemic control. The latter may be of particular importance in the acutely hyperglycemic patient, given the potential for high blood glucose concentrations to impair gastric motility, exacerbate symptoms, and inhibit the effects of prokinetic drugs.

Much of the evidence concerning treatment of diabetic gastroparesis is suboptimal and based on poorly controlled data. Emerging therapies should ideally be evaluated with randomized controlled trials due to the potential for substantial placebo responses.

Nutritional guidelines are not well evidence-based, but in malnourished patients with refractory diabetic gastroparesis (> 5% weight loss in 3 months), a trial of nasojejunal tube feeding should be considered[3]; such an approach also allows the potential benefit of a more permanent percutaneous jejunal feeding tube to be evaluated. Glycemic control should be optimized, and there are uncontrolled data to support the use of insulin pumps in patients with diabetic gastroparesis for improving glycemia and reducing hospitalizations.[13]

Efforts to develop more effective pharmacological therapies for diabetic gastroparesis have been driven by the limited efficacy of existing agents, concerns about adverse effects including tardive dyskinesia with metoclopramide, and the withdrawal of drugs, particularly cisapride, from the market. The motilin agonists have been an ongoing focus of drug development, despite the lack of efficacy of alemcinal (ABT-229) in clinical trials, possibly as a result of tachyphylaxis. Another motilin agonist, mitemcinal, has demonstrated persisting acceleration of gastric emptying over 3 months in patients with diabetic gastroparesis, but symptom improvement was no greater than with placebo.[13]

There has been considerable interest in the potential for ghrelin agonists to accelerate gastric emptying in diabetic gastroparesis, and both intravenous TZP-101 and RM-131 have shown improvements in the rate of gastric emptying and symptoms when given acutely, although in more prolonged studies of the oral ghrelin agonist TZP-102, symptoms did not improve more than with placebo.[35] Therefore, further trials with other ghrelin agonists appear to be required to determine whether this class holds any promise for therapy.

The 5HT-4 agonists prucalopride and velusetrag have been shown to accelerate gastric emptying in patients with constipation—for whom they were primarily developed—but there is a lack of evidence as to whether they are beneficial in diabetic gastroparesis.[13]

Key issues for future clinical trials of prokinetic drugs include not only appropriate patient selection and trial design (including choosing the most relevant endpoints), but also the need for better understanding of drug actions and optimal dosing.[36] Motilin agonists, for example, can stimulate gastric smooth muscle contraction directly in a manner that fades with prolonged use or they can facilitate cholinergic transmission, which tends to be a longer-lasting effect; the latter is observed with the nonpeptide motilin receptor agonist camicinal (GSK962040).[37] Different drugs may potentially bind to different regions of the motilin receptor to elicit varying responses—a concept known as *biased agonism*.[36] For ghrelin receptor agonists, much less is known about the mechanism of action (eg, whether vagal or central). A deeper understanding of mechanisms is needed to guide the logical development of new prokinetic drugs.

Aside from accelerating gastric emptying, pharmacological therapy directed at specific symptoms is often used in diabetic gastroparesis. This includes antiemetics such as phenothiazines, 5HT-3 antagonists, cannabinoids, and the H1 receptor antagonist diphenhydramine, none of which have been specifically evaluated in clinical trials for their effects in patients with diabetes. A similar caveat applies to agents used to treat abdominal pain, including low-dose antidepressants, gabapentin, and pregabalin.[3]

Intrapyloric injection of botulinum toxin appeared to be a promising therapy for gastroparesis in initial open-label reports. However, two sham-controlled trials, each of which included patients with diabetic gastroparesis, failed to demonstrate a difference between toxin and saline injections for improving either symptoms or gastric emptying.[19]

Gastric electrical stimulation using the Enterra device (Medtronic) has appeared in open-label studies to deliver better symptom relief in patients with diabetic rather than idiopathic gastroparesis. In the only sham-controlled trial of this treatment in patients with diabetic gastroparesis, there was considerable reduction in vomiting frequency in the initial open-label phase of the study, but no difference in the subsequent blinded phase between periods when the stimulator was on or off,[38] indicating the need for better controlled clinical trials, ideally randomized from the outset, before the efficacy of this therapy can be established.

Modulation of Gastrointestinal Motility to Improve Glycemic Control

In considering disordered upper gastrointestinal function in diabetes, a key consideration is the interrelationship between the rate of gastric emptying and glycemia. Not only can acute changes in blood glucose affect motility, as discussed, but the motor function of the upper gut is a key determinant of the postprandial rise in blood glucose concentrations.[39] The latter predominates over fasting glycemia in its contribution to overall glycemic control—and therefore the risk of diabetic complications—in patients with a glycated hemoglobin in the lower range (less than about 7.5%), which accounts for a majority of type 2 patients in the community. Modulation of gastric emptying by pharmacological or dietary approaches can have a profound impact on glycemic control in patients with diabetes by influencing the rate at which carbohydrates are released to the small intestine for absorption. For example, slowing gastric emptying with morphine or prior consumption of a nutrient "preload" reduces the glycemic excursion in patients with type 2 diabetes after a subsequent meal, while acceleration of emptying with erythromycin substantially increases postprandial blood glucose concentrations. Patients with type 2 diabetes who are not treated with insulin may, therefore, benefit from slowing of gastric emptying, provided symptoms are not induced. Indeed, newer therapies that target postprandial glycemic control may act predominantly by retarding emptying, including the "short acting" glucagon-like peptide-1 (GLP-1) agonists exenatide BD and lixisenatide, and the amylin agonist pramlintide. Recent evidence indicates that sustained GLP-1 receptor stimulation is associated with tachyphylaxis for the initial effect to slow gastric emptying, so "long-acting" agonists (eg, liraglutide) probably do not have a major effect on gastric emptying with ongoing use.[40] Moreover, the efficacy of these drugs to improve postprandial glycemia is related to the magnitude of slowing of gastric emptying, which is, in turn, dependent on the rate of gastric emptying at baseline, so that patients who already have relatively slow gastric emptying are unlikely to benefit further from these agents. These considerations are of relevance to the increasing use of the combination of basal insulin with a GLP-1 agonist in the management of type 2 diabetes,[40] and may provide a rationale for the measurement of gastric emptying to select the appropriate therapy.

In patients with type 1 or insulin-treated type 2 diabetes, an additional consideration must be to coordinate the emptying of nutrients from the stomach with the onset of the action of exogenous insulin.[39] This may require the use of prokinetic drugs to make the former more predictable.

Changes in gastrointestinal transit of nutrients also appear to be implicated in the improvement or resolution of type 2 diabetes—independent of weight loss—that follows bariatric surgery, particularly Roux-en-Y gastric bypass (RYGB)[41]; rapid emptying of nutrients from the gastric pouch and greater access to more distal regions of the small intestine enhance the secretion of "hindgut" hormones, including GLP-1, with associated improvement in insulin secretion. It should be recognized, however, that numerous additional mechanisms potentially contribute to the amelioration of type 2 diabetes after RYGB, including exclusion of the foregut, changes in intestinal microbiota and bile acid metabolism, and shifts in small intestinal glucose metabolism.[42]

SMALL AND LARGE INTESTINE

Symptoms of diarrhea, constipation, and/or fecal incontinence are all reported substantially more frequently in people with diabetes than in controls in surveys of community-dwelling individuals,[1] as well as in the tertiary referral setting. "Diabetic diarrhea"—first described by Dooley in 1936—typically occurs in patients with a long history of type 1 diabetes, associated with peripheral and cardiac autonomic neuropathy, and with intermittent bouts of explosive, voluminous stool, which occur nocturnally as well as during the day.[43]

Pathophysiology

The rate of small intestinal transit in patients with diabetes is frequently abnormal but may be either rapid or slow[44]; the latter can contribute to diarrhea by predisposing to small bowel bacterial overgrowth. Small bowel motility is abnormal in up to 80% of patients with diabetic gastroparesis,[45] with the most characteristic feature being an early return of phase III of the migrating motor complex after a meal. Loss of adrenergic innervation of the small intestine has been reported in rodent models of diabetes, and may contribute to the etiology of diarrhea.[43]

Colonic motility has not been well studied in diabetes, but colonic transit is reported to be delayed, particularly in patients with evidence of cardiac autonomic neuropathy.[44] Analysis of tissue from patients with diabetes undergoing colectomy indicates a loss of myenteric neurons and decrease in ganglion size when compared to nondiabetic controls, with preferential loss of inhibitory nitrergic neurons associated with oxidative stress.[46] Defects of anorectal function in patients with diabetes include impaired rectal sensation to distension and dysfunction of the external anal sphincter.[44]

As in other segments of the gastrointestinal tract, lower gut function is acutely influenced by changes in blood glucose concentrations, with colonic reflexes being inhibited, rectal compliance increased, and anal sphincter pressures potentially reduced during acute hyperglycemia.[10]

Diagnosis

Medications should be specifically considered as a cause of diarrhea in patients with diabetes (Table 23-2), with metformin frequently being implicated, possibly due to its capacity to inhibit disaccharidases at the brush border. Other drug classes that should be considered as potentially contributing to diarrhea include alpha-glucosidase inhibitors (acarbose and miglitol), GLP-1 agonists, lipase inhibitors (orlistat), and sugar alcohols (sorbitol, mannitol, and xylitol).[43] The possibility of small intestinal bacterial overgrowth should be specifically considered. While jejunal fluid aspiration and culture has been considered a gold standard, it is far from perfect and generally requires endoscopy. Hydrogen breath tests, using lactulose or other substrates, lack sensitivity, but are relatively practical. Celiac disease affects around 5% of patients with type 1 diabetes, compared to perhaps 1% of the general population, and serological screening appears to be justified in this group even in the absence of gut symptoms. Up to 50% of patients with type 1 and type 2 diabetes have low levels of fecal elastase, possibly as a result of loss of trophic effects of insulin or changes in the levels of other islet hormones on the pancreas, autoimmunity, autonomic neuropathy, or because the diabetes may be a consequence of otherwise unrecognized chronic pancreatitis.[47] Many such patients may not have clinically meaningful pancreatic exocrine insufficiency,[43] and an evidence base to support the use of pancreatic enzyme replacement in this situation is currently lacking. Other diagnoses to be considered in patients with diarrhea include microscopic colitis, the incidence of which may be increased in the setting of diabetes,[43] as well as all causes of diarrhea that affect the general population, including irritable bowel syndrome. The diagnosis of diabetic diarrhea, as described earlier, is a clinical one. Finally, fecal incontinence should always be considered in patients presenting with diarrhea, and may need to be specifically elicited in the history.

The diagnostic approach to constipation and fecal incontinence in diabetes does not differ from that in nondiabetic patients. After excluding "alarm features" for malignancy and medications that may cause constipation (such as anticholinergics, opiates, or calcium channel antagonists), a therapeutic trial of a laxative is indicated, with subsequent specific evaluation for a defecatory disorder or slow colonic transit if this proves ineffective.[48]

Epidemiology

In tertiary referral populations of patients with diabetes, the prevalence of diarrhea has been reported as about 20%, and that of constipation as high as 60%.[44] These symptoms appear less common in community-based patients, albeit still increased when compared to controls—in one survey, around 15% reported diarrhea compared to 10% of controls, while symptoms of constipation were only slightly increased (11% vs. 9%). Fecal incontinence was reported by 2.6% of respondents with diabetes but only 0.8% of controls.[1]

TABLE 23-2
POTENTIAL CAUSES OF DIARRHEA IN PATIENTS WITH DIABETES

- Medications
  - Metformin
  - Acarbose or miglitol
  - GLP-1 agonists
  - Orlistat
  - Sorbitol, mannitol, or xylitol
- Small intestinal bacterial overgrowth
- Celiac disease (especially in type 1 diabetes)
- Pancreatic exocrine insufficiency
- Microscopic colitis
- Diabetic diarrhea (especially in type 1 diabetes)
- Fecal incontinence

Treatment

Treatment for diarrhea will depend on the specific cause. Antibiotic therapy, such as with rifaximin, is indicated when there is evidence of small intestinal bacterial overgrowth. Pancreatic enzyme replacement should be tried in patients with evidence of pancreatic exocrine insufficiency; this can potentially be associated with substantial improvements in postprandial glycemia in those with fat malabsorption due to the restoration of normal hormonal feedback (including the "incretin" hormones) from the small intestine.[49] In refractory cases of diabetic diarrhea, subcutaneous octreotide or oral clonidine (an alpha-2 agonist) may be effective, and there are case reports indicating benefit from 5HT-3 antagonists.[43]

Few treatments for constipation have been specifically evaluated in patients with diabetes. Recent evidence indicates that the cholinesterase inhibitor pyridostigmine improves colonic transit during 7 days of therapy[50] and the 5HT-4 agonist mosapride increases bowel frequency over 8 weeks of treatment[51] in patients with diabetes who suffer from constipation, but longer-term studies are needed.

Anorectal dysfunction in diabetes can potentially respond to biofeedback therapy.[52]

CONCLUSION

The gastrointestinal tract is increasingly recognized as being central to diabetes management. Not only does each region of the gut have the potential for dysfunction in diabetes, with consequent symptoms and impaired quality of life, but it is now appreciated that the motility of the upper gut is central to blood glucose homeostasis, particularly in the postprandial phase. Moreover, the modulation of gastric function can be used therapeutically to improve postprandial glycemic control, as reflected in the widespread adoption of drugs acting on the incretin axis.

Gastrointestinal symptoms are prevalent in diabetes, but their origin is multifactorial and their relationship to disordered motility is relatively weak. Priorities for future research include the development of a better understanding of the etiology of symptoms to develop more targeted therapies and the undertaking of well-designed randomized controlled trials to establish the efficacy and optimum use of new treatments.

REFERENCES

1. Bytzer P, Talley NJ, Leemon M, Young LJ, Jones MP, Horowitz M. Prevalence of gastrointestinal symptoms associated with diabetes mellitus: a population-based survey of 15,000 adults. *Arch Intern Med.* 2001;161:1989-1996.

2. Horowitz M, Maddox AF, Wishart JM, Harding PE, Chatterton BE, Shearman DJ. Relationships between oesophageal transit and solid and liquid gastric emptying in diabetes mellitus. *Eur J Nucl Med.* 1991;18(4):229-234.

3. Kashyap P, Farrugia G. Diabetic gastroparesis: what we have learned and had to unlearn in the past 5 years. *Gut.* 2010;59(12):1716-1726.

4. Lluch I, Ascaso JF, Mora F, et al. Gastroesophageal reflux in diabetes mellitus. *Am J Gastroenterol.* 1999;94:919-924.

5. Lee SD, Keum B, Chun HJ, Bak YT. Gastroesophageal reflux disease in type ii diabetes mellitus with or without peripheral neuropathy. *J Neurogastroenterol Motil.* 2011;17(3):274-278.

6. Mandelstam P, Lieber A. Esophageal dysfunction in diabetic neuropathy-gastroenteropathy. Clinical and roentgenological manifestations. *JAMA.* 1967;201:582-586.

7. Holloway RH, Tippett MD, Horowitz M, Maddox AF, Moten J, Russo A. Relationship between esophageal motility and transit in patients with type I diabetes mellitus. *Am J Gastroenterol.* 1999;94:3150-3157.

8. Frokjaer JB, Brock C, Brun J, et al. Esophageal distension parameters as potential biomarkers of impaired gastrointestinal function in diabetes patients. *Neurogastroenterol Motil.* 2012;24(11):1016-e1544.

9. Brock C, Graversen C, Frokjaer JB, Softeland E, Valeriani M, Drewes AM. Peripheral and central nervous contribution to gastrointestinal symptoms in diabetic patients with autonomic neuropathy. *Eur J Pain.* 2013;17(6):820-831.

10. Rayner CK, Samsom M, Jones KL, Horowitz M. Relationships of upper gastrointestinal motor and sensory function with glycemic control. *Diabetes Care.* 2001;24(2):371-381.

11. Iyer PG, Borah BJ, Heien HC, Das A, Cooper GS, Chak A. Association of Barrett's esophagus with type II diabetes mellitus: results from a large population-based case-control study. *Clin Gastroenterol Hepatol.* 2013;11(9):1108-1114, e1105.

12. Kassander P. Asymptomatic gastric retention in diabetics (gastroparesis diabeticorum). *Ann Intern Med.* 1958;48:797-812.

13. Stevens JE, Jones KL, Rayner CK, Horowitz M. Pathophysiology and pharmacotherapy of gastroparesis: current and future perspectives. *Expert Opin Pharmacother.* 2013;14(9):1171-1186.

14. Jones KL, Russo A, Stevens JE, Wishart JM, Berry MK, Horowitz M. Predictors of delayed gastric emptying in diabetes. *Diabetes Care.* 2001;24:1264-1269.

15. Parkman HP, Yates K, Hasler WL, et al. Similarities and differences between diabetic and idiopathic gastroparesis. *Clin Gastroenterol Hepatol.* 2011;9(12):1056-1064.

16. Parkman HP, Yates KP, Hasler WL, et al. Dietary intake and nutritional deficiencies in patients with diabetic or idiopathic gastroparesis. *Gastroenterology.* 2011;141(2):486-498, 498, e481-487.

17. Horowitz M, Jones KL, Rayner CK, Read NW. "Gastric" hypoglycaemia: an important concept in diabetes management. *Neurogastroenterol Motil.* 2006;18(6):405-407.

18. Jones KL, Tonkin A, Horowitz M, et al. Rate of gastric emptying is a determinant of postprandial hypotension in non-insulin-dependent diabetes mellitus. *Clin Sci.* 1998;94:65-70.

19. Thazhath SS, Jones KL, Horowitz M, Rayner CK. Diabetic gastroparesis: recent insights into pathophysiology and implications for management. *Expert Rev Gastroenterol Hepatol.* 2013;7(2):127-139.

20. Grover M, Farrugia G, Lurken MS, et al. Cellular changes in diabetic and idiopathic gastroparesis. *Gastroenterology.* 2011;140(5):1575-1585, e1578.

21. Faussone-Pellegrini MS, Grover M, Pasricha PJ, et al. Ultrastructural differences between diabetic and idiopathic gastroparesis. *J Cell Mol Med.* 2012;16(7):1573-1581.

22. Grover M, Bernard CE, Pasricha PJ, et al. Clinical-histological associations in gastroparesis: results from the Gastroparesis Clinical Research Consortium. *Neurogastroenterol Motil.* 2012;24(6):531-539, e249.

23. Kashyap P, Farrugia G. Oxidative stress: key player in gastrointestinal complications of diabetes. *Neurogastroenterol Motil.* 2011;23(2):111-114.

24. Mazzone A, Bernard CE, Strege PR, et al. Altered expression of Ano1 variants in human diabetic gastroparesis. *J Biol Chem.* 2011;286(15):13393-13403.

25. Laway BA, Malik TS, Khan SH, Rather TA. Prevalence of abnormal gastric emptying in asymptomatic women with newly detected diabetes and its reversibility after glycemic control: a prospective case control study. *J Diabetes Complications.* 2013;27(1):78-81.

26. Shin AS, Camilleri M. Diagnostic assessment of diabetic gastroparesis. *Diabetes.* 2013;62(8):2667-2673.

27. Quan C, Talley NJ, Cross S, et al. Development and validation of the Diabetes Bowel Symptom Questionnaire. *Aliment Pharmacol Ther.* 2003;17(9):1179-1187.

28. Revicki DA, Camilleri M, Kuo B, Szarka LA, McCormack J, Parkman HP. Evaluating symptom outcomes in gastroparesis clinical trials: validity and responsiveness of the Gastroparesis Cardinal Symptom Index-Daily Diary (GCSI-DD). *Neurogastroenterol Motil.* 2012;24(5):456-463, e215-456.

29. Choung RS, Locke GR, 3rd, Schleck CD, Zinsmeister AR, Melton LJ, 3rd, Talley NJ. Risk of gastroparesis in subjects with type 1 and 2 diabetes in the general population. *Am J Gastroenterol.* 2012;107(1):82-88.

30. Jung HK, Choung RS, Locke GR, 3rd, et al. The incidence, prevalence, and outcomes of patients with gastroparesis in Olmsted County, Minnesota, from 1996 to 2006. *Gastroenterology.* 2009;136(4):1225-1233.

31. Wang YR, Fisher RS, Parkman HP. Gastroparesis-related hospitalizations in the United States: trends, characteristics, and outcomes, 1995-2004. *Am J Gastroenterol.* 2008;103(2):313-322.

32. Hyett B, Martinez FJ, Gill BM, et al. Delayed radionucleotide gastric emptying studies predict morbidity in diabetics with symptoms of gastroparesis. *Gastroenterology.* 2009;137(2):445-452.

33. Chang J, Rayner CK, Jones KL, Horowitz M. Prognosis of diabetic gastroparesis: a 25-year evaluation. *Diabet Med.* 2013;30(5):e185-188.

34. Chang J, Russo A, Bound M, Rayner CK, Jones KL, Horowitz M. A 25-year longitudinal evaluation of gastric emptying in diabetes. *Diabetes Care.* 2012;35(12):2594-2596.

35. Camilleri M, Acosta A. A ghrelin agonist fails to show benefit in patients with diabetic gastroparesis: let's not throw the baby out with the bath water. *Neurogastroenterol Motil.* 2013;25(11):859-863.

36. Sanger GJ. Ghrelin and motilin receptor agonists: time to introduce bias into drug design. *Neurogastroenterol Motil.* 2014;26(2):149-155.

37. Depoortere I. Can small non-peptide motilin agonists force a breakthrough as gastroprokinetic drugs? *Br J Pharmacol.* 2012;167(4):760-762.

38. McCallum RW, Snape W, Brody F, Wo J, Parkman HP, Nowak T. Gastric electrical stimulation with Enterra therapy improves symptoms from diabetic gastroparesis in a prospective study. *Clin Gastroenterol Hepatol.* 2010;8(11):947-954.

39. Marathe CS, Rayner CK, Jones KL, Horowitz M. Relationships between gastric emptying, postprandial glycemia, and incretin hormones. *Diabetes Care.* 2013;36(5):1396-1405.

40. Horowitz M, Rayner CK, Jones KL. Mechanisms and clinical efficacy of lixisenatide for the management of type 2 diabetes. *Adv Ther.* 2013;30(2):81-101.

41. Salehi M, D'Alessio DA. Effects of glucagon-like peptide-1 to mediate glycemic effects of weight loss surgery. *Rev Endocr Metab Disord.* 2014;15(3):171-179.

42. Rubino F, Amiel SA. Is the gut the "sweet spot" for the treatment of diabetes? *Diabetes.* 2014;63(7):2225-2228.

43. Gould M, Sellin JH. Diabetic diarrhea. *Curr Gastroenterol Rep.* 2009;11(5):354-359.

44. Phillips LK, Rayner CK, Jones KL, Horowitz M. An update on autonomic neuropathy affecting the gastrointestinal tract. *Curr Diab Rep.* 2006;6(6):417-423.

45. Camilleri M, Malagelada JR. Abnormal intestinal motility in diabetics with the gastroparesis syndrome. *Eur J Clin Invest.* 1984;14(6):420-427.

46. Chandrasekharan B, Anitha M, Blatt R, et al. Colonic motor dysfunction in human diabetes is associated with enteric neuronal loss and increased oxidative stress. *Neurogastroenterol Motil.* 2011;23(2):131-138, e126.

47. Hardt PD, Ewald N. Exocrine pancreatic insufficiency in diabetes mellitus: a complication of diabetic neuropathy or a different type of diabetes? *Exp Diabetes Res.* 2011;2011:761950.

48. Bharucha AE, Dorn SD, Lembo A, Pressman A. American Gastroenterological Association medical position statement on constipation. *Gastroenterology.* 2013;144(1):211-217.

49. Kuo P, Stevens JE, Russo A, et al. Gastric emptying, incretin hormone secretion, and postprandial glycemia in cystic fibrosis - effects of pancreatic enzyme supplementation. *J Clin Endocrinol Metab.* 2011;96(5):E851-E855.

50. Bharucha AE, Low P, Camilleri M, et al. A randomized controlled study of the effect of cholinesterase inhibition on colon function in patients with diabetes mellitus and constipation. *Gut.* 2013;62(5):708-715.

51. Ueno N, Inui A, Satoh Y. The effect of mosapride citrate on constipation in patients with diabetes. *Diabetes Res Clin Pract.* 2010;87(1):27-32.

52. Wald A, Tunuguntla AK. Anorectal sensorimotor dysfunction in fecal incontinence and diabetes mellitus. Modification with biofeedback therapy. *N Engl J Med.* 1984;310:1282-1287.

24

Scleroderma and the Gut

Deborah M. Bethards, MD and Ann Ouyang, MD

KEY POINTS

- Involvement of the gastrointestinal (GI) tract is very common in scleroderma.
- Symptoms resulting from GI involvement should be queried, as they are present in almost 90% of patients.
- Management of reflux to prevent complications, as well as management of gastroparesis and small bowel bacterial overgrowth, is recommended.
- Malnutrition is a common complication in scleroderma.

INTRODUCTION AND DEFINITION

Scleroderma and other connective tissue diseases, such as systemic lupus erythematosus (SLE), rheumatoid arthritis, dermatomyositis, Behcet disease, and polyarteritis nodosa, as well as other vasculitides, are uncommon but have the potential to be profoundly life altering to patients. Most of these chronic inflammatory autoimmune disorders result in multisystem disease, including abnormalities in the GI tract. Motility disorders have been most clearly associated with systemic sclerosis (SSc), but have been described in other collagen vascular disorders. This chapter will focus on the effects of SSc on the GI tract, especially as it relates to motility issues. Gut involvement impacts morbidity and mortality in patients with SSc and can occur in as many as 90% of these patients.[1]

Systemic sclerosis results from three pathologic processes: cellular, humoral autoimmunity, and specific vascular changes. The pathophysiology of GI dysmotility is still incompletely understood, but is felt to result from vascular ischemia followed by fibrosis of the lamina propria, as well as neural dysfunction, which may involve antibody inhibition of muscarinic enteric cholinergic neurotransmission.[2] Sclerodermatous GI involvement is a major source of morbidity but is the cause

Rao SSC, Parkman HP, McCallum RW, eds.
Handbook of Gastrointestinal Motility and Functional Disorders (pp 303-321).
© 2015 Taylor & Francis Group.

of death in only 11% of cases.[3] Early occurrence of severe gut dysmotility in SSc is associated with a poor outcome, with a 9-year cumulative survival rate of only 15%.[2] If questioned directly, almost all patients with SSc have some GI symptoms Not only does SSc result in GI, renal, cardiac, skin, pulmonary, and immunologic abnormalities, but also is associated with an increased risk of malignancy, the most common of which are of lung and breast.[5]

Scleroderma is a rare, complex, fibrosing disease with an insidious onset and unknown etiology, occurring most frequently in females from 35 to 65 years old; there is evidence for etiologic factors related to genetics and the environment.[1] It is generally described in two forms: limited cutaneous SSc and diffuse SSc, with a common feature being ultimately a fibrosing disease. The GI tract is commonly involved in both subsets of SSc. Systemic or organ involvement in the limited cutaneous form develops later and frequently involves the esophagus, but not as often the heart or kidneys, and is more frequent in adults than in children. Characteristic antibodies found in the limited cutaneous form include antinuclear antibodies (ANA) and anticentromere antibodies (anti-CENP). Patients with diffuse SSc may have early diffuse fibrosis of the esophagus, lungs, heart, and kidneys. Characteristic serologies in this group also include a positive ANA (found in >90% SSc patients overall), as well as Scl-70, otherwise known as antitopoisomerase I. Other SSc-related antibodies are anti-RNA polymerase III.[6]

Pathophysiology

Although the definitive pathogenic course of SSc remains unknown, studies from animal models indicate a sequence of pathogenic events involving a complex interaction between multiple cell types during the evolution of SSc.[2] This sequence starts with microvascular change and endothelial activation followed by immune cell activation (B-cells, T-cells, and macrophages), with the development of autoantibodies and release of cytokines and growth factors. This vasculopathy results in repeated ischemic events; the reparative and immunological events are "inappropriate" and result in collagen deposition. Subsequently, through presumed mediator interaction, profibrotic fibroblastic cell proliferation occurs with ensuing fibrosis.

Genetic factors are probably important in the pathogenesis of SSc, and there is increasing evidence to support this, although no gene has yet been identified. That there is a genetic predisposition is suggested by the fact that familial aggregation (multiple families with 2 or more members affected with SSc) is a risk factor for developing the disease even though the frequency is low (1.2% to 1.5% of SSc families), and there is the higher prevalence of autoimmune diseases and antibodies in relatives of patients with SSc. There is also interest in whether extracellular matrix genes such as fibrillin-1 can contribute to the inheritance of the disease.

Possible environmental etiologies are always intriguing. One hypothesis is that exposure to chemicals (including silica, solvents, silicone, and epoxy resins) and viruses (high prevalence of cytomegalovirus [CMV] antibodies have been found) may activate mononuclear cells, resulting in the release of cytokines and connective tissue growth factor.

CLINICAL FEATURES AND PATHOPHYSIOLOGY

The GI tract is one of the most commonly involved organs in SSc, with progressive changes throughout the GI tract. Collagen replaces vascular and enteric smooth muscle and results in autonomic dysfunction with consequent smooth muscle changes resulting in reduction or loss of motility and luminal dilatation, as well as "tensile rigidity" and eventual organ failure. Abnormalities of the esophagus and anorectum are most commonly reported (in up to 80% of patients).[1] These changes also occur in other connective tissue disorders. Diseases of the pancreas and liver have also been described. Gastrointestinal involvement is subclinical in about 30% of patients with SSc, but can result in high morbidity and can even be life threatening.[7] It has been reported that sleep disturbance is worse in patients with GI symptoms, mostly due to symptoms related to reflux, but also those with abdominal bloating, early satiety, nausea and vomiting, and changes in bowel habits. Survival rates are probably lower in SSc patients with GI disease than those without. Although GI involvement is common, severe GI tract involvement is less frequent (8%) than the presence of severe skin thickening (24%), severe heart disease (15%), and severe pulmonary fibrosis (15%).[8]

Esophagus

Table 24-1 summarizes the motility changes seen with SSc. More than 50% of SSc patients have esophageal disease, specifically in the distal two-thirds of the esophagus where the pathologic lesion is atrophy of the smooth muscle (muscularis propria). The function of the upper esophageal sphincter (UES), pharynx, and proximal skeletal muscle is spared. Later, collagen deposition results in fibrosis and thickening of the serosal layer.[1] Although definite changes occur in the vasculature as well as the nerves, there is controversy about the order of involvement. One hypothesis is that hypoperfusion occurs initially and ischemia results in microvascular changes (fibrotic cuffing around the artery), as well as concurrent collagen infiltration. Once fibrosis occurs, the smooth muscle function is compromised. Autonomic dysfunction also impacts esophageal and lower esophageal sphincter (LES) function. When asked directly, up to 80% of patients with SSc complain of heartburn, and nearly 60% of nausea.[4] Esophageal motility disorders have also been described in other connective tissue disorders. Dysphagia in a patient with lupus has been described from vagal nerve dysfunction secondary to brainstem vasculitis.[9] Amyloid deposits in the esophagus may affect swallowing in patients with long-standing rheumatoid arthritis. Involvement of other organs by amyloid and the presence of amyloidosis on biopsies from the GI tract correlate highly with finding amyloid deposits on renal biopsies. Dysphagia from esophageal hypomotility has been reported in up to 35% of patients with dermatomyositis/polymyositis in a retrospective study of 79 consecutive patients with these disorders.[10]

Patients' symptoms closely mirror these esophageal changes and include dysphagia for liquids and solids, heartburn, and regurgitation in as many as 82% of SSc patients. Patients may have esophageal involvement with SSc without symptoms.[1] Esophageal motility studies may demonstrate low amplitude but peristaltic contraction in the distal two-thirds of the esophagus initially, with loss of peristalsis as the disease progresses. The LES pressure is often low and can be found before the clinical diagnosis of scleroderma is made (see Figure 24-1). Dysphagia is usually related to esophageal dysmotility with abnormal bolus transit, as well as esophageal reflux, but can also be from secondary esophagitis and strictures. Heartburn is normally worse at night or postprandially. The lack of buffering capacity of saliva resulting from Sjogren syndrome in scleroderma increases the potential for mucosal damage from acid reflux. As the disease worsens, patients can experience early satiety, regurgitation of food, malnutrition, and even food bolus impaction requiring intervention. Impaired esophageal clearance may result in drug-induced esophagitis with drugs such as quinidine, potassium chloride, bisphosphonates, and nonsteroidal anti-inflammatory drugs (NSAIDs).

As a result of these esophageal dysfunctions, SSc patients are at risk for associated complications that include gastroesophageal reflux disease (GERD) with secondary esophagitis, Barrett's esophagus, and strictures (seen in approximately 40%). Dysfunction of the LES and delayed gastric emptying contribute to GERD, and loss of esophageal clearance increases the risk of subsequent complications. In the setting of acid suppression and immunosuppressive therapy, infectious esophagitis related to *Candida*, CMV, or herpes virus is seen. There is no evidence that GERD is caused by excess transient lower esophageal sphincter relaxations (TLESRs).[1]

Complications of GERD are the same as those found in non-SSc patients: erosive esophagitis (seen in about 60%), GI bleeding (usually secondary to telangiectasias, which are more common in CREST than SSc), Barrett's metaplasia (prevalence estimates range from 2% to 37%),

---

TABLE 24-1
PATHOPHYSIOLOGIC PROCESSES SEEN IN THE GASTROINTESTINAL TRACT IN SYSTEMIC SCLEROSIS

I. Esophageal dysfunction

    A. Esophageal dysmotility — see Figures 24-1 and 24-2 low-amplitude but peristaltic contractions (especially distally) absent peristalsis

    B. Lower esophageal sphincter (LES) dysfunction — see Figure 24-2

        1. Abnormal LES relaxation as well as closure

        2. Reduced LES pressure

        3. Total LES incompetence

    C. Impaired coordination between the distal esophagus and LES[7]

    D. Shortening of the esophagus

    E. Hiatal hernia secondary to esophageal shortening

    F. Decreased esophageal mucosal resistance

    G. Loss of normal esophageal clearance secondary to dysmotility and reflux[3,7]

    H. Loss of buffering by saliva secondary to Sjogren syndrome

II. Gastric dysfunction: Delayed gastric emptying/gastroparesis: autonomic dysfunction results in abnormal tonic contraction of the proximal stomach and antroduodenal incoordination. Antroduodenal incoordination may result in delayed emptying of solids as well as liquids.

    A. Alteration in gastric accommodation: autonomic dysfunction may result in impaired gastric compliance

    B. Abnormal gastric myoelectric activity and motility secondary to the following:

        1. Phases I and II of the interdigestive MMCs are less frequent and of lower amplitude.

        2. Phase III MMCs are decreased in frequency and amplitude, resulting in decreased antral contractility and impaired antral "pump."

        3. Reduced frequency of slow waves (bradygastria) and decreased slow-wave amplitude postprandially are found. Tachygastria may also occur.

III. Small bowel dysfunction

    A. Decreased/abnormal small bowel motility, both fasting and postprandially (decreased motility index, ie, small-amplitude contractions)

    B. Increased bowel wall stiffness (probably due to collagen)

    C. Low wall tension (due to atrophy of the muscularis)

    D. Duodenal dilatation

(continued)

---

and carcinoma. Other maladies such as mouth ulcers, cough, hoarseness, asthma, and pneumonia occur. Gastroesophageal reflux disease has been postulated to play a role in the pathogenesis of lung fibrosis in SSc.[2] In patients with severe esophageal dysmotility, dysphagia results primarily from the motility disorder and not from stricture and may not improve after esophageal dilatation or medical therapy.

TABLE 24-1 (CONTINUED)

PATHOPHYSIOLOGIC PROCESSES SEEN IN THE GASTROINTESTINAL TRACT IN SYSTEMIC SCLEROSIS

E. Absent MMCs (in 25%), reduced-amplitude MMCs (100%), slow propagation of MMCs (83%)[13]

F. Lack of phase III of the IMMC is associated with stasis of the small bowel contents, which contributes to small bowel bacterial overgrowth

IV. Colonic dysfunction

A. Loss of gastrocolonic response

B. Colonic dilatation, loss of haustrations

C. Formation of wide-mouthed diverticula (all 3 layers of bowel involved, ie, "true" diverticula); these diverticula seem to resolve with worsening atrophy and rigidity of the colonic wall

D. Delay in whole gut transit time

E. Fluid residuals in colonic lumen

F. Antibodies to muscarinic M3 receptor[2]

V. Rectoanal dysfunction

A. Internal anal sphincter resting tone is decreased (mostly smooth muscle)

B. There is usually normal EAS/skeletal muscle function, and thus a normal or slightly decreased maximal squeeze pressure

C. Rectoanal inhibitory reflex (RAIR) is decreased or absent in 12% to 80% of patients, suggesting neuronal abnormality

D. Imaging indicates a thin hyperechoic IAS (fibrotic)

E. Antibodies to muscarinic M3 receptor[2]

Stomach

Table 24-1 summarizes the changes seen with SSc. Similar pathologic changes are found in the stomach in about 50% of patients with SSc, with collagen and elastic fibers surrounding edematous nerves and smooth muscle cells as seen on electron microscopy. The lumen of the microvasculature may be partly or completely occluded by red blood cells and neutrophils, contributing to ischemic damage.[1-3] These histological changes are associated with significant morbidity and mortality.

The symptoms are similar to those found in patients with gastroparesis from any cause and include nausea, vomiting, bloating, heartburn, regurgitation, epigastric or retrosternal pain, and early satiety. All of these symptoms can lead to significant weight loss and malnutrition. Interestingly, patients with a low body mass index (BMI) have delayed gastric emptying, especially if the BMI is less than 20.[3]

In one study of 38 SSc patients, dyspepsia was described as "gastric fullness," and these patients complained of epigastric pain/burning, belching/burping, and fullness; epigastric fullness was the main symptom and was found in both the fasting and the postprandial state. In those with normal

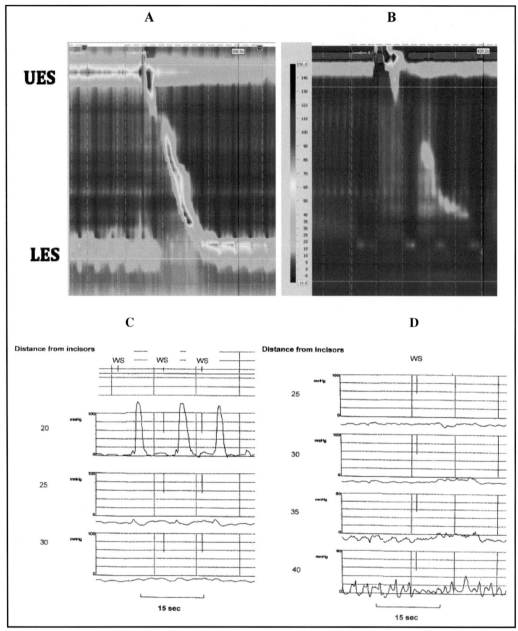

Figure 24-1. Esophageal motility in scleroderma. (A) High-resolution manometry in a normal subject. Relaxation of upper esophageal sphincter (UES) with a wet swallow, followed by a peristaltic contraction down the body of the esophagus and accompanied by relaxation of the lower esophageal sphincter. (B) High-resolution manometry in a patient with scleroderma. Normal UES relaxation and proximal esophageal contraction. Low-amplitude contractions in esophageal body. Very low resting LES pressure. (C) Pressure tracing in the esophagus of a patient with scleroderma. Normal contraction in upper esophageal body. (D) Loss of peristalsis and low-amplitude contractions in mid and distal body and low LES pressure.

gastric emptying, there was still dyspepsia in 35% of the patients. The investigators attributed the symptom to the patients having a "small and stiff antral area" rather than gastric emptying abnormality and hypothesized an altered smooth muscle basal tone.[1-2]

In addition to the motility disorders seen commonly in SSc, patients may develop gastric antral vascular ectasia (GAVE) involving the antrum that may result in melena and anemia.[12]

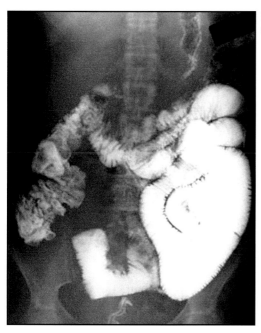

Figure 24-2. Small bowel x-ray in patient with scleroderma showing hide-bound thickened folds in jejunum.

This is usually treated endoscopically using argon plasma coagulation. Gastrointestinal bleeding in scleroderma can occur as a result of erosive esophagitis, GAVE, or wide-mouthed colonic diverticula.

Small Bowel

Table 24-1 summarizes the changes seen with SSc. The small bowel has been less well studied than other areas of the GI tract. The same pathological changes of smooth muscle atrophy and replacement with collagen and fibrotic tissue are found (Figure 24-2). Reports indicate that between 17% and 57% of patients are affected by small bowel sclerodermatous disease.[1-3] Again, there is significant morbidity attached to small bowel disease, and up to 12% may die from related complications.

Systemic sclerosis patients with small bowel involvement have a variety of symptoms and possible complications, but have rapid progression and subsequent deterioration if followed over 5 years.[13] Symptoms related to small bowel disease in SSc are generally very severe and difficult to manage, although many patients with delayed small bowel transit may be asymptomatic, leading to an underdiagnosis or delayed diagnosis of small bowel involvement. The most common symptoms are bloating, nausea, vomiting, and abdominal pain. A study of the distensibility of the duodenum in patients with SSc demonstrated that the duodenal wall is stiffer in patients compared to controls, and patients complained of greater pain at any given strain, where strain is a measure of the fractional increase in radius.[14] Due to the altered small bowel motility with loss of the interdigestive motor complex, small bowel bacterial overgrowth occurs, resulting in diarrhea, and later may contribute to complications including malabsorption. Protein-losing enteropathy may ensue. There is concern that chronic proton pump inhibitor (PPI) treatment may result in achlorhydria and predispose patients to bacterial overgrowth.[1] Small bowel bacterial overgrowth is reported in up to 40% of SSc patients. Thus, diarrhea can result from abnormal motility, bacterial overgrowth, or perhaps even vascular insufficiency.

Iron deficiency results from the dysmotility, leading to small bowel bacterial overgrowth, abnormal absorptive surface (although some report only minimal villous atrophy), and vascular destruction; ascorbic acid and folate are absorbed normally, but B_{12} is not (the bacteria ingest the vitamin).[3] Where there is smooth muscle atrophy and replacement with fibrotic tissue, there can be the development of small bowel (jejunal) diverticula. These diverticula consist of all layers of the bowel wall and can be a rare cause of perforation and bleeding. Associated celiac disease can also be a cause of malabsorption.[15]

A rare GI complication of SSc is pneumatosis cystoides intestinalis (PCI) in which multiple air-filled cysts develop in the small bowel wall (probably related to fibrotic changes, especially in the jejunum) and can rupture, causing pneumoperitoneum.[1] Pneumoperitoneum can also occur without concurrent PCI and can be found radiologically without evidence of peritonitis. Although PCI is often considered a benign condition, its finding in SSc is felt to be a poor prognostic sign.

Probably the most difficult complication to manage is chronic intestinal pseudoobstuction (CIPO) that can occur in the small or large bowel as a result of SSc and other mixed connective tissue diseases such as SLE. By definition, there is no mechanical obstruction to the flow of bowel contents, despite radiologic changes of segmental bowel dilatation, in contrast to functional small bowel disorders in which there is no radiologic dilatation.[16] It is important to exclude mechanical obstruction before making this diagnosis. Symptoms referable to CIPO include bloating, abdominal fullness, nausea, malaise, and abdominal pain; acute exacerbations may require hospitalization due to severe intractable vomiting, pain, and resulting dehydration. Once smooth muscle atrophy and fibrosis have developed in SSc, medical treatment of CIPO with prokinetics is ineffective. Chronic intestinal pseudoobstuction has been described in dermatomyositis and polymyositis and is rare in SLE. Case reports in SLE suggest that small intestine involvement results from vasculitis and may be reversible with treatment.

Colon

Table 24-1 summarizes the changes seen with SSc. Colonic involvement in SSc occurs in between 10% and 50% of patients and usually affects the entire colon (pancolonic). Reduced colonic motility correlates with a longer duration of SSc and with aperistalsis in the esophagus.[17]

Patients can present with diarrhea or constipation, and therefore sclerodermatous colonic disease can be overlooked and is probably underreported.[4] Colonic involvement of SSc can result in CIPO, as was noted earlier with small bowel disease. Whether patients develop diarrhea or constipation with diffuse intestinal dysmotility in SSc depends on which is more predominant: small bowel dysmotility and bacterial overgrowth or colonic inertia. Other factors contributing to diarrhea include decrease in colonic surface area and permeability, lymphatic fibrosis (through the same mechanism as other GI tract involvement), and reduced blood flow due to vascular involvement. Colonic inertia and delayed colonic transit result in constipation.[1]

Complications of SSc in the colon include perforation, which is rare but can be asymptomatic and found only at autopsy and is thought to be secondary to an atrophic thin bowel wall with possible ischemia. Severe constipation can result in stercoral ulcers (from stool impaction, especially in the rectosigmoid area), rectal prolapse, volvulus (secondary to dilated and elongated bowel), PCI (resulting in pain, diarrhea/constipation, mucus/bloody rectal drainage), and bowel ischemia/infarction (rare). Pneumoperitoneum from ruptured cysts in PCI is usually benign, but can be confused with colonic perforation. Disordered motility is not commonly described in SLE, where colonic involvement usually results from ischemia and results in ulceration and can proceed to perforation.[17] Colonic dysmotility is not a complication of dermatomyositis/polymyositis. It should be remembered that an underlying malignancy is found in almost 50% of older patients developing these connective tissue disorders (particularly dermatomyositis), with colon cancer being one of the most common.

Rectum and Anus

Table 24-1 summarizes the changes seen with SSc. SSc involvement of the rectum results from atrophy and fibrosis of the circular and longitudinal muscles, and sclerosis of small arteries and arterioles that supply the muscles and nerves. The internal anal sphincter (IAS) is a continuation of the smooth circular muscle of the rectum and is responsible for 85% of the resting pressure, whereas the external anal sphincter (EAS) is skeletal muscle and contributes about 15% of the resting pressure. In SSc, the smooth muscle of the IAS is abnormal, eventually resulting in fibrosis.[2,3] Interestingly, the sphincter pressures, although lower than normal, are similar between patients with scleroderma with symptoms and those without symptoms. Endoanal ultrasound shows atrophy of the IAS in patients with scleroderma, again in both symptomatic and asymptomatic patients,[2] suggesting that muscle atrophy is not the primary cause of incontinence. Others have found circulating autoantibodies to the cholinergic muscarinic M3 receptor on both nerves and muscles. Pooled IgG from patients with scleroderma inhibits the response of the internal anal muscle from the rat IAS and colon to bethanechol, an inhibition that is prevented by pooled IgG from normals.[2]

Clinical sequelae of these changes include fecal incontinence in up to 40% of patients and rectal prolapse from straining and submucosal weakness. Fecal incontinence is quite disabling and may be underreported by patients.

Liver, Biliary, Gallbladder, and Pancreas

Eighteen percent of patients with primary biliary cirrhosis (PBC) have SSc; it is usually found in the limited cutaneous form and most often begins after the onset of SSc. Nodular regenerative hyperplasia of the liver has also been described and may lead to portal hypertension.[18]

In a small study, fasting gallbladder volumes and gallbladder emptying were no different in patients with SSc compared to healthy controls, while gallbladder refilling was delayed in patients with SSc and dyspepsia patients, with a delayed refilling time being found only in those patients with delayed gastric emptying.[11] No such correlation was found in dyspeptic patients. Reduced exocrine pancreatic function may be found in 30% of SSc patients, but the clinical significance of this is unclear; it does appear that levels of amylase and lipase are reduced postprandially.[19]

NUTRITIONAL IMPACT OF SYSTEMIC SCLEROSIS

Malnutrition and weight loss have been reported in up to 56% of SSc patients with GI tract involvement (usually with severe or end-stage disease), although BMI and serum albumin do not seem to be accurate parameters to follow in them. Two tools, the Subjective Global Assessment (SGA) and the Malnutrition University Screening Tool (MUST), may be helpful in predicting patients at risk for malnutrition. Nutritional supplementation and support may impact not only quality of life, but also progression of debilitation.[2,20] Two percent of patients may eventually become dependent on parenteral nutrition because of intestinal failure, although there is not much information about the rate of nutritional decline in these patients. It has also been recognized that other SSc-related organ diseases (cardiac, pulmonary), mood disorders, and other functional issues affect oral intake and nutrition.[21]

Diagnostic Testing

The current and "future" diagnostic modalities available for motility testing related to SSc and other connective tissue diseases is ever expanding and becoming a topic unto itself. There is much ongoing research investigating testing methods for a better understanding of GI dysmotility. Details of the methodology of the studies that are available are outlined in early chapters in this book. Tables 24-2 to 24-6 summarize expected findings on these studies in patients with SSc and other connective tissue disorders where data are available. Studies are organized by area of the GI tract involved and clinical problem associated with SSc. Where available, comparisons have been made with the findings in other collagen vascular disorders.

Appropriate studies should be chosen based on symptom complex and the likelihood that the results of the study will impact treatment. For example, all patients complaining of dysphagia should undergo an endoscopy to evaluate for stricture, esophagitis, and Barrett's. If no stricture is found, an esophageal motility study is helpful to determine the severity of dysmotility in the patient. Evidence of poor esophageal clearance by scintigraphy or barium study may also help in decisions about methods of enteral feeding. Gastric emptying studies will be important in patients in whom enteral feeding options are being considered and if promotility agents beyond metoclopramide are being considered, as these would involve off-label use of medications. Small intestine motility studies are still primarily research tools, but may be important in determining whether a patient is likely to respond to promotility agents. Finding loss of contractile activity with or without motilin agonists or cholinesterase inhibitors suggests that there is smooth muscle atrophy or fibrosis, and it is unlikely that any pharmacologic agents will improve the contractility of the end organ, the smooth muscle. Tests of bacterial overgrowth, such as breath tests, may be helpful to determine bacterial overgrowth, but if not readily available, a trial of antibiotics and evaluation of clinical response is an acceptable approach.

It should be remembered that many patients might be asymptomatic early on but still have evidence of dysmotility on testing. Early treatment may alter progression of the clinical course, such as targeting the inflammatory sequences that lead to a fibrotic response. A similar approach has been reported to be successful in a very limited number of patients with SLE.[3] As future treatments become available, we should be challenged to determine what disease processes are occurring in the event that we can intervene early on and perhaps improve morbidity in these patients (see the "Treatment" section later).

Epidemiology

The epidemiology of SSc is difficult to study because of its variable presentation and geographical variation.[22] Prevalence is strongly influenced by early diagnosis and prolonged survival, which have improved in SSc over the last decades. The reported prevalence ranges widely from 7/million to 489/million. It is higher in the United States (240/million) and Australia than in many other countries and may rise with improved survival.

The annual incidence of SSc in the United States is 1 to 2/100,000 adults and may be increasing. It occurs more frequently in women (3 to 4:1), with initial symptoms presenting in the third to fifth decade.[23]

Several studies indicate an ethnic difference with a higher incidence of SSc and more serious disease in the Black population, with Black women developing the disease earlier than white women. Whether there is a genetic basis for SSc is not yet clear, but studies suggest an association of the disease with chromosome 15 near the fibrillin locus. Supporting a possible genetic or environmental determinant is a recent Canadian study of North American natives, suggesting that this group has a distinct clinical phenotype, with presentation at a younger age, more severe Raynaud

TABLE 24-2

ESOPHAGUS: MOTILITY STUDIES IN SCLERODERMA AND OTHER COLLAGEN VASCULAR DISORDERS (WHERE AVAILABLE)[2,3,35]

TEST/STUDY	POSSIBLE/EXPECTED RESULTS IN SCLERODERMA	DIFFERENTIAL DIAGNOSIS AND FINDINGS IN OTHER COLLAGEN VASCULAR DISORDERS
Upper endoscopy (EGD)	Dilatation of esophagus Changes of reflux/esophagitis Stricture Barrett's esophagus Candida esophagitis Pill-induced esophagitis Retained food	Achalasia: dilated esophagus and esophagitis from food retention GERD: Barrett's and/or stricture/esophagitis Pill-induced esophagitis Amyloid complicating rheumatoid arthritis Dermatomyositis/polymyositis esophageal hypomotility
Esophagram/radiologic studies	Dilatation and shortening of esophagus Hiatal hernia Reflux Stricture/rings Perforation Delayed emptying Air in esophagus without A/F level	Achalasia: dilated esophagus with tapering at gastroesophageal junction ("bird beak"); delayed emptying; esophageal A/F level Myasthenia gravis — pharyngeal weakness SLE myopathy involving pharyngeal and laryngeal muscles SLE vasculitis involving brainstem and affecting vagal nerves
Esophageal manometry (traditional or high resolution)	Upper esophageal sphincter (UES) pressure can be low, normal, or high Preserved proximal contraction and amplitudes Absent or decreased amplitude contraction in distal two-thirds of esophagus Aperistalsis of mid and distal esophagus Low or normal LES pressure Abnormal LES opening and incomplete closure	Achalasia: no preservation of proximal esophageal contraction; aperistalsis; often elevated LES pressure with incomplete or poorly coordinated relaxation Mixed connective tissue disease and SLE (lupus): decreased LES pressure; normal proximal contractions; low-amplitude simultaneous contractions in distal two-thirds of esophagus Amyloidosis: low LES pressure; low-amplitude contractions in distal esophagus Dermatomyositis/polymyositis: decreased amplitude of contraction of esophageal body

(*continued*)

TABLE 24-2 (CONTINUED)

ESOPHAGUS: MOTILITY STUDIES IN SCLERODERMA AND OTHER COLLAGEN VASCULAR DISORDERS (WHERE AVAILABLE)[2,3,35]

TEST/STUDY	POSSIBLE/EXPECTED RESULTS IN SCLERODERMA	DIFFERENTIAL DIAGNOSIS AND FINDINGS IN OTHER COLLAGEN VASCULAR DISORDERS
pH/impedance	Normal bolus transit until amplitude of contraction is <30 mm Hg Abnormal bolus transit Increase in aperistalsis with more frequent/longer reflux events Decrease in esophageal pH due to loss of salivary bicarbonate (in 50% to 80% of patients) Delayed clearance from distal esophagus	Achalasia: delayed bolus clearance from proximal esophagus GERD: variable dysfunction of LES and increased frequency of TLESR
Scintigraphy	Abnormal in >50%	
Endoluminal ultrasound	Hyperechoic changes in muscularis propria (fibrosis)	
High-resolution CT	Esophageal dilatation	Esophageal dilatation and air/fluid level in esophagus in achalasia

phenomenon, and greater severity of GI symptoms other than esophageal dysmotility, which was similar to that found in White and non-White, non-North American natives.[24]

About 10% of adults with SSc note the onset of symptoms during childhood. A review of patients less than 16 years of age in 270 pediatric rheumatologic centers worldwide noted less internal organ involvement in pediatric disease than in adults.[25] Specifically, involvement of the heart, kidneys, and brain were rare, whereas pulmonary and GI disease were most common. In children, the female to male ratio is 3.6:1, the mean age of onset of disease is 8 years, and a family history of autoimmune or rheumatologic disease has been identified in 11.5% of childhood SSc. Raynaud's and musculoskeletal system disease occur in 75% and 30%, respectively, in childhood (juvenile) SSc. In terms of serologic testing, ANA as well as Scl-70 were more likely to be found than anti-CEMP (81%, 34%, and 7%, respectively). From a GI perspective, gastroesophageal reflux (GER) and/or dysmotility was less frequent in children, occurring in only 8% of juvenile SSc compared with 79% of adult patients.

It appears that patients who do not develop severe organ involvement in the first 5 years of disease have a better survival rate, but the overall mortality in SSc is clearly higher than in the general population. The organ involvement may be associated with specific autoantibodies, as GI involvement also appears to be less in patients with anti-PM/Scl antibodies.[26]

Table 24-3

Stomach: Motility Studies in Scleroderma and Other Collagen Vascular Disorders (Where Available)[2,3,35]

TEST/STUDY	POSSIBLE/EXPECTED RESULTS IN SCLERODERMA	DIFFERENTIAL DIAGNOSIS AND RESULTS IN OTHER COLLAGEN VASCULAR DISORDERS
Upper endoscopy (EGD)	Food/debris/bezoar NSAID ulcers Gastric outlet obstruction Decreased gastric contractility Minimal relaxation with glucagon	SLE and vasculitides— ulceration in stomach and duodenum
Gastric scintigraphy	Decreased emptying of solids and liquids (solids slower) Decreased antral distention (increased stiffness)	Decreased rate of emptying of solids in all conditions with severe antral ulcerations
SmartPill (Given Imaging)	Prolonged gastric dwell time	
UGI/radiologic study	Delayed contrast emptying	
Antroduodenal manometry	Antral hypomotility Decreased number of MMCs Decreased amplitude of MMCs	
EGG	Abnormal electrical activity Bradygastria	

TREATMENT

Although the evaluation of dysmotility in SSc, other collagen vascular diseases, and all other motility disorders has improved dramatically over the last 15 years, the treatment regimens unfortunately remain limited. Testing and treatment of neurogastroenterology and motility disorders can be a challenging area for both patients and physicians; this is no less true in SSc and the collagen vascular diseases. An attempt to "reset autoimmunity" by hematopoietic stem cell transplantation is being investigated.[27] Guidelines for management of patients with scleroderma have been proposed by some European organizations, and with respect to the GI tract include PPIs to prevent SSc-related complications; prokinetics for the management of motility disturbances such as GERD, delayed gastric emptying, bloating, and pseudoobstruction; and management of small bowel bacterial overgrowth with antibiotics.[28]

In the GI tract, the possible and proposed treatments of scleroderma are specific to symptoms, and they can be outlined as follows:

TABLE 24-4
SMALL BOWEL: MOTILITY STUDIES IN SCLERODERMA AND OTHER COLLAGEN VASCULAR DISORDERS (WHERE AVAILABLE)[2,3,35]

TEST/STUDY	POSSIBLE/EXPECTED RESULTS IN SCLERODERMA	DIFFERENTIAL DIAGNOSIS AND RESULTS IN OTHER COLLAGEN VASCULAR DISORDERS
Small bowel follow-through	Duodenal dilatation Thickened small bowel folds "Hide-bound" sign (diffuse dilatation due to inner circular muscle fibrosis) Pooling of barium Pneumatosis in bowel wall Jejunal diverticula	Similar findings on small bowel follow-through in SLE as seen in scleroderma
Small bowel manometry	Absent/abnormal MMCs Decreased amplitude of contractions Decreased fasting and postprandial contractility	Similar manometric findings in any cause of chronic intestinal pseudoobstruction: includes SLE
Plain film of abdomen or computed tomography (CT) scan	CIPO (see text) Volvulus	SLE: small and large bowel wall thickening on CT scan Henoch-Schonlein: ileo-ileal intussusception
Lactulose hydrogen breath test	Sustained rise in hydrogen consistent with small bowel bacterial overgrowth	Bacterial overgrowth seen in all causes of small bowel dysmotility, including SLE, idiopathic, and paraneoplastic syndromes
Oral cecal transit time (OCTT)/ lactulose hydrogen breath test Cine-MRI wireless motility capsule	Abnormal with decreased OCTT Assesses motility of entire small bowel; in CIPO, luminal diameter is increased and contraction ratio is decreased[36] Delayed small bowel transit time	

TABLE 24-5
COLON: MOTILITY STUDIES IN SCLERODERMA AND OTHER COLLAGEN VASCULAR DISORDERS (WHERE AVAILABLE)[2,3,35]

TEST/STUDY	POSSIBLE/EXPECTED RESULTS IN SCLERODERMA	DIFFERENTIAL DIAGNOSIS AND RESULTS IN OTHER COLLAGEN VASCULAR DISORDERS
Plain abdominal film	Lack of haustrations Dilatation of bowel Volvulus (transverse, sigmoid, splenic flexure) PCI (see text) Pneumoperitoneum without peritonitis	
Radioactive markers (Sitzmarks) study	Increased whole gut transit time (normal: expel >80% markers by day 5)	
Barium enema	Postevacuation residual Wide-mouthed diverticula Stercoral ulceration Rectal prolapse Perforation (rare) Colonic infarction (rare)	SLE: "collar button" ulceration (mucosal ulceration with underlying rigid muscle wall) Behcet: diffuse colonic ulcers (in 15% of patients) frequently involving ICV Dermatomyositis/polymyositis: increased incidence of colonic malignancies
Colonic manometry	Absent gastrocolonic response Decreased postprandial motility compared to normals	
Bristol Stool Scale	More solid stool form (secondary to increase in colonic transit time)	
MRI	Buckling of anterior rectal wall	

1. Dysphagia
   - Endoscopically guided stricture dilation
   - Pilocarpine (for dry mouth): 5 mg orally 4 times daily
   - Facial exercises to increase oral aperture
2. Reflux
   - Small, frequent meals; sit upright after eating; do not eat before bedtime; and/or raising the head of the bed at night

TABLE 24-6

RECTUM/ANUS: MOTILITY STUDIES IN SCLERODERMA AND OTHER COLLAGEN VASCULAR DISORDERS (WHERE AVAILABLE)[2,3,35]

TEST/STUDY	POSSIBLE/EXPECTED RESULTS IN SCLERODERMA	DIFFERENTIAL DIAGNOSIS AND RESULTS IN OTHER COLLAGEN VASCULAR DISORDERS
Anorectal manometry (ARM)	Abnormal IAS (smooth muscle) with decreased resting tone Normal or decreased maximal squeeze pressure (skeletal muscle) RAIR may be decreased or absent Low tolerance for balloon distention	
Plain film	Fecal impaction	
Endoanal ultrasound	Thinning of IAS	
MRI	Thinning of IAS	
Colonoscopy	Stercoral ulcer Solitary rectal ulcer	Multiple discrete ulcers in Beçhet's
Anal exam	Rectal prolapse	

- Avoidance of certain food (eg, fatty foods, peppermint, chocolate, alcohol) and medication that can lower LES pressure (eg, calcium channel blockers)

- Avoid smoking

- H2 blockers or PPI therapy, usually twice daily (and often in higher doses)

- Consider partial fundoplication (Toupet) for selected patients with severe refractory GERD only.[29] This is controversial, as the success reported in the literature may not be reproducible at all surgery centers, and preselection of patients cannot be determined from the reports.

3. Gastroparesis

- Gastroparesis diet (low residue, low fat)

- Metoclopramide: 10 mg 4 times orally daily, 30 minutes before meals

  ○ Mechanism: dopamine receptor antagonist

  ○ Potential problems: risk of extrapyramidal symptoms; less effective in SSc patients with small bowel disease as well. There is currently a warning from the Food and Drug Administration (FDA) about the risk of neurologic side effects of metoclopramide.

- Erythromycin (for 4 to 8 weeks): 50 to -100 mg orally 4 times a day. Most studies showing improvement in gastric emptying use IV erythromycin.[30]

  ○ Mechanism: motilin receptor agonist

- ◦ Potential problems: tachyphylaxis after several weeks; avoid using with digoxin and Coumadin (warfarin)
- Domperidone: 10 to 20 mg orally 4 times daily (useful if patient is intolerant of metoclopramide)
  - ◦ Mechanism: peripheral dopamine receptor antagonist
  - ◦ Problem: not approved in United States
- Jejunal feeding via jejunostomy or jejunal extension. Patients may also need a venting gastrostomy if gastroparesis is severe to allow some oral intake for improved quality of life.

4. Duodenal/jejunal/ileal involvement leading to malabsorption and intestinal pseudoobstruction.

- Monitor vitamin levels: B_{12}, A, D, E, and K; supplement as needed
- Diet: low fat, low residue, low lactose
- Medium-chain triglyceride (MCT) supplements
- Polymeric diet formulas are more palatable and less expensive than elemental diets
- Elemental nutritional supplement via jejunal feeding tube
- Octreotide: 50 to 100 mcg subcutaneously daily at bedtime or long-acting-release (LAR) 20 mg subcutaneously monthly[31]
  - ◦ Mechanism: somatostatin analogue – induces a small intestinal phase III of the migrating motor complex (MMC)
  - ◦ Use alone or in combination with erythromycin, which prevents the impaired gastric motility that results from octreotide
  - ◦ Potential problems: hyper-/hypoglycemia, bradycardia, cholelithiasis
- Bowel transplantation reported in severe cases of intestinal involvement in children. High mortality.[32]

5. Diarrhea

- Lactose avoidance
- Antibiotics if breath test is positive for small intestinal bacterial overgrowth (SIBO) (see later)

6. Small intestinal bacterial overgrowth (SIBO)

- Octreotide (see earlier)
- Rotating schedule of antibiotics, 7 to 10 days each month:
  - ◦ Ciprofloxacin 500 mg twice daily
  - ◦ Doxycycline 100 mg twice daily
  - ◦ Metronidazole 250 mg 3 times a day
  - ◦ Amoxicillin/clavulanic acid 125 to 500 mg twice daily
  - ◦ Rifaximin 200 to 400 mg 3 times a day, or 550 mg twice a day (currently not approved for this diagnosis)

7. Chronic intestinal pseudo-obstruction (CIPO)

- Octreotide (see earlier)
- Metoclopramide (see earlier)
- Erythromycin: 500 mg IV every 8 hours for acute obstruction (in setting of CIPO) in hospital use

- Neostigmine: 0.2 to 2 mg IV every 6 hours as needed for acute exacerbations of CIPO (no controlled trials)
- Endoscopically/surgically placed tubes (gastrostomy or jejunostomy) for venting and/or enteral feeding (enteral feeding always preferable if possible)
- Total parenteral nutrition (TPN) if unable to manage oral/enteral feeding (may be especially effective if used with decompression tube as well)

8. Pneumatosis cystoides intestinalis (PCI)

- Oxygen, antibiotics, observation

9. Constipation

- Laxatives and stool softeners: bisacodyl, docusate sodium (fiber supplements may worsen symptoms)
- Polyethylene glycol 3350 if needed (Golytely, Miralax)
- Lubiprostone, a chloride channel activator
  ○ Dosing would be for idiopathic constipation, 24 mcg orally twice daily with food and water
- Linaclotide, a guanylate cyclase-C (GC-C) agonist
  ○ Dosing would be for idiopathic constipation, that is, 145 mcg orally once daily at least 30 minutes prior to the first meal of the day
- Surgical (literature consists of case reports)
  ○ Bowel resection with ileostomy
  ○ Segmental colectomy (diseased bowel only), preserving the ileocecal valve if possible[33]

10. Fecal Incontinence (see diarrhea earlier)

- Solidify liquid stool
- Biofeedback
- Sacral nerve stimulation. May not be successful once there is atrophy and fibrosis of the muscle. Unknown efficacy in fecal incontinence in scleroderma.[34]
- Surgical repair of rectal prolapse

Nontraditional alternative therapies have been reported, including para-aminobenzoic acid purported to be antifibrotic, vitamin E (antioxidant and antifibrotic), vitamin D (inhibition of collagen synthesis and fibroblast growth), evening primrose oil/gamma-linolenic acid (anti-inflammatory), and others whose mechanisms are unknown. Also, acupressure and gastric pacing may be helpful in certain patients. Clearly, preventive strategies would be ideal.

REFERENCES

1. Sallam H, McNearney TA, Chen JD. Systematic review: pathophysiology and management of gastrointestinal dysmotility in systemic sclerosis (scleroderma). *Aliment Pharmacol Ther.* 2006;23:691-712.
2. Gyger G, Baron M. Gastrointestinal manifestations of scleroderma: recent progress in evaluation, pathogenesis and management. *Curr Rheumatol Rep.* 2012;14:22-29.
3. Ebert EC. Gastric and enteric involvement in progressive systemic sclerosis. *J Clin Gastroenterol.* 2008;42(1):5-12.
4. Schmeiser T, Saar P, Jin D, et al. Profile of gastrointestinal involvement in patients with systemic sclerosis. *Rheumatol Int.* 2012;32:2471-2478.
5. Wooten M. Systemic sclerosis and malignancy: a review of the literature. *South Med J.* 2008;101(1):59-62.
6. Van den Hoogen F, Khanna D, Fransen J, et al. 2013 classification criteria for systemic sclerosis: an American College of Rheumatology/European League against Rheumatism collaborative initiative. *Arthritis Rheum.* 2013;65:2737-2747.

7. Di Caula A, Covelli M, Berardino M, et al. Gastrointestinal symptoms and motility disorders in patients with systemic scleroderma. *BMC Gastroenterol.* 2008;8:7-17.

8. Muangchan C, Canadian Scleroderma Research Group, Baron M, Pope J. The 15% rule in scleroderma: the frequency of severe organ complications in systemic sclerosis: a systematic review. *J Rheumatol.* 2013;40:1545-1556.

9. Yu K-H, Yang C-H, Chu C-C. Swallowing disturbance due to isolated vagus nerve involvement in systemic lupus erythematosus. *Lupus.* 2007;16:746-748.

10. Marie I, Hatron PY, Levesque H, et al. Influence of age on characteristics of polymyositis and dermatomyositis in adults. *Medicine.* 1999;78:139-147.

11. Di Caula A, Covelli M, Berardino M, et al. Gastrointestinal symptoms and motility disorders in patients with systemic scleroderma. *BMC Gastroenterol.* 2008;8:7-17.

12. Hung EW, Mayes MD, Sharif R, et al. Gastric antral vascular ectasia and its clinical correlates in patients with early diffuse systemic sclerosis in the SCOT trial. *J Rheumatol.* 2013;40:455-460.

13. Marie I, Ducrotte P, Denis P, et al. Outcome of small-bowel motor impairment in systemic sclerosis: a prospective manometric 5-year follow-up. *Rheumatology.* 2007;46:150-153.

14. Pedersen J, Gao C, Egekvist H, et al. Pain and biomechanical responses to distention of the duodenum in patients with systemic sclerosis. *Gastroenterology.* 2003;124:1230-1239.

15. Gomez-Puerta JA, Gil V, Cervera R, et al. Coeliac disease associated with systemic sclerosis. *Ann Rheum Dis.* 2004;63:104-105.

16. Lyford G, Foxx-Orenstein A. Chronic intestinal pseudoobstruction. *Curr Treatment Options Gastroenterol.* 2004;7:317-325.

17. Alva S, Abir F, Longo WE. Colorectal manifestations of collagen vascular disease. *Am J Surg.* 2005;189:685-693.

18. Riviere E, Vergniol J, Reffet A, et al. Gastric variceal bleeding uncovering a rare association of CREST syndrome, primary biliary cirrhosis, nodular regenerative hyperplasia and pulmonary hypertension. *Eur J Gastroenterol Hepatol.* 2010;22:1145-1148.

19. Hendel L, Worning H. Exocrine pancreatic function in patients with progressive systemic sclerosis. *Scand J Gastroenterol.* 1989;24:461-466.

20. Murtaugh MA, Frech TM. Nutritional status and gastrointestinal symptoms in systemic sclerosis patients. *Clin Nutr.* 2013;32:130-135.

21. Harrison E, Herrick AL, McLaughlin JT, Lal S. Malnutrition in systemic sclerosis. *Rheumatology.* 2012;51:1747-1756.

22. Chifflot H, Fautrel B, Sordet C, et al. Incidence and prevalence of systemic sclerosis: a systematic literature review. *Semin Arthritis Rheum.* 2008;37:223-235.

23. Lawrence RC, Helmick CG, Arnett FC, et al. Estimates of the prevalence of arthritis and selected musculoskeletal disorders in the United States. *Arthritis Rheum.* 1998;41:778.

24. Bacher A, Mittoo S, Hudson M, et al. Systemic sclerosis in Canada's North American native population: assessment of clinical and serological manifestations. *J Rheumatol.* 2013;40:1121-1126.

25. Martini G, Foeldvari I, Russo R, et al. Systemic sclerosis in childhood. *Arth Rheum.* 2006;54(12):3971-3978.

26. D'Aoust J, Hudson M, Tatibouet S, et al. Clinical and serological correlates of anti-PM/Scl antibodies in systemic sclerosis: a multicenter study of 763 patients. *Arth Rheumatol.* 2014;accepted article. doi:10.1002/art.38428.

27. Tyndall A, Furst DE. Adult stem cell treatment of scleroderma. *Curr Opin Rheumatol.* 2007;19:604-610.

28. Kowal-Bielecka O, Landewi R, Avouac J, et al. EULAR recommendations for the treatment of systemic sclerosis: a report from the EULAR Scleroderma Trials and Research group (EUSTAR). *Ann Rheum Dis.* 2009;68:620-628.

29. Watson DI, Jamieson GG, Bessel JR, Devitt PG. Laparoscopic fundoplication in patients with an aperistaltic esophagus and gastroesophageal reflux. *Dis Esophagus.* 2006;19:94-98.

30. Arts J, Caenepeel P, Verbeke K, Tack J. Influence of erythromycin on gastric emptying and meal related symptoms in functional dyspepsia with delayed gastric emptying. *Gut.* 2005;54:455-460.

31. Perlemuter G, Cacoub P, Chaussade S, et al. Octreotide treatment of chronic intestinal pseudoobstruction secondary to connective tissue diseases. *Arth Rheum.* 1999;42:1545-1549.

32. Loinaz C, Rodríguez MM, Kato T, et al. Intestinal and multivisceral transplantation in children with severe gastrointestinal dysmotility. *J Pediatr Surg.* 2005;40(10):1598-1604.

33. Lindsey I, Farmer CR, Cunningham IG. Subtotal colectomy and cecosigmoid anastomosis for colonic systemic sclerosis. *Dis Colon Rectum.* 2003;46:1706-1711.

34. Leroi AM, Damon H, Faucheron JL, et al. Consensus statement: sacral nerve stimulation in faecal incontinence: position statement based on a collective experience. *Colorectal Dis.* 2009;11:572-583.

35. Paine P, McLaughlin J, Lai S. Review article: the assessment and management of chronic severe gastrointestinal dysmotility in adults. *Alimentary Pharmacol Ther.* 2013;38:1209-1229.

Opiate-Induced Bowel Dysfunction

Eva Szigethy, MD, PhD; Marc Schwartz, MD;
and Douglas A. Drossman, MD

KEY POINTS

- Given limited evidence to support its use in chronic noncancer pain, opioid pain medication should be used with great care by experienced physicians when nonopioid approaches to pain control fail.

- Early laxative therapy should be employed in patients on opioids to prevent and treat opioid-induced constipation (OIC). Those who fail to respond to laxative therapy can be treated with agents such as lubiprostone, tapentadol, oxycodone/naloxone, and methylnaltrexone.

- Clinicians need to have a high index of suspicion for narcotic bowel syndrome (NBS) in patients who have persistent or worsening abdominal pain in the presence of opioids.

- An empathic doctor–patient relationship is essential in treating NBS so that education about this condition can occur in a nonjudgmental manner and patient concerns can be addressed.

- While different behavioral and nonopioid medication strategies can be used to treat chronic abdominal pain, opioid detoxification is the most critical step in NBS treatment.

Over the past decade opioid consumption has shown a dramatic rise throughout the world, particularly in the United States.[1] This rise in usage may relate to increased access, both legally and illegally, along with professional mandates, such as from the Joint Commission, to treat pain more aggressively. Opioids have long been used for acute pain and cancer pain with benefit; however, recently, there has been increased opioid use for noncancer chronic pain.[2] In most patients, opioids alleviate pain by their actions at receptors in the central and peripheral nervous systems. With chronic use, however, tolerance can develop, with reduction in the analgesic benefit and increased risk for gastrointestinal (GI) side effects. There are primarily 2 opioid-related bowel syndromes: opioid-induced bowel dysfunction (OBD) and NBS that are the focus of this chapter. The former

Rao SSC, Parkman HP, McCallum RW, eds.
Handbook of Gastrointestinal Motility and Functional Disorders (pp 323-337).
© 2015 Taylor & Francis Group.

TABLE 25-1

DEFINITION OF OPIOID-INDUCED CONSTIPATION

A change from baseline bowel habits after initiation of opioid therapy that is characterized by any of the following:

- Reduced bowel movement frequency
- Development or worsening of straining to pass stools
- A sense of incomplete rectal evacuation
- Harder stool consistency

---

is due to opioid-mediated changes in the GI tract, while the latter is mediated by central nervous system processes.

OPIOID-INDUCED BOWEL DYSFUNCTION

Definition

Opioid-induced bowel dysfunction refers to the GI side effects of prescription opioids. The most common symptoms are constipation, abdominal discomfort, nausea, and vomiting, but gastroparesis, ileus, and colonic pseudo-obstruction can also occur. The hallmark of OBD is that symptoms occur or exacerbate after starting opioids and resolve after discontinuation. A multinational working group formulated an operational definition for OIC, the most prevalent GI symptom caused by opioid use (Table 25-1).[3]

Epidemiology

Opioid prescriptions in the United States have quadrupled over the past decade, resulting in proportional increases in drug treatment admissions and unintentional deaths from prescription opioid overdose.[4] Nine million Americans are on opioids for chronic noncancer pain—a majority of them with low back pain.[5] In a population-based study of 2055 Americans taking chronic daily opioids for noncancer pain, 36% complained of worsening constipation over the past 4 weeks as a result of opioid use, while 57% complained of constipation exacerbated by opioids at any point. Over the past 4 weeks opioid-induced abdominal pain occurred in 22%, nausea in 23%, bloating in 17%, and increased gas in 24%. One-third of patients report constipation as the most bothersome opioid-induced symptom, while nausea, abdominal pain, and flatulence were each reported by 10% of respondents.[6]

Pathophysiology

Mu-opioid receptors are expressed throughout the GI tract and are most responsible for the motility effects of opioids, while activation of central mu receptors in the brain and spinal cord account for most of the pain relief. The kappa and gamma receptors are involved in pain pathways, but to a lesser degree and have little effect on the GI tract.

Opioid binding to the mu receptor alters GI motility by slowing gastric emptying, decreasing propulsive contractions of the small intestine and colon, decreasing pancreaticobiliary and intestinal secretion, and increasing pyloric and anal sphincter tone, while reducing the defecatory

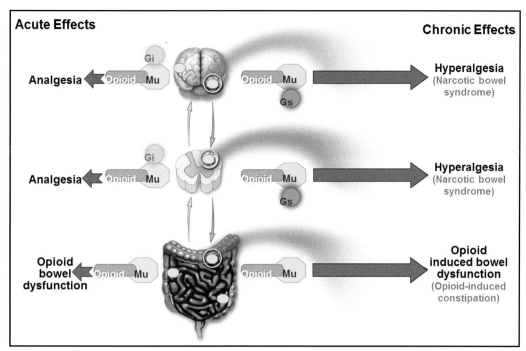

Figure 25-1. Acute and chronic effects of opioids in the central nervous system and GI tract.

reflex. This combination of effects leads to constipation and other GI symptoms such as nausea and vomiting.[7] Figure 25-1 illustrates the proposed opioid actions at mu-opioid receptors in the context of acute and chronic opioid use. Such diagrams can be useful in explaining symptoms to patients.

Diagnosis

Making a diagnosis of OBD begins with a thorough history focusing on stool pattern and the timing of GI symptoms. A stool diary is ideal. Other causes of constipation, nausea, and vomiting must be excluded. A differential diagnosis for OIC is listed in Table 25-2, although there can be overlap. For a diagnosis of OBD, symptoms must occur after starting opioids or be exacerbated by opioid use and resolve with discontinuation. The presentation of OBD forms a continuum of severity, with more severe OBD causing a diminished quality of life.[8]

Bloating is a common complaint in various GI disorders, including constipation, irritable bowel syndrome (IBS), carbohydrate malabsorption, and small intestinal bacterial overgrowth (SIBO). Typically, SIBO and carbohydrate malabsorption, both causes of IBS-D, cause diarrhea. The incidence of SIBO in IBS-D ranges from 4% to 78%, with the true incidence is likely in the middle.[9] Although it is conceivable that constipation results in retrograde movement of colonic bacteria into the small bowel, no evidence shows that it leads to SIBO. Given the limitations of hydrogen breath testing,[9] we find a 2-week course of empiric antibiotics (eg, neomycin, metronidazole, norfloxacin, or rifaximin) is often just as helpful as a hydrogen breath test for diagnosing and treating SIBO, but we have not used this approach in OIC.

Treatments

Since OIC is the most common symptom of OBD and has the greatest effect on quality of life, its treatment will be the primary focus of this review. It is also the primary endpoint in most clinical trials assessing OBD. While other OBD symptoms, such as nausea and vomiting, can respond to

TABLE 25-2
DIFFERENTIAL DIAGNOSIS FOR OPIOID-INDUCED CONSTIPATION

- Bowel obstruction
- Side effects of other medications (eg, tricyclic antidepressants)
- Functional constipation
- Diabetic gastrointestinal complications
- Intestinal pseudoobstruction
- Diverticulitis
- Idiopathic gastroparesis
- Irritable bowel syndrome
- Parkinson's disease

the treatments discussed later, they are usually treated symptomatically, for example, with antiemetics such as ondansetron and phenergan.

Laxatives

Osmotic laxatives are effective for the treatment of functional constipation, but have not been studied in randomized controlled trials (RCTs) to treat OIC. The presence of untreated OIC can exacerbate other GI symptoms such as nausea, vomiting, and abdominal pain. Polyethylene glycol 3350 (PEG) is the most effective therapy for functional constipation and appears to be similarly effective in OIC. It is inexpensive and has few side effects. Aggressive programs to increase the use of laxatives in palliative care populations produce a corresponding decrease in the incidence and severity of OIC. When used appropriately, laxatives can adequately treat at least half of OIC patients.[10,11]

Lubiprostone is a locally acting chloride channel activator approved for functional constipation in addition to OIC. In one large RCT, after 8 weeks of treatment, lubiprostone (24 mg twice daily) increased the frequency of spontaneous bowel movements (SBMs) by 3.3 per week, compared to 2.4 additional SBMs per week with placebo ($p=0.005$). There were small, but statistically significant, improvements in symptoms such as stool consistency, constipation, straining, and abdominal discomfort, but no improvement in abdominal bloating and bowel habit regularity.[12] A dose-ranging study in chronic constipation identified no significant difference in efficacy between doses of 24, 48, and 72 mcg per day, since by 3 weeks none of the dosing regimens were superior to placebo.[13] Linaclotide, a chloride channel activator like lubiprostone, is approved for idiopathic constipation and could be of benefit in OIC. Doses of 145 and 290 mcg daily have been shown to be similarly effective.[14]

Peripheral Acting Mu-Opioid Receptor Antagonists

Recent drug development for OIC has emphasized peripheral acting mu-opioid receptor antagonists (PAMORAs), including methylnaltrexone, alvimopan, and naloxegol. These agents bind to mu receptors on the GI tract without activating them, which prevents opioid binding and the resulting altered motility. The central opioid receptors, which are responsible for pain control, are not blocked, permitting unaffected activity. Methylnaltrexone, alvimopan, and naloxegol have completed phase 3 studies in OBD for patients with noncancer chronic pain. Methylnaltrexone is approved by the Food and Drug Administration (FDA) for use in OIC unresponsive to laxatives.

Alvimopan is approved for postoperative ileus but not OIC. Alvimopan and naloxegol are taken by mouth, while methylnaltrexone is a subcutaneous injection. Study results for OIC have been similar across the PAMORAs. Taken daily for 4 to 12 weeks, they induce 1 to 1.5 additional SBMs/week than placebo. Treatment increases the relative response rates by about 30% for the endpoint of > 3 SBMs/week, but improvements in symptoms and overall quality of life have been elusive. These endpoints are not consistently evaluated, but when they are, the results have been small and often fail to meet statistical or clinical significance. The number needed to treat (NNT) with PAMORAs for one responder ranges from 6 to 8 patients.[15]

Daily methylnaltrexone (12 mg) provides a greater benefit than every-other-day dosing, although the dosing frequency does not alter the frequency of an SBM within 4 hours of a dose. While quality of life is higher in patients receiving daily or every-other-day treatment compared to placebo, it is highest with daily dosing. Compared to placebo, every-other-day dosing of methylnaltrexone produces an additional 0.5 SBMs per week (NS) and requires rescue laxatives in 49% ($p = 0.03$) of patients, while daily dosing induces an extra 1.5 SBMs/week ($p < 0.001$), with 39% ($p < 0.001$) using rescue laxatives. Abdominal pain, nausea, vomiting, and hyperhydrosis were common side effects of methylnaltrexone, but occurred less frequently at the higher dose.[16] When the methylnaltrexone dose was doubled from 0.15 mg/kg to 0.3 mg/kg each day in patients with advanced illness, the rate of laxation within 4 hours increased from 15% to 24%.[17]

There have been 4 RCTs assessing alvimopan in OIC including a total of 1693 patients. A meta-analysis of the 4 studies found alvimopan to be more effective than placebo. Twice-daily dosing of 0.5 mg may be more effective than 0.5 mg once daily with NNT of 5 and 10, respectively.[15]

Naloxegol is a pegylated derivative of naloxone, a mu-opioid receptor antagonist. Pegylation prevents it from crossing the blood–brain barrier. Naloxegol is not approved by the FDA, but a phase 2 dose-ranging study found the 25- and 50-mg daily doses to be more effective than 5 mg daily and placebo.[18] A recently published pair of phase 3 studies compared 12.5 and 25 mg of daily naloxegol to placebo and found the 25-mg dose to be superior to placebo in both studies, while the 12.5-mg dose was only superior to placebo in one of the 2 studies. Based on these two studies, the NNT for 12.5 mg is 11, while the NNT is 8 for the 25-mg dose. The higher dose led to 10% more adverse events (6% greater abdominal pain) and a 6% higher rate of treatment discontinuation.[19]

Mu-receptor Antagonists

The combination of oxycodone with naloxone, a pure opioid receptor antagonist, offers similar pain control to oxycodone alone, but with fewer GI side effects. Constipation was improved in 66% of patients receiving OxyNal (oxycodone with naloxone) compared to only 44% on placebo ($p < 0.005$).[20]

Investigational Treatments

There are several medications in development to treat OIC, including additional PAMORAs. Two agents with novel mechanisms are prucalopride and tapentadol. Prucalopride is a selective 5-HT4 agonist that enhances cholinergic activity and is marketed as a prokinetic motility agent. In functional constipation and OIC, it increases motility of the stomach, small bowel, and colon without affecting the anorectal defecatory complex.[21] Although there was a statistically significant increase in several measures of bowel movement frequency, treatment just failed to meet its primary endpoint, an increase of > 1 SCBM per week for 4 weeks. Thirty-eight percent of patients on 4 mg of prucalopride found it to be "quite or extremely effective" for constipation compared to 17% who received placebo ($p < 0.05$), but treatment produced no improvement in quality of life.[22]

Tapentadol is a centrally acting analgesic that provides mu-receptor agonism and norepinephrine reuptake inhibition. Taken instead of traditional opioids, tapentadol (up to 500 mg/day) consistently provided pain control similar to oxycodone, while decreasing constipation, nausea, and vomiting by about half. Although superior to placebo, tapentadol has not been shown to be any more effective than typical short- or long-acting opioids used in conjunction with PEG.[23]

It can be a particular challenge treating gastroparesis in the setting of chronic opioid use. Nausea and vomiting are common symptoms of gastroparesis, as well as OBD. The use of opioids to treat chronic noncancer pain may exacerbate gastroparesis since gastric emptying is slowed by opioids. Because the symptoms of gastroparesis are nonspecific, they can be difficult to attribute to a particular etiology. Gastric emptying studies are rarely helpful in the setting of opioid use since gastric emptying will be delayed, making it impossible to identify underlying gastroparesis.[24] Mu-receptor agonists may improve gastric emptying in gastroparetics who are also on opioids, but this subgroup of patients has not been identified in any clinical trials. If symptoms of gastroparesis are exacerbated by opioid use, the opioid dose should be minimized. Mu-receptor antagonists might be helpful, but there is no evidence to support this approach.

Treatment Approach

There is inadequate evidence to offer a definitive treatment algorithm for OIC, but we propose the following approach as both effective and cost conscious. The most effective way to prevent OIC, and all morbidity and mortality caused by opioids, is to minimize their unnecessary use. While this can be difficult in chronic cancer pain, the approach has been implemented successfully in the management of chronic noncancer pain. A prime example is chronic low back pain, the most common indication for chronic opioid use, for which the "STarT Back" approach was developed. By using nonopioid pain medications, patient education, psychiatric interventions, and physical therapy opioid use was decreased while improving outcomes.[25]

Opioid-induced constipation requires treatment when symptoms are severe enough to have a negative effect on the patient's quality of life. When opioids are used, prophylactic or early PEG can prevent up to half of all OIC cases. While PEG may be the most effective laxative, other osmotic (magnesium, sorbitol) and stimulant (senna, bisacodyl) agents can be used to tailor a safe regimen for long-term use.

Laxatives are ideal first-line therapy for OIC because they are safe, effective, and inexpensive, but require adequate treatment doses. Based upon the authors' experience, reports that approximately 50% of patients with OIC "fail" laxatives may be due to underdosing of laxatives and/or pain and functional symptoms that are unrelated to OIC. While all of the prescription therapies reviewed in this chapter for the treatment of OIC have proven to be more effective than placebo, none has been tested head-to-head against PEG or other laxatives.

Opioid-induced constipation that does not respond adequately to laxatives requires treatment with one of the novel therapies. All of these treatments appear to be similarly effective, with comparable side effect profiles and an NNT of 6 to 8. Due to its high cost, approximately $18,000 per year, methylnaltrexone, the only PAMORA approved for use in OIC, is ideal for episodic bouts of severe constipation, while lubiprostone, tapentadol, and OxyNal (available only in Europe), which have similar efficacy at less than one-quarter the cost, are better suited for chronic daily use if an opioid taper is not feasible. Most of the treatments have a 2-dose range of therapeutic effect, for example, 12 mg of methylnaltrexone every day or every other day. It is reasonable to start at either dose and then titrate up or down as tolerated.

There are several medications for OIC in various stages of development, so additional therapeutic options will soon be available (Table 25-3). Future RCTs will be of greatest value if they compare new medications with both standard care (laxatives) and placebo, and offer valid measures of quality of life.

TABLE 25-3
MEDICATIONS FOR OPIOID-INDUCED CONSTIPATION

MEDICATION	MECHANISM	FDA APPROVAL	INDICATIONS	DOSE
PEG 3350	Osmotic laxative	Y	Constipation	17 gm BID
Methylnaltrexone	PAMORA	Y	OIC	12 mg QD
Alvimopan	PAMORA	Y	Post-op ileus	0.5 mg BID
Naloxegol	PAMORA	Y	OIC	25 mg QD
OxyNal	Nonselective opioid antagonist	N (Eur/Can)	Chronic pain	40/20 mg QD
Tapentadol	Mu-agonist and NRI	Y	Chronic pain	250 mg BID
Lubiprostone	Chloride channel activator	Y	OIC	24 mcg BID
Linaclotide	Chloride channel activator	Y	Chronic Constipation	145 to 290 mcg QD
Prucalopride	5-HT4 antagonist	N (Eur/Can)	Chronic Constipation	2 to 4 mg QD

PAMORA = peripheral acting mu-opioid receptor antagonist; OIC = opioid-induced constipation; BID = twice a day; QD = once a day.

NARCOTIC BOWEL SYNDROME

Definition

NBS is characterized by the development or worsening of abdominal pain with chronic or escalating dosages of exogenous opioids, which paradoxically were prescribed to alleviate the pain (Table 25-4). Pain improves when opioids are withdrawn.[26]

Pathophysiology

Grunkemeier et al defined NBS as abdominal pain due to central hyperalgesia that occurs in response to high-dose or chronic opioids.[26-29] The exact neurobiological mechanisms underlying the paradoxical increase in abdominal pain in NBS, even with escalating doses of opiates, is not known. Features of NBS are similar to the concept of opioid-induced hyperalgesia (OIH) of somatic pain, which is well studied in animal and experimental human models.[30,31] While there is some question as to whether OIH exists as a unique entity,[44] NBS has distinguishing features that make it a more plausible entity: the low rates in spite of very high rates of opioid use for noncancer

---

TABLE 25-4
NARCOTIC BOWEL SYNDROME CRITERIA[27, 35]

Chronic or frequently recurring abdominal pain that is treated with acute high-dose or chronic narcotics and at least 3 of the following:

- Pain worsens or incompletely resolves with continued or escalating dosages of narcotics.
- There is marked worsening of pain when the narcotic dose wanes and improvement when narcotics are reinstituted.
- There is a progression of the frequency, duration, and intensity of pain episodes.
- The nature and intensity of the pain is not explained by a current or previous gastrointestinal diagnosis (eg, may have a diagnosis of inflammatory bowel disease, but the activity of the disease process is not sufficient to explain the pain).

---

pain suggesting possible genetic vulnerability and its occurrence even after relatively acute use in postoperative patients who are previously naïve to pain.[35] There is growing evidence for genetic polymorphisms mediating opioid-related hyperalgesia.[45] It is still unclear if NBS is a component of OIH or a separate clinical entity; however, the putative mechanisms of glial cell activation leading to dorsal horn release of cytokines that upregulate pain transmission and bimodal opioid modulation (both excitatory and inhibitory) in the spinal cord have been postulated for both. Another putative mechanism underlying OIH is related to glutamate at N-methyl-D-aspartate (NMDA) receptors mediated by increases in phosphokinase C. Other neuroactive mediators of opioid-related hyperalgesia have also been explored, including cholecystokinin, bradykinin, and dynorphin, and may serve as substrates for future pharmacological agents to treat chronic pain that is caused or exacerbated by narcotics (see Figure 25-1).[32] Finally, there is also interest in exploring genetic vulnerability to opioid-related hyperalgesia, particularly in individuals who develop NBS early in the course of opioid treatment or with relatively small doses.

At the behavioral level, an ineffective patient–doctor interaction can inadvertently perpetuate the use of opioids and the development of NBS.[26] The patient may only view opioids as the treatment for their pain, since that is what they have been prescribed, and thus may feel that the physician who refuses opioids does not believe that the pain is "real" or that they are drug seeking. This frustrates the patient and leads to increased health care utilization as they struggle to find a physician who will "help" them. In turn, the physician, in an effort to avoid conflict or to save time, may choose to prescribe the opioids rather than undertake a more appropriate, and more time consuming, treatment strategy, which in our health care system, is less readily reimbursed. This vicious cycle can only be interrupted if a diagnosis of NBS is made and then successful treatment is undertaken to detoxify them and provide more effective nonopiate treatment options (eg, behavioral and nonopioid pain-reducing agents) in order to engage the patient in the treatment process, improve symptoms, and reduce recidivism.

Diagnosis

For a positive NBS diagnosis, paradoxical abdominal pain related to escalating doses of opioids is the hallmark feature. There may be other or overlapping factors and diagnoses to consider. It is important to assess whether the escalating pain is due to nonopioid-related causes (eg, an underlying GI disease, infection, or obstruction) or not due to the development of tolerance.

Opioid tolerance is defined as reduced analgesic effects with repeated exposure. Tolerance can be innate (genetic insensitivity) or acquired (due to pharmacokinetic and pharmacodynamic effects). Tolerance is one of the symptom criteria for opioid dependence, which additionally includes withdrawal symptoms and continued substance use despite substance-related problems in functioning. While patients have little tolerance for the GI effects of opioids (eg, constipation), tolerance for analgesic effects are common. Abdominal pain can worsen during physiological withdrawal from opioids, but this pain is usually accompanied by lacrimation, rhinorrhea, yawning, restlessness, and diarrhea. Further, NBS can resemble other GI disorders such as IBS or other functional gastrointestinal disorders (FGID),[42] or can be referred from musculoskeletal pain from the abdominal area. The pain in NBS is above and beyond that of these other structural or functional conditions and often of a different quality.

NBS can also be challenging to diagnose when it is comorbid with somatization disorders, the psychiatric correlates of FGIDs. Somatic symptom disorder, predominantly pain type, a new diagnostic entity replacing somatoform disorders in the *Diagnostic and Statistical Manual of Mental Disorders* (DSM)-5,[33] is characterized by excessive thoughts, feelings, or behaviors associated with a somatic symptom ("pain") for at least 6 months that disrupt daily life and are associated with one of the following: "1) Disproportionate and persistent thoughts about the seriousness of one's symptoms; 2) Persistently high level of anxiety about health or symptoms; and 3) Excessive time and energy devoted to these symptoms or health concerns." Comorbid somatoform disorder is found in over one-third of adults with irritable bowel syndrome.[34] In one small study characterizing patients with NBS, risk factors included female gender, middle aged, psychosocial impairment, high rates of anxiety and depression, and tendency to catastrophize (cognitively view a situation worse than it is).[35] Larger-scale studies are needed to confirm these findings. Longitudinal tracking of pain severity, physical and psychological symptoms, opioid timing, and dosage can best confirm the diagnosis of NBS.

Epidemiology

While case reports of opioid-induced visceral hyperalgesia were described several decades ago, reports of NBS have increased across chronic pain conditions, possibly due to increased opioid prescriptions for pain unrelated to cancer. In fact, the dramatic increase in opioid use and prescribing has been termed a national "epidemic" due to associated morbidity and even mortality.[25] It has also been reported in patients without previous pain histories who were given high narcotic doses for postsurgical pain. In one study, 146 patients at a pain management center were evaluated for NBS (mean opioid dose of 127.5 mg/day morphine equivalent with a range of 7.5 to 600 mg/day and mean duration of 365 days). NBS was defined as very severe abdominal pain of at least 3 months duration and greater than 100 mg/day morphine equivalent. In this setting, 6.4% of patients met criteria for NBS.[36] In another study, 2913 randomly selected patients were identified, with 117 taking opioids and 5 with probable NBS—defined as new abdominal pain not explained by a GI diagnosis and at least 2 weeks on opioids. This is consistent with a rate of 0.17% of total sample and 4.2% of opioid users.[37] It is estimated that over 142,000 people in the United States have NBS. While this prevalence in pain clinics is relatively low, it may be an artifact due to a lack of recognition of NBS by many clinicians and the fact that many of these patients are seen in GI clinics and not pain clinics. These rates are alarming given that there is no evidence that opioids are efficacious for chronic abdominal pain.

Treatment

A strong therapeutic alliance with opioid-using patients is a critical first step in treatment, as it creates an empathic, nonjudgmental environment that facilitates honest and open interaction. As with OBD, avoiding opioids is the best way to prevent NBS, particularly given the lack of evidence

TABLE 25-5

FACTORS ASSOCIATED WITH DETOXIFICATION FAILURE OR RECIDIVISM AFTER DETOXIFICATION[35]

- Prior history of substance abuse (opioids, sedative-hypnotics, or illicit drugs)
- Diagnosis of opioid use disorder (DSM-5)
- High rates of catastrophizing (negative cognitive distortions)
- History of opioid use for other somatic complaints
- Associated personality disorder (eg, borderline, antisocial, dependent—DSM-5)
- Extreme negativity and/or unwillingness to engage in discussion of protocol
- Creating barriers to successful detoxification (hiding opioids or bargaining, [eg, "just one more dose"])
- Enablement from family (ie, bringing in opioids)

for efficacy of narcotics for chronic abdominal pain. The mainstay of NBS treatment is a taper of opioids, which can often require inpatient hospitalization to avoid withdrawal complications. Drossman et al[35] published findings on an inpatient detoxification program with taper using intravenous morphine or hydromorphone equivalents reduced by 15% to 33%/day. The duration of this taper was 4 to 10 days, and patients received nonopioid medications for pain control (eg, serotonin-norepinephrine reuptake inhibitors [SNRI] or tricyclic antidepressants [TCA]), as well as long-acting benzodiazepines for anxiety and clonidine for withdrawal symptoms. Using this approach, almost 90% of patients successfully stopped opioids, with improved pain reported in over 60%. However, there was no systematic follow-up of these patients and within 3 months, half of the patients had returned to opioid use. For those who stayed off opioids, the reduction in pain severity persisted. This high rate of recidivism may be reduced with more intensive psychosocial follow-up after hospital discharge.

In this study, patients with NBS who had evidence of opioid abuse, personality disorders, emotional distress, or catastrophizing (eg, pervasive negative cognitions) had higher rates of recidivism.[35] It may be worthwhile to administer validated screening instruments for aberrant substance use, personality traits, and negative cognitive traits as part of treatment so that these additional factors can also be addressed. The Common Opioid Misuse Measure (COMM) is one such measure that has been used in patients with NBS to predict recidivism after opioid detoxification (Table 25-5).[35]

Patients in this withdrawal study who returned to opioid use had a rapid return of their pain.[35] In fact, there is no evidence that a drug holiday from narcotics, lower dosing of opioids, or switching to a different class (eg, morphine to fentanyl) leads to less recurrence of NBS. While there is some support that switching from oral to transdermal or transmucosal administration of opioids or using partial agonists (eg, buprenorphine)[46] or mixed combinations of opioids and opioid antagonists (eg, slow-release oxycodone plus slow-release naloxone)[47] can reduce constipation, there is no evidence that NBS-related pain would improve.

A biopsychosocial approach anchored by a solid doctor–patient relationship is critical for success of managing NBS both before and after detoxification. This effective communication needs to be combined with a consistent plan for opioid withdrawal and nonopioid treatments to manage presenting complaints such as bowel symptoms, pain, and emotional distress (eg, anxiety, depression). Building from an empathic therapeutic alliance, the rationale and benefits for stopping opioids must be explained. During this precontemplation stage, it is important to utilize positive motivational techniques and process resistance thoughtfully, all while teaching cognitive behavioral coping strategies. After successful detoxification, continued follow-up therapy is essential, since patients are at an especially high risk for relapsing to opioid use 6 months after detoxification. The neurochemical basis for such empathic interpersonal connection still remains to be elucidated. Hypnotherapy and meditation have also been associated with reduced chronic visceral pain and may have anti-inflammatory and genomic effects.

Antidepressants with a noradrenergic substrate such as TCAs (eg, desipramine, nortriptyline) and SNRIs (eg, duloxetine, milnacipran) have shown the greatest promise in reducing abdominal pain in these patients.[43] Selective serotonin reuptake inhibitors (SSRIs) or bupropion can be effective for comorbid mood symptoms. If pain persists, agents such as pregabalin and gabapentin have shown efficacy for central pain syndromes and visceral pain and may reduce inflammation.[38] Glutaminergic agonists such as memantine act at the NMDA receptor and have analgesic effects.[39] Recent evidence suggests that ketamine could have direct analgesic effects via both NMDA receptor antagonism and inhibition of tumor necrosis factor alpha and interleukin 6.[40] It likely prevents sensitization of nociceptive pathways within the central nervous system and attenuation of opioid tolerance and OIH[41] and also antidepressant effects. Several limitations of ketamine in the United States are that it is only available intravenously and serious side effects have been reported, such as cognitive changes, psychosis, and urinary symptoms, although many of these subjects were substance abusers; thus, it is unclear whether these symptoms were directly caused by ketamine versus other agents.[41] Clearly, many of these agents have complex mechanisms of action affecting multiple neurochemical substrates, and further research is needed to determine how the hyperalgesia of NBS is mediated.

Table 25-6 represents an algorithm for approaching the diagnosis and treatment of NBS. The following case example demonstrates how adherence to such a multifaceted treatment approach can successfully treat NBS and improve patient quality of life.

Case example: Mary is a 64-year-old married female with long-standing Crohn's disease that required significant resection and subsequent ostomy 8 years ago. Since that time, she has had significant rectal pain without a clear organic cause, which was treated with escalating doses of narcotics for the past 6 years. She worked part-time in a secretarial job but had stopped most other activities. Despite escalating doses of narcotics (oxycodone, hydromorphone, and fentanyl), her pain persists and over the past year has been worsening. She has had several organic workups for inflammation, masses, and other mechanical causes for pain, with all being negative. She has diagnoses of major depression and generalized anxiety disorder. She also reported frequent fatigue and memory deficits that did not meet criteria for separate diagnoses. Mary was started on an SNRI, duloxetine (up to 60 mg), and gabapentin (up to 2700 mg) with only minimal relief of pain and no improvement in mood symptoms. She was tapered off the duloxetine and started on bupropion (for fatigue and depression) with improvement in mood symptoms but continued significant rectal pain. Opioid doses were increased per patient request, but her pain continued to worsen. A TCA, desipramine (50 mg), was started, which improved her sleep (insomnia) but had minimal effects on pain. In psychotherapy sessions, she was taught cognitive behavioral techniques (behavioral activation to distract her from pain and cognitive reframing to alter negative cognitions or pervasive pessimism about pain and her life (catastrophizing), as well as relaxation and guided imagery techniques (hypnosis) to distract her from her pain. These techniques, along with her medications, collectively reduced her pain severity by 20% but her pain-related disability remained. She agreed to hospitalization for an opioid detoxification (25% reduction of total opioid dose/day) and over the next 5 days, she was tapered with clonidine and clonazepam available to reduce side effects of the detoxification. Sertraline (100 mg/day) was started for her extreme anxiety about the pain. Over the next month, her pain improved an additional 40% and she continued with regular psychotherapy to reinforce her coping skills. Her fatigue and cognitive deficits significantly improved soon after being off the opioids, and she was able to increase her daily activities. Although improved,

TABLE 25-6

ALGORITHM AND RATIONALE OF STAGES FOR OPIOID DETOXIFICATION FOR PATIENTS WITH NARCOTIC BOWEL SYNDROME WITH ELEMENTS DRAWN FROM MULTIPLE SOURCES

PROTOCOL	RATIONALE
Build empathic relationship with patients and listen to their illness experience. Education about the neurophysiology of opioid-induced effects and nonopioid treatment options available. Teach behavioral techniques such as distraction and cognitive reframing and hypnosis for reduction of pain intensity and suffering. Treat comorbid psychiatric conditions such as anxiety, depression, and somatization disorders. Initiate alternative nonopioid pain medications such as TCAs, SNRIs, SSRIs, and other second-line psychoactive medications. Screening for opioid misuse.	Break the frustration cycle of anger and feeling unheard. Reduce misperceptions about pain drivers and treatment. Improve a sense of control and self-efficacy in pain management. Target predisposing and maintaining pain factors. Risk–benefit profile of nonopioid psychotropic agents favor their use. Opioid misuse is a predictor of opioid use relapse and requires more intensive interventions.
If outpatient taper of opioids is not effective, then medical hospitalization may be necessary with 10% to 33% daily reduction of intravenous morphine equivalent of outpatient opioid dosage. Clonidine and benzodiazepines for acute anxiety reduction and withdrawal symptoms. Continue titrating nonopioid pain medications. Management of bowel problems (constipation/diarrhea). Psychosocial support with empathy and reinforcement of behavioral strategies.	All aspects of the plan are negotiable to help patients with a sense of control, except the daily reduction in opioid dosage. Careful attention to reducing withdrawal and increasing comfort will help patients tolerate this stage. Medical and lifestyle management.
As outpatient, continue behavioral interventions. Consider peer support and group therapy options. Continue nonopioid pain medications with consideration of other psychoactive agents, such as pregabalin, quetiapine, memantine, and ketamine, as appropriate. Continue to treat comorbid conditions.	Behavioral conditioning, empathy, and motivational techniques to prevent recidivism are key. Social support can alter pain perception. Alternative medications to reduce pain severity and suffering with ultimate goal of the simplest nonopioid regimen to prevent persistent pain.

a low-grade constant pain persisted, and thus she was started on a glutaminergic agent, memantine (14 mg/day)[39,40] and continued monthly maintenance psychotherapy. Over the next several months, her pain improved an additional 20% with an overall 80% improvement in her baseline pain 9 months after her initial assessment as measured by a pain visual analogue scale, remaining off opioids and fully reengaged in her life.

This case illustrates the importance of a strong therapeutic alliance and the opioid detoxification when NBS is suspected. Further, it shows the importance of following an algorithm of nonopioid medication changes until maximum relief is obtained. In this case, the patient was started on more traditional noradrenergic agents first (SNRI, TCA) and gabapentin for pain, treated with other antidepressant agents for persistent psychiatric comorbidity (SSRI and bupropion), and only when pain persisted, started on newer, less empirically supported pharmacotherapy (memantine). The importance of ongoing psychosocial intervention is also highlighted by this case. With significant pain relief and the provision of coping skills from psychotherapy, it may be possible to begin to taper medications for anxiety and depression to simplify her psychopharmacological regime while maintaining her symptomatic and functional gains.

CONCLUSION

Chronic opioid use for noncancer pain is on the rise and increasingly leading to higher rates of morbidity and mortality. Such chronic use commonly causes GI side effects, particularly constipation. When laxatives fail to control symptoms, chloride channel activators, mu-receptor agonists/NRIs, opioid antagonists, and PAMORAs can be helpful. Less frequently, opioid use will also cause central nervous system changes leading to visceral hyperalgesia, known as NBS. Due to the significant side effects of opioids, it is important that clinicians carefully weigh risks and benefits before prescribing for noncancer pain on a chronic basis. When OIC or NBS occur, opioid detoxification and multidisciplinary approaches combining psychosocial and nonopioid pharmacological interventions will lead to the best outcomes. Strategies to prevent opioid recidivism are also critical to longer-term treatment benefits.

REFERENCES

1. Mehendale AW, Goldman MP, Mehendale RP. Opioid overuse pain syndrome (OOPS): the story of opioids, Prometheus unbound. *J Opioid Manage.* 2013;9(6):421-438.
2. Manchikanti L, Helm S, 2nd, Fellows B, et al. Opioid epidemic in the United States. *Pain Physician.* 2012;15(3 Suppl):Es9-38.
3. Camilleri M, Drossman DA, Becker G, Webster LR, Davies AN, Mawe GM. Emerging treatments in neurogastroenterology: a multidisciplinary working group consensus statement on opioid-induced constipation. *J Neurogastroenterol Motil.* 2014;in press.
4. Centers for Disease Control and Prevention (CDC). Vital signs: overdoses of prescription opioid pain relievers: United States, 1999-2008. *Morb Mortal Wkly Rep.* 2011;60(43):1487-1492.
5. Dunn KM, Saunders KW, Rutter CM, et al. Opioid prescriptions for chronic pain and overdose: a cohort study. *Ann Int Med.* 2010 Jan 19;152(2):85-92.
6. Cook SF, Lanza L, Zhou X, et al. Gastrointestinal side effects in chronic opioid users: results from a population-based survey. *Aliment Pharmacol Ther.* 2008;27(12):1224-1232.
7. Holzer P. Opioids and opioid receptors in the enteric nervous system: from a problem in opioid analgesia to a possible new prokinetic therapy in humans. *Neurosci Lett.* 2004;361(1-3):192-195.
8. Camilleri M. Opioid-induced constipation: challenges and therapeutic opportunities. *Am J Gastroenterol.* 2011;106(5): 835-842.
9. Pyleris E, Giamarellos-Bourboulis EJ, Tzivras D, Koussoulas V, Barbatzas C, Pimentel M. The prevalence of overgrowth by aerobic bacteria in the small intestine by small bowel culture: relationship with irritable bowel syndrome. *Dig Dis Sci.* 2012;57(5):1321-1329.

10. Dipalma JA, Cleveland MV, McGowan J, Herrera JL. A randomized, multicenter, placebo-controlled trial of polyethylene glycol laxative for chronic treatment of chronic constipation. *Am J Gastroenterol.* 2007;102(7):1436-1441.

11. Ishihara M, Ikesue H, Matsunaga H, et al. A multi-institutional study analyzing effect of prophylactic medication for prevention of opioid-induced gastrointestinal dysfunction. *Clin J Pain.* 2012;28(5):373-381.

12. Cryer B, Katz S, Vallejo R, Popescu A, Ueno R. A randomized study of lubiprostone for opioid-induced constipation in patients with chronic noncancer pain. *Pain Med.* 2014 Apr 9. [Epub ahead of print].

13. Johanson JF, Ueno R. Lubiprostone, a locally acting chloride channel activator, in adult patients with chronic constipation: a double-blind, placebo-controlled, dose-ranging study to evaluate efficacy and safety. *Aliment Pharmacol Ther.* 2007;25(11):1351-1361.

14. Lembo AJ, Schneier HA, Shiff SJ, et al. Two randomized trials of linaclotide for chronic constipation. *N Engl J Med.* 2011;365(6):527-536.

15. Ford AC, Brenner DM, Schoenfeld PS. Efficacy of pharmacological therapies for the treatment of opioid-induced constipation: systematic review and meta-analysis. *Am J Gastroenterol.* 2013;108(10):1566-1574.

16. Michna E, Blonsky ER, Schulman S, et al. Subcutaneous methylnaltrexone for treatment of opioid-induced constipation in patients with chronic, nonmalignant pain: a randomized controlled study. *J Pain.* 2011;12(5):554-562.

17. Thomas J, Karver S, Cooney GA, et al. Methylnaltrexone for opioid-induced constipation in advanced illness. *N Engl J Med.* 2008;358(22):2332-2343.

18. Webster L, Dhar S, Eldon M, Masuoka L, Lappalainen J, Sostek M. A phase 2, double-blind, randomized, placebo-controlled, dose-escalation study to evaluate the efficacy, safety, and tolerability of naloxegol in patients with opioid-induced constipation. *Pain.* 2013;154(9):1542-1550.

19. Chey WD, Webster L, Sostek M, Lappalainen J, Barker PN, Tack J. Naloxegol for opioid-induced constipation in patients with noncancer pain. *N Engl J Med.* 2014;370(25):2387-2396.

20. Simpson K, Leyendecker P, Hopp M, et al. Fixed-ratio combination oxycodone/naloxone compared with oxycodone alone for the relief of opioid-induced constipation in moderate-to-severe noncancer pain. *Curr Med Res Opin.* 2008;24(12):3503-3512.

21. Bouras EP, Camilleri M, Burton DD, Thomforde G, McKinzie S, Zinsmeister AR. Prucalopride accelerates gastrointestinal and colonic transit in patients with constipation without a rectal evacuation disorder. *Gastroenterology.* 2001;120(2):354-360.

22. Sloots CE, Rykx A, Cools M, Kerstens R, De Pauw M. Efficacy and safety of prucalopride in patients with chronic noncancer pain suffering from opioid-induced constipation. *Dig Dis Sci.* 2010;55(10):2912-2921.

23. Hartrick C, Van Hove I, Stegmann, J-U, Oh C, Upmalis D. Efficacy and tolerability of tapentadol immediate release and oxycodone HCl immediate release in patients awaiting primary joint replacement surgery for end-stage joint disease: a 10-day, phase III, randomized, double-blind, active- and placebo-controlled study. *Clin Ther.* 2009;31(2):260-271.

24. Camilleri M, Parkman HP, Shafi MA, Abell TL, Gerson L. Clinical guideline: management of gastroparesis. *Am J Gastroenterol.* 2013;108(1):18-37.

25. Hill JC, Whitehurst DG, Lewis M, et al. Comparison of stratified primary care management for low back pain with current best practice (STarT Back): a randomised controlled trial. *Lancet.* 2011;378(9802):1560-1571.

26. Grunkemeier DM, Cassara JE, Dalton CB, Drossman DA. The narcotic bowel syndrome: clinical features, pathophysiology, and management. *Clin Gastroenterol Hepatol.* 2007;5(10):1126-1139.

27. Kurlander JE, Drossman DA. Diagnosis and treatment of narcotic bowel syndrome. *Nat Rev Gastroenterol Hepatol.* 2014;11(7):410-418.

28. Hutchinson MR, Bland ST, Johnson KW, Rice KC, Maier SF, Watkins LR. Opioid-induced glial activation: mechanisms of activation and implications for opioid analgesia, dependence, and reward. *Sci World J.* 2007;7: 98-111.

29. Farmer AD, Ferdinand E, Aziz Q. Opioids and the gastrointestinal tract: a case of narcotic bowel syndrome and literature review. *J Neurogastroenterol Motil.* 2013;19(1):94-98.

30. Lee M, Silverman SM, Hansen H, Patel VB, Manchikanti L. A comprehensive review of opioid-induced hyperalgesia. *Pain Physician.* 2011;14(2):145-161.

31. Chu LF, Angst MS, Clark D. Opioid-induced hyperalgesia in humans: molecular mechanisms and clinical considerations. *Clin J Pain.* 2008;24:479-496.

32. Drossman DA, Szigethy E. Narcotic bowel syndrome: a recent update. *Am J Gastroenterol Suppl.* 2014;2:22-30.

33. American Psychiatric Association. *Diagnostic and Statistical Manual of Mental Disorders* (5th ed.) Arlington, VA: American Psychiatric Publishing; 2013.

34. Miller AR, North CS, Clouse RE, Wetzel RD, Spitznagel EL, Alpers DH. The association of irritable bowel syndrome and somatization disorder. *Ann Clin Psychiatry.* 2001;13(1):25-30.

35. Drossman DA, Morris CB, Edwards H, et al. Diagnosis, characterization, and 3-month outcome after detoxification of 39 patients with narcotic bowel syndrome. *Am J Gastroenterol.* 2012;107(9):1426-1440.

36. Tuteja AK, Biskupiak J, Stoddard GJ, Lipman AG. Opioid-induced bowel disorders and narcotic bowel syndrome in patients with chronic non-cancer pain. *Neurogastroenterol Motil.* 2010;22(4):424-430, e496.

37. Choung RS, Locke GR, 3rd, Zinsmeister AR, Schleck CD, Talley NJ. Opioid bowel dysfunction and narcotic bowel syndrome: a population-based study. *Am J Gastroenterol.* 2009;104(5):1199-1204.

38. Clarke H, Bonin RP, Orser BA, et al. The prevention of chronic postsurgical pain using gabapentin and pregabalin: a combined systematic review and meta-analysis. *Anesth Analg.* 2012;115:428-442.

39. Hackworth RJ, Tokarz KA, Fowler IM, Wallace SC, Stedje-Larsen ET. Profound pain reduction after induction of memantine treatment in two patients with severe phantom limb pain. *Anesth Analg.* 2008;107(4):1377-1379.

40. Grande LA, O'Donnell BR, Fitzgibbon DR, Terman GW. Ultra-low dose ketamine and memantine treatment for pain in an opioid-tolerant oncology patient. *Anesth Analg.* 2008;107(4):1380-1383.

41. Hocking G, Cousins MJ. Ketamine in chronic pain management: an evidence-based review. *Anesth Analg.* 2004;97:1730-1739.

42. Drossman DA. *Rome III: The Functional Gastrointestinal Disorders.* Degnon Associates; 2006.

43. Drossman DA. Beyond tricyclics: new ideas for treating patients with painful and refractory functional gastrointestinal symptoms. *Am J Gastroenterol.* 2009;104:2897-2902.

44. Tompkins DA, Campbell CM. Opioid-induced hyperalgesia: clinically relevant or extraneous research phenomenon. *Curr Pain Headache Rep.* 2011;15:129-136.

45. Jensen KB, Lonsdorf TB, Schalling M, Kosek E, Ingvar M. Increased sensitivity to thermal pain following a single opiate dose is influenced by the COMT val (158)met polymorphism. *PLoS One.* 2009;4:e6016.

46. Pergolizzi JV, Jr, Mercadante S, Echaburu AV, et al. The role of transdermal buprenorphine in the treatment of cancer pain: an expert panel consensus. *Curr Med Res Opin.* 2009;25:1517-1528.

47. Mueller-Lissner S. Fixed combination of oxycodone with naloxone: a new way to prevent and treat opioid-induced constipation. *Adv Ther.* 2010;27:581-590.

FINANCIAL DISCLOSURES

Dr. Abimbola O. Aderinto-Adike has not disclosed any relevant financial relationships.

Mr. Patrick Berg has not disclosed any relevant financial relationships.

Dr. Deborah M. Bethards has not disclosed any relevant financial relationships.

Dr. Wojciech Blonski has no financial or proprietary interest in the materials presented herein.

Dr. Lin Chang has served on advisory committees or review panels for Takeda, Salix Pharmaceuticals, Forest, Ironwood, Drais Pharmaceuticals, and QOL Medical.

Dr. Giuseppe Chiarioni has not disclosed any relevant financial relationships.

Dr. Jeffrey L. Conklin is a consultant and speaker for Covidien.

Dr. Chad J. Cooper has no financial or proprietary interest in the materials presented herein.

Dr. Sameer Dhalla has not disclosed any relevant financial relationships.

Dr. Douglas A. Drossman has been a consultant for AstraZeneca.

Dr. Ronnie Fass is a speaker for Takeda, AstraZeneca, and Eisai; has conducted research for Mederi Therapeutics; and has consulted for Given Imaging.

Dr. Mark R. Fox has received funds for research from Nestle Research International, AstraZeneca R&D, Given Imaging, and Reckitt Benckiser. He has received support for educational events from Given Imaging, Medical Measurement Systems, and Sandhill Scientific Instruments. He has received honoraria for presentations and/or reimbursement for attending symposia and/or is a member of advisory boards for Given Imaging, AstraZeneca, Reckitt Benckiser, Shire, Almirall, and Sucampo.

Dr. Andrew J. Gawron has not disclosed any relevant financial relationships.

Dr. Kevin A. Ghassemi has no financial or proprietary interest in the materials presented herein.

Dr. C. Prakash Gyawali has not disclosed any relevant financial relationships.

Dr. William L. Hasler has received grant support from Given Imaging.

Dr. Steve Heymen has not disclosed any relevant financial relationships.

Dr. Michael Horowitz has participated on advisory boards and/or symposia for AstraZeneca, Boehringer Ingelheim, Eli Lilly, Merck Sharp & Dohme, Novartis, Novo Nordisk and Sanofi and has received honoraria for this activity.

Dr. Karen L. Jones has received funding and/or trial medication from Merck, Sharp and Dohme, and Sanofi. Her salary is funded via a fellowship provided by the National Health and Medical Research Council of Australia.

Dr. Carolina Malagelada has received a research grant from Given Imaging.

Dr. Juan R. Malagelada is an advisory board member for Shire Pharmaceuticals, has received a research grant from Given Imaging, and is a consultant for Almirall.

Dr. Richard W. McCallum has not disclosed any relevant financial relationships.

Dr. Baha Moshiree has no financial or proprietary interest in the materials presented herein.

Dr. Ann Ouyang has no financial or proprietary interest in the materials presented herein.

Dr. John E. Pandolfino is a lecturer, advisory board member, and consultant for Given Imaging and Sandhill Scientific, from which he as also received grants. He has spoken for AstraZeneca and Takeda.

Dr. Henry P. Parkman has not disclosed any relevant financial relationships.

Dr. Pankaj Jay Pasricha has not disclosed any relevant financial relationships.

Dr. Eamonn M. M. Quigley has not disclosed any relevant financial relationships.

Dr. Satish S.C. Rao has not disclosed any relevant financial relationships.

Dr. Kulthep Rattanakovit has not disclosed any relevant financial relationships.

Dr. Christopher K. Rayner has received research funding from AstraZeneca, Merck, and Novartis.

Dr. Jose M. Remes-Troche has not disclosed any relevant financial relationships.

Dr. Joel E. Richter has no financial or proprietary interest in the materials presented herein.

Dr. Yehuda Ringel has no financial or proprietary interest in the materials presented herein.

Dr. Richard J. Saad has no financial or proprietary interest in the materials presented herein.

Dr. Gina Sam has not disclosed any relevant financial relationships.

Dr. Erica A. Samuel has not disclosed any relevant financial relationships.

Dr. Maria Samuel has not disclosed any relevant financial relationships.

Dr. Lawrence R. Schiller has no financial or proprietary interest in the materials presented herein.

Dr. Marc Schwartz has not disclosed any relevant financial relationships.

Dr. Robert M. Siwiec has not disclosed any relevant financial relationships.

Dr. Joseph K. Sunny, Jr. has not disclosed any relevant financial relationships.

Dr. Rami Sweis has received funds for research from Reckitt Benckiser. He has received honoraria for presentations and/or reimbursement for attending symposia from Given Imaging/Covidien.

Dr. Eva Szigethy has received a research grant from Crohn and Colitis Foundation of America, and has been a consultant and advisory board member for Merck, and a consultant for AbbVie. She has also received royalties from APPI as a book editor.

Dr. Jan Tack has not disclosed any relevant financial relationships.

Dr. Thangam Venkatesan has not disclosed any relevant financial relationships.

Dr. Elizabeth J. Videlock is supported by NIH grant T32 NIH-NIDDK AM 41301.

Dr. William E. Whitehead has not disclosed any relevant financial relationships.

Dr. John M. Wo has no financial or proprietary interest in the materials presented herein.

Index

Printed in the United States
by Baker & Taylor Publisher Services